Running Out of Time

RUNNING RAW AROUND AUSTRALIA

Running Out of Time
RUNNING RAW AROUND AUSTRALIA

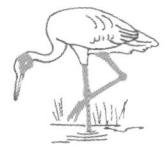

JANETTE MURRAY-WAKELIN

PLEASE NOTE

The information and suggestions in this book pertaining to imagery and meditation are presented only as material of general interest and not as a prescription for any specific person or any condition in a specific case. the reader is advised and encouraged to seek the aid of a qualified health practitioner for advice pertaining to his or her particular conditions and needs.

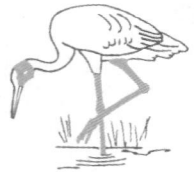

Published by Brolga Publishing Pty Ltd
ABN 46 063 962 443
PO Box 12544
A'Beckett St
Melbourne, VIC, 8006
Australia

email: markzocchi@brolgapublishing.com.au

All rights reserved. No part of this publication may be reproduced, stored in a retrieval system or transmitted in any form or by any means electronic, mechanical, photocopying, recording or otherwise without prior permission from the publisher.

Copyright © 2014 Janette Murray-Wakelin

National Library of Australia
Cataloguing-in-Publication data

Running Out Of Time
Janette Murray-Wakelin

ISBN 9781922175588

Cover credits:
Front: Kohi Love Photography-Melissa Kilkelly
Back: John Kilkelly
Insert (3rd image): Alan & Janette Cecil Bodnar

Printed in China
Cover design & Typesetting by Wanissa Somsuphangsri

BE PUBLISHED

Publish through a successful publisher. National distribution, Macmillan & International distribution to the United Kingdom, North America. Sales Representation to South East Asia
Email: markzocchi@brolgapublishing.com.au

To Alan
For being there...every step of the way

Dedicated to
The Children and All HumanKind
The Animals and All Creatures Great and Small
The Earth and Mother Nature

In Honour of
The Ancient Wisdom of the Indigenous Peoples
of This Sacred Land called Australia

In Hope for
A Time of Kindness and Compassion
For All Living Beings and This Planet we call Home

ACKNOWLEDGEMENTS

During the three years before Running Raw Around Australia, while we were planning, organising and training for the Run, and of course, during the year 2013 while we were on the Road, there were many people who offered their assistance and support, without whom it would have been much more of a challenge. We would like to acknowledge and thank everyone who helped make the Run possible. There were those who volunteered their time and expertise, those who gave free and discounted items including food from their own gardens, those who offered showers, laundry and a 'real' bed, those who prepared shared meals in their own homes. There were those who sent messages of thanks, encouragement and love through our website and on our Facebook Page, there were those who stopped us on the Road to give donations and have a chat, and there were those who joined us on the road, running alongside for part of the way. There were those who organised speaking events and there were those who attended, wishing us well and donating to the Charities. Everyday we met and were encouraged by people who were willing to help make RunRAW2013 happen, because they cared. Their kindness and compassion kept us going, day after day, for 366 days all the way around Australia. There are so many that we cannot mention them all by name, but you know who you are and we know that you care enough to be sharing the positive message that we shared while Running Raw Around Australia and that with your help, we have inspired countless others worldwide to live a more conscious lifestyle. Together, we will make a difference, thank you. However, we would like to acknowledge and give special thanks to the following people for their love, help and support throughout 2013 while we were Running Raw Around Australia. Without you, we truly would have been Running Out of Time! Thank you.

SPECIAL THANKS

To our Family
Kaje and Clelia, Alana and Michael
Kieran, Liam, Lily, Flynn and Marlo
Thank you for your love and support and for being with us all the way.

To our Support Crew - Thank you for being there.
Melbourne Day 1 - Graeme Ward
Melbourne to Sydney - Maureen Foster and Ping Chan
Melbourne to Canberra - Tabitha Hobbins
Canberra to Bulehdulah - Graeme Ward
Sydney to Townsville - Francine Maas
Bulehdula to Currumbin - Bradley Cope
Currumbin to Townsville - Michaela Olsen
Townsville to Mt Isa - John and Marleen Kilkelly
Mt Isa to Katherine - Rose Berry and Narelle Chesworth
Katherine to Perth - Myke Tran and Melissa Kilkelly
Perth to Ceduna - Graeme Ward
Perth to Albany - Margit Magi
Norseman to Adelaide - Narelle Chesworth
Ceduna to Melbourne - Michael Gillan
Adelaide to Hobart - Sylvia Pringle
Melbourne to Hobart - Keith Pringle
Hobart to Launceston - Anne Milligan
Melbourne to Warrandyte - Graeme Ward

MANY THANKS TO OUR SPONSORS, WITHOUT WHOM RUNRAW2013 WOULD NOT HAVE BEEN POSSIBLE:

Eileen Sims, noodle HQ Australia

RunRAW2013 Sponsor Eileen Sims of noodle HQ Australia, used her trans-Tasman network of media contacts to guarantee media exposure for RunRAW2013. Eileen brought valuable insight with an impressive background including the direction of Bronson and Jacobs business units in both New Zealand and Australia. She executes PR and copywriting for a number of noodle's other clients including fashion designer Jill Main, super yacht Vertigo, Sir Michael Hill and his golf course 'The Hills' and many more. A health, food and fitness enthusiast rolled into one, Eileen relishes opportunities to write about food, health & well-being, sustainability, environmental issues and anything that will make a difference. www.noodlehq.com.au

Philip Wollen OAM, Australia.

Philip Wollen OAM provided much appreciated financial support for RunRAW2013. Through his kindness and generosity as a philanthropic humanitarian, Philip brings crucial help to many charitable causes and inspires others to share his humanitarian values and ideals. His achievements in the business world mark him as a man of action and he channels this energy into practical outcomes for the causes he champions through the Winsome Constance Kindness Trust.

Philip received the *Medal of the Order of Australia 2005* for service to international humanitarian relief and to animal welfare, particularly through the establishment of the Winsome Constance Kindness Trust. Philip received *The Australian Humanitarian Award 2006* and was awarded *Australian of the Year Victoria 2007* at Government House in Melbourne, Australia. Philip promotes kindness towards all other living beings and strives to enshrine this as a recognisable trait in the Australian character and culture. The measure of his support can be seen in the extraordinary list of organisations the Winsome Constance

Kindness Trust supports, benefiting children, animals, the ill, the environment and aspiring youth. www.kindnesstrust.com

Dr Douglas Graham, FoodnSport, UK & USA

Dr. Douglas Graham has been living a raw conscious lifestyle for many years and established the low fat raw vegan diet which we follow and which sustained us during RunRAW2013. Dr. Graham was our nutrition and fitness adviser for RunRAW2013. He is the director of Health & Fitness Weeks which provide Olympic class training and nutritional guidance to people of all fitness levels around the world. Dr. Graham is the author of several highly acclaimed books including 'Nutrition and Athletic Performance' and the best-selling book 'The 80/10/10 Diet.' He is the raw foods and fitness adviser for VegSource.com (the largest vegetarian site on the internet). Through his boundless energy and joy for living, Dr. Graham emanates living proof that eating whole, fresh, ripe, raw plant food is the nutritional way to vibrant health and vitality. A professional speaker since 1980 at many national health, animal rights, environmental, and sports performance seminars, Dr. Graham seeks to make a point while making a friend. www.foodnsport.com

Barefoot Inc Vibram Australia

Barefoot Inc is a proud sponsor of RunRAW2013 for Vibram Five Finger barefoot shoes and clothing. Based in Sydney Australia, Barefoot Inc are stockists and distributors throughout Australia and New Zealand of a wide range of inspired products for ultra athletes. Barefoot Inc offers an extensive range of minimal footwear, clothing and accessories that set the standards of excellence in comfort, design and application, while also offering barefoot running clinics in Sydney and Melbourne. Running in Vibram Barefoot shoes enables us to experience the freedom and joy of running 'barefoot' while reducing the risk of exposure to obstacles that may cause injury. Running 'barefoot' around Australia in Vibram Five Finger shoes is a conscious lifestyle choice to tread softly on the earth. www.barefootinc.com.au

Coles

Coles generously sponsored fresh fruit and vegetables throughout RunRAW2013. Coles are committed to helping Australia grow and provide fresh Australian grown fruit and vegetables. They are dedicated to sourcing as much fresh fruit and veg from Aussie growers as possible and their supply of fresh Australian fruit and veg is something that Coles is extremely proud of. coles.com.au

Alive Organics Perth and Healthy Valley Organics

When we arrived in Perth, WA we were graciously hosted by the owners of Alive Organics and Healthy Valley Organics. They also generously offered to sponsor our food for the entire time that we were in Western Australia, which included fresh fruit and veg and dried fruit, nuts and seeds, all certified organic. They went out of their way to supply us when we were on the road, and made sure we had enough food supply to get across the Nullarbor and into South Australia. Alive Organics is an organic food shop located in Morley, WA, and specialises in organic raw, living foods. They offer the freshest in-season certified organic, bio-dynamic and chemical-free fruits & vegetables, a great range of organic dried fruits, nuts & seeds, as well as other organic products. They also have an in-store cafe providing fresh juices, smoothies and delicious raw, vegan food. Alive Organics is supplied by Healthy Valley Organics, owned and operated by the same health conscious family for over 10 years, providing organic outlets throughout WA. www.healthyvalleyorganics.com.au

Costa

Based in Victoria, Costa is Australia's largest private producer, marketer and exporter of premium quality fresh fruit and vegetables. Costa's banana category is based in North Queensland where they and their joint venture partners manage four farms, growing and marketing Cavendish and Lady Finger bananas to their customers 52 weeks per year. The Costa Group Goes Bananas for RunRAW2013 and was proud to donate $3,000 worth of bananas in support of our year long run around Australia. "To see people like Janette and

Alan promoting the benefits of a healthy lifestyle, with a focus on eating plenty of fresh fruit and vegetables, really highlights the importance of preventative health measures for all Australians, especially in reducing the incidence of chronic diseases, such as type 2 diabetes", said Frank Costa AO, Chairman of the Costa Group "The Costa Group is honoured to help them on their journey and we wish them all the best in their efforts to complete 365 marathons in 365 days by running around Australia," said Frank Costa AO. www.costagroup.com.au

Orbital Autogas Australia

Orbital Autogas Australia supplied and serviced LPG systems on our vehicles for RunRAW2013, as well as contributing to LPG fuel supply through Gas Energy Australia. The range of Orbital Liquid LPG systems have been tested in accordance with ADR 79 emissions requirements (the same as required by vehicle manufacturers). These tests show that Liquid LPG systems on average reduce climate changing CO_2 vehicle emissions by 13%. That's a big plus for the environment. www.liquidlpg.com.au

Gas Energy Australia

Sponsors Gas Energy Australia in conjunction with Unigas LPG and Orbital Autogas supplied LPG fuel for RunRAW2013 vehicles. LP Gas is a highly efficient clean, green source of energy. Vehicle emissions are recognised as one of the main contributors to climate change, but LPG is recognised for its inherent environmental benefits and offers an immediate reduction of up to 15% in carbon dioxide emissions compared to a petrol powered vehicle, while more than 90% of damaging particulates are eliminated by replacing a diesel engine with LPG powered equivalent. Filling an LPG tank is a fully sealed process so it also benefits the environment during refueling with no chemical vapours escaping into the atmosphere. Using LP Gas as a sustainable fuel is a conscious lifestyle choice. www.poweredbygas.com.au

Marlin Signs

A Victoria based company, Marlin Signs generously provided the signs on the RunRAW2013 vehicles and the safety road signs. www.marlinsigns.com.au

'botanical cuisine'

'botanical cuisine' generously supplied their delicious raw products to enhance our meals when fresh produce was in short supply or unavailable in some of the more remote areas of our Run Around Australia. 'botanical cuisine' is handmade in Melbourne by chefs using locally grown quality ingredients, creating flavours and textures with a commitment to beautiful artisan inspired gourmet, organic sustainable products. 'botanical cuisine' products are made with minimal processing at low temperatures and are sugar, dairy and gluten free with no artificial additives. www.botanicalcuisine.com

Froothie

RunRAW2013 Sponsors Froothie supplied the commercial-grade Optimum 9200 blender to emulsify fruits and vegetables which were used to make smoothies, soups and sauces for us and our Support Crew. We used the Optimum 9200 Blender approximately 3 times a day, over 1000 times during RunRAW2013 and it never missed a beat! We highly recommend the use of blenders and juicers supplied by Froothie. www.froothie.com.au

Garmin Australasia

Garmin creates navigation and communication devices that record accurate performance through satellite technology. Accurate navigation and distance recording of RunRAW2013 daily running was assured with Garmin Automotive GPS in the RunRAW2013 vehicles and with Garmin Running Watches that we wore while on the Run, all sponsored by Garmin Australasia. www.garmin.com

FOREWORD

Many years ago I received a letter from a married couple I didn't know, asking if they could use "Kindness House" to teach the benefits of fresh, organic, raw vegan food.

It was Janette and Alan.

My policy is always, if possible, to say YES to everything.

Imagine my joy to see tables with tablecloths, immaculately adorned by massive arrays of colourful fruit, nuts, vegetables and flowers. A gastronomic Harrods!

More recently they asked for an appointment, and tentatively described their idea to "Run around Australia". One marathon a day for 365 consecutive days.

Before they had finished their introduction; before I discovered that Janette was a "cancer survivor"; before I had learned that they had run from the Northern to the Southern tip of New Zealand; before they had asked me for a penny, I jumped the gun and said "I want to sponsor it".

I "flagged" them off at Federation Square early on New Year's Day and nervously followed their footsteps on facebook and radio. A year later, I spoke at the packed welcome dinner at Kindness House.

Their journey reminded me of the journey of two great heroes in Australian history - and the ironies that life plays on us.

Burke and Wills, two intrepid Australian explorers, departed from Royal Park, a few hundred yards from Kindness House. They intended to travel to the Gulf of Carpentaria. Janette and Alan departed from Federation Square, also a few hundred yards from Kindness House, and intended to traverse the entire coast of Australia.

Burke and Wills travelled 3,000 kilometres. Janette and Alan travelled 15,782 kilometres.

In the time it took Janette and Alan to reach the Victorian border, Burke and Wills had reached Essendon, a nearby suburb.

Burke and Wills had the backing of the Governor, the Chief Justice, Knights of the Realm and powerful political interests. Janette and Alan had the backing of friends.

Burke and Wills used 23 horses and 26 camels. Janette and Alan used their own two feet – and were often barefoot.

Burke and Wills ran out of meat and were hungry. So they killed and ate their horses, bullocks and camels. Janette and Alan ran on fruit, nuts and vegetables and were never hungry. And they never killed anyone.

Burke and Wills shot native animals on the way. Janette and Alan stopped and watched them at play.

Burke and Wills burned timber to cook their food. Janette and Alan ate fresh, raw vegan food.

Burke and Wills failed tragically. Janette and Alan succeeded admirably.

Burke and Wills died half way. Janette and Alan are here today.

Nothing diminishes the great achievement of Burke and Wills. But one cannot help but wonder. A softer, gentler journey along the road less travelled brings enlightenment too.

Janette and Alan have helped us lift the blinding methane fog caused by the animal industrial complex. It has made us sick, cruel and violent. It has also caused massive deforestation, climate change and the world's worst record of species extinction.

Veganism is the Swiss Army Knife of the future. One implement solves our ethical, moral, financial, environmental, water, health problems and ends animal cruelty forever.

Traveling through pretty Australian countryside is like passing Potemkin Villages, erected to fool Empress Catherine II during her visit to Crimea in 1787. Fake villages, built to impress gullible passers-by that all is sweet and peaceful. But every sheep, cow, and pig in this bucolic scene is really just another innocent murder victim on death row.

I admire Janette and Alan for running past these gulags without getting physically ill.

I thank them for giving us the privilege of sponsoring their run; for being a shining example to millions; But most of all, for giving us another reason to get off the meat and dairy drug, for inspiring others to reclaim their health and live their lives as if their ethics really mattered. We are deeply indebted to them.

Philip Wollen. OAM
www.kindnesstrust.com

CONTENTS

A Journey of Discovery 1

Running Raw Around Australia Route and Schedule 25

January 2013 27

February 2013 43

March 2013 63

April 2013 81

May 2013 107

June 2013 127

July 2013 149

August 2013 175

September 2013 195

October 2013 213

November 2013 233

December 2013 253

Marathon #366, January 1, 2014 273

Running Out of Time - Recipes from the Road 283

Author's Bio 295

A Journey of Discovery

Throughout the year 2013, as veteran raw vegan runners, my husband Alan and I ran together around Australia: 15,782 kilometres, averaging 43 kilometers, a marathon everyday. Step for step, stride for stride all the way. We started in Melbourne, Victoria on January 1, 2013, following Highway 1 around the perimeter of the country running through every State Capital and finished running 365 marathons in 365 days back in Melbourne December 31, 2013. On January 1, 2014, we ran one more marathon (number 366) from Melbourne to Warrandyte along the Yarra River Trail, thereby setting a new World Record for running the most consecutive marathons as the oldest and only couple to run around Australia, fueled entirely by fruit and vegetables and wearing barefoot shoes.

We wanted to inspire and motivate others to make more conscious lifestyle choices, to promote kindness and compassion for all living beings and to raise environmental awareness for a sustainable future. The truth is, the most endangered species on this planet is Humankind. As a species, we have become obsessed with speed, the Human Race is on, but we are not winning. Through misinformation and misleading marketing, we are disregarding the innate intelligence of our own bodies and have become a malnourished species, while the sickness industry flourishes. Due to our poor food choices we have become a species of (non) survivors. The majority of us are spending most of our lives dying instead of thriving. The amount of money and time spent on 'scientific research' to find a cure for our ill health would be better spent on prevention and returning to our natural way of being. Our obsession with technology has us careering down a path of self destruction. In our rush to become technically advanced we have lost sight of the importance of Being. Our poor lifestyle choices are creating our own demise, we are spiraling into oblivion, and we are Running Out of Time.

We believe that the Human Race needs to slow down and heed what one of our greatest teachers, Gandhi in his wisdom told us, "There is more to life than increasing it's speed." We need to revisit who we are and why we are here. We need to understand the consequences of the choices we make in life and how they can affect our very being.

By doing so, we can make a difference. Awareness comes through being informed with truth, understanding the information and acting on it, but knowledge requires action to become conscious awareness.

We wanted to share a positive message of truth and hope from the experiences and knowledge that we had gained through living consciously during the previous decade, so that others may make their own informed lifestyle choices that will make a difference. We k So many times we've been asked, "

new the best way to do that was to lead by example, walk (or in this case) run the talk. Inspiration is what motivates people to never stop pushing for what they believe in and for what they want to achieve. By running a marathon distance together every day for a year around Australia, we hoped to inspire others to think more consciously about the choices they make in life, to believe in themselves, to follow their dreams, and to achieve their goals. While we were Running around Australia during the year 2013, we had the opportunity to show that by eating raw living plant based foods, we are healthier, more physically fit and have unlimited energy at beyond 60 years of age than in our earlier years, including when we ran the length of New Zealand 13 years previously.

We have been enjoying unlimited energy for over 12 years due primarily to our 100% Low Fat Raw Vegan Diet. A vegan diet is based on fresh, ripe, organic fruits and vegetables with NO animal products. A 100 percent low fat, raw, vegan diet is based on the 80/10/10 principle of 80 percent carbohydrates, 10 percent protein and 10 percent fat derived from fresh, ripe, organic fruits and vegetables. A low fat, raw vegan 80/10/10 diet does NOT include any animal products, processed or junk foods and does NOT include any stimulants, drugs, supplements nor 'superfoods'. By eliminating all acid-forming foods (everything other than fresh ripe fruits and vegetables) and increasing the amount of alkaline foods in our diet, (obtained only from fresh, ripe fruits and vegetables) we have attained a higher level of optimum health, improved our physical fitness and increased our performance level.

In our experience, unlimited Raw Energy is attained by consuming an abundance of high nutrient- laden, fresh, ripe, organic fruits and vegetables. It is also our experience that true happiness is attained through making conscious lifestyle choices for one's own health, the health of the environment, and all living beings with whom we share the planet. We are living proof of what can be achieved by making conscious lifestyle choices.

So many times we've been asked, "Where do you get your protein?" The answer is simple: "The same place that the cow gets it from - greens." Protein from plant based sources is healthier than the protein derived from animal sources and does not contribute to health issues such as heart dis-ease and cancer. It is much more efficient for people to consume the plant food directly. We are also asked where we get our calcium, or iron, or any other nutrients a person thinks to name. Again, the answer is that we get all our necessary nutrients from the food we eat, just the same as animals in their natural habitat do. Malnutrition is unknown in people and animals who eat raw living food in abundance. We live in a world where over 790 million people are chronically undernourished and over 27,000 children under the age of five die of malnutrition every day. The world's cattle consume enough plant food to feed 8.7 billion people, more than the entire human population. Available protein from plants that the animals eat and 80-95 percent of food energy is wasted when converted to meat for human consumption. Cooking food also reduces the available nutrients and enzymes essential for optimum health. By nourishing our bodies with raw living vegan foods, humans not only can achieve optimal physical, mental and spiritual health, but can also acquire unlimited Raw Energy which enables us to achieve our goals and follow our dreams. Raw Energy is already achieved by every other free animal on the planet. The good news is that Raw Energy is readily available to humans just by making informed conscious lifestyle choices. Living a conscious lifestyle is a safe, sure way to get back on track with your health and ensures optimal health and happiness, the two things that everyone is ultimately striving for. Everyone can benefit from learning how to take control of their own health and therefore feel good about themselves. It is immensely gratifying to see how even small changes can make such a difference in one's life and having the right information empowers one to make conscious life choices. All dis-ease and related health issues are reversible through maintaining all aspects of a conscious living lifestyle. Becoming conscious of the lifestyle choices we make personally and collectively as a community and a species, will help to bring about the change to a more sustainable future for ourselves, our children and future generations."

Our personal lifestyle throughout 45+ years of marriage and raising a family, operating a successful business partnership and extensive world travel, has always been centered on health and wellness and sharing our consciousness with others. From sailing in our 40' sailboat with our two young children throughout New Zealand, the South Pacific and Papua New Guinea, to working our 400-ton freight boat on the inland waterways of Europe; from traveling in our converted bus from Holland to Portugal while home schooling our children, to residing on Vancouver Island Canada while our children went to University; and from operating a 100' hotel boat in France taking guests on health oriented canal cruises, to running the length of New Zealand with the support of our two (adult) children, Alan and I enjoyed a physically active, healthy lifestyle throughout our traveling years with our family.

We married young and our two children were born while we were still in our early twenties. We then spent most of their childhood traveling together worldwide. In search of a more healthy lifestyle for our little family, we sailed from our home country of New Zealand when our children were still very small. Our sailboat was completely self-sufficient, relying on the four winds to take us throughout the South Pacific; visiting, living and working in places like the Tongan Islands, Micronesia and Papua New Guinea. It was fun home-schooling our children and as a family we grew very close. It was a carefree life with very little stress, our food was mostly locally grown fresh fruit and vegetables and our environment was clean and green. Our time on the ocean was incredible. We learned a lot about ourselves from living on the sea. Most of the time it was beautiful and serene, but there were moments of awe when the storms and seas raged around us!

However a few years later while we were living in Canada, the next chapter in our lives created a much greater challenge....I was diagnosed with highly aggressive carcinoma breast cancer and was 'given' six months to live. I was alerted to the possibility of cancer being present when my little grandson inadvertently found the tumour. I had been carrying him all day as we walked around a local festival and he had fallen asleep in my arms. When we finally got home and I put him down, I noticed some pain in the breast area where he had been holding on to me. It was then that I discovered the lump. I was not too perturbed as I had always done regular self breast examinations and had never had any sign of a problem. Apart from a bout of scarlet fever and measles as a tiny child, I had never been sick in my life. I had never had so much as a cold and I'd never taken any drugs, not even an aspirin! I thought it was just bruising to the tissue from being held onto for hours by my grandson. It was my daughter who suggested I should have it looked at and the following day I had an ultrasound and biopsy, which proved the diagnosis. The tumour was 3 cm and the cancer had spread into the chest wall and the lymph nodes. It was recommended that I undergo conventional chemotherapy and radiation treatment, which may extend my life a further 6 months.

At 52 years, a mother of two and grandmother of one, I was not willing to accept this prognosis. The power of intention is far greater than that of fear and I had every intention of staying around for a long time! I believed I had lived a very healthy lifestyle, being vegetarian for 25 years and vegan for the previous 15 years. I had also been extremely physically active all my life, so I was quite shocked with the diagnosis.

It was hard for me to think of what the cause may have been, given the healthy lifestyle we had been living. Then I recalled that during a maintenance refit for the sailboat, I did suffer an accident which exposed me to a high dose of toxins. I was painting the boat when the scaffolding collapsed under me. It happened so fast that I was still holding the can of paint when I hit the ground!

I was completely covered in marine paint that has toxic antifouling properties; it was in my hair, my eyes, nose, ears and mouth. I ingested a large amount and most of my skin was covered in paint. It took 3 months before my normal skin colour came back and, since the skin is the largest organ of the body, overexposure of toxins for me was inevitable. After four years sailing in the South Pacific, we embarked on a new adventure for a further four years; living and working on a cargo ship on the inland waterways throughout Europe. This adventure is another story in itself, but during that time I was also exposed to toxic fallout from the Chernobyl disaster. Looking back over my life and remembering those two times when I was overexposed to toxins, I realized that my body must have been highly compromised. Whether it was one incident or the other, or perhaps the combination of both, I was sure that the toxic overload in my body predisposed me to the onset of cancer. I could think of no other explanation, but once I had established the cause, I felt more empowered to do something about it. I was no longer guessing, taking a gamble on treatment, nor in fear of the outcome. I knew that I could take control of the situation myself, doing 100% the best I could for my body.

My intuitive response to the recommended treatment was that it did not make sense to compromise the body's system further. It seemed obvious to me that I should be helping the body to rejuvenate and rebuild, thereby reversing the problem. My instinct told me that treating the symptoms would not address the cause. I was also convinced that I was not meant to die of cancer, so I treated the diagnosis as a challenge. It seemed to me that this was just a message from my body that there was a problem I needed to deal with. A year earlier, I had been present at my grandson's birth and had held his little hand for his first 24 hours of life. I promised him that we would have many wonderful times together over the years and that I would always be there for him. Now he had brought this to my attention so that I could take care of the problem and be able to keep my promise.

My family's initial reaction to the diagnosis was to research all they could about breast cancer, the possible causes and the treatments that were recommended, as well as looking into natural holistic therapies and making lifestyle changes that would be most likely to result in a positive outcome. We needed to know all the possibilities so that I could make an informed choice as to the best course of action to take. I knew that it made sense to do everything I could to give the body the tools it needed to take me on my journey to optimum health. Our extensive research not only gave me the knowledge to do just that, but also the confidence to know that I had made the right choice.

Environmentally, my immune system had been compromised and to compromise it further didn't make sense to me. I chose to help my body heal itself of cancer, by boosting the immune system with the natural nutrients it needed and increasing the oxygen in the blood through exercise and juicing fresh fruits and vegetables. The path that I took with the support of Alan and my family, resulted in an inevitable journey to a more healthy conscious way of living and the passion to share our extensive knowledge and experience with others.

With the help of my naturopathic physician, we established a regime that focused on the holistic approach of mind, body and spirit. This intensive regime included intravenous immune therapy; Infrared detoxification therapy; increasing the amount of oxygen to the body through ozone treatment, conscious breathing and aerobic exercise; visualization, meditation, positive thinking and spiritual awareness; and maximizing the amount of nutrients taken into the body through juicing, wheatgrass and living food nutrition.

For the following six months after receiving the diagnosis, I spent 3 hours a day, 5 days a week at the naturopathic clinic having therapy to help boost the immune system. I used the time sitting hooked up to the intravenous drip to relax and it gave me time to do more research.

I also increased the amount of exercise that I was already doing on a daily basis, incorporating yoga and long distance running. With yoga I was able to reunite with myself. I came to know my inner self and to love myself unconditionally. My running became more meditative. I chose to run on trails in the mountains or barefoot in the sand along the beach. I could feel again the sense of freedom that I remembered when I ran as a child. I visualized achieving personal goals that I had long since put aside; perhaps I would paint, perhaps I would write. I visualized myself proudly looking on at my grandson's wedding; perhaps going full circle and being present at his child's birth. Daily sessions in the infrared sauna maximized the detoxification process. I could feel the body ridding itself of toxins while enjoying the feeling of complete relaxation during the sessions.

My nutritional intake took a huge leap. I started juicing in earnest. It made sense that I could consume more nutrients by juicing because I just wouldn't be able to eat that amount of food. If it takes 4 cups of carrots to produce 1 cup of juice and I could drink 4 cups of juice per day, I knew I was way ahead of the game. I think I was close to consuming a truckload of carrots every week during those 6 months! My hands turned orange, but I didn't care, I was alive and running!

I also started drinking wheatgrass juice. When I learned that one ounce of wheatgrass juice has the equivalent nutritional value of 2 pounds of green leafy vegetables, (that's more than most people eat in a week), I didn't hesitate. Apart from having all the vitamins and most of the minerals the body needs to be healthy, wheatgrass juice also has all the amino acids making it a complete protein. Like all greens, wheatgrass is also very high in chlorophyll, which is pure oxygen to the body. When taken, the juice goes directly to the bloodstream, oxygenating the blood and the whole body. I knew from the research we had done, that this was a crucial factor in stopping the mutation of cancer cells. Cancer cannot survive in an oxygenated environment, therefore the more oxygen I could pump into the body through exercise, conscious breathing and drinking wheatgrass, the better!

Although I had been vegetarian and vegan for most of my life, I decided that if I was going to 'give it 100%' I would also eliminate all cooked food, thereby getting the maximum amount of nutrients from all foods I consumed. I couldn't believe the difference in the way I felt within only one week of changing to 100% raw plant based food. The first thing I noticed was that my clarity of mind was intensely heightened. I no longer had to think about decision making. Everything became very clear, there was no longer any hesitation. I lost 15 pounds within the first month of eating 100% raw vegan food, which took me just below my recommended weight per height ratio. The following month my weight came back up a few pounds and stayed there.

During the first 6 months, my body revisited old injuries that had clearly not completely healed. For example, during my accident with the paint, I sustained an injury to my elbow that had left me unable to straighten my arm. During the healing process when I 'went raw' I experienced ten days of pain in the elbow, similar to that which I had endured at the time of the accident, but when the pain stopped I could straighten my arm again! Several other accidents that had caused injuries throughout my life healed in a similar manner. I also found I had much more energy than before and that it lasted longer. It was especially evident during my long training runs and, as a result, my physical performance level increased.

There is absolutely no doubt in my mind that consuming 100% raw plant based food made a huge difference to my recovery time and to my overall healing. It is interesting that although the lifestyle changes I made were minimal, the positive results were profound. I really only had to stop eating the odd muffin, a sandwich now and then, eliminate the pasta and rice, and stop cooking my vegetables. I had already eliminated meats as a child, dairy in my teens and I had never eaten processed or junk food. So the change to 100% raw food for me was not that big, but the change to my overall health was huge. Not only did I immediately experience clarity of mind, increased energy, specific injury healing and a feeling of well-being, but I cured myself of cancer!

Within the six months that I was 'given' to live after my diagnosis, I received a clean bill of health. There was no longer any sign of cancer cells in my body. Those crucial six months were also filled with love, laughter and much support from my family and friends. I am blessed with a loving family who rallied for me with the research, with physical and mental support, and most of all, with their unwavering conviction that the path I had chosen was mine to choose. I believe having unconditional support is also paramount in healing the body. I now have four more grandchildren whom I believe I would never have known had I not made these informed choices to follow a conscious lifestyle.

My diagnosis of cancer and resulting journey to optimum health has been an experience I am truly grateful for. I finished the immune therapy regime, but have continued with all other aspects of the raw conscious lifestyle. Now, I am living proof that the body is capable of healing itself. I know for certain that I will continue on the raw path, as I continue to experience more health benefits and an ever-increasing enlightened consciousness.

Following a conscious lifestyle with raw plant based diet and regular exercise also made a huge difference in Alan's life, who fifteen years earlier was a 2-pack-a-day smoker, was overweight, often sick and would get several colds a year, he always felt tired having little or no energy. When he changed his eating habits, stopped smoking and started exercising, he completely turned his life around. In the space of one year he lost 70 pounds, he went from being unable to run one city block to completing his first marathon and he hasn't been sick since. Now he feels twenty years younger than his 68+ years and his energy level has increased so that he can run faster and further now than when he was in his twenties. "Every day is exciting when you are RAW!"

As a result of our life changing experiences, Alan and I founded a Centre for Optimum Health in Canada, where our focus was on encouraging healthy conscious lifestyles through living nutrition and exercise for the mind, body and spirit. Our approach to healthy living is as simple and clear as nature itself. Our vision was to share our knowledge gained through our multitude of life experiences, and to encourage natural, healthy conscious lifestyles within our community. Education and learning is an all important factor in the growing process, both for individuals and for a community, and we believe healthy minds create a healthy community. On a weekly basis we offered health presentations, seminars and workshops by over 40 holistic practitioners affiliated with the Centre, and international health educators spoke monthly. The Centre had a Raw Vegan Restaurant, a Raw Lifestyle Store, a Book, Film & Internet Library, a Fitness Studio, and an Infrared Sauna Spa. We offered Raw Food Preparation Classes and monthly Raw Food Dinners. We also established a highly successful Living Food & Conscious Lifestyle Program and shared our secrets of good health through a series of inspirational presentations both at the Centre and internationally during the following eight years. Learning how to live a healthy conscious lifestyle with an emphasis on nutrition and exercise, gave people the possibility to prevent disease, or reverse health issues they may be struggling with; such as being overweight, having addictions ranging from sugar to smoking and dealing with dis-ease as serious as diabetes and cancer. The response was overwhelming with hundreds of people being encouraged to make their own informed choices regarding diet, exercise and maintaining a healthy and conscious lifestyle. Many attested to experiencing positive changes to their health and overall well being.

However, I still felt that we were not reaching enough people with the positive message, and had an overwhelming feeling that we (as a species) were Running Out of Time.

After six years of operating the Centre in Canada, we decided to move to Australia to live, and at the same time, came up with the idea of sharing the positive message worldwide by Running Raw Around Australia. The idea developed into a project that we felt committed to complete. We knew that we were physically and mentally capable of completing the Run and felt sure that in doing so, we would also achieve our goal on a global scale of inspiring and motivating many more people to think more consciously about the choices they make in life.

I also decided it was time to write my first book entitled 'Raw Can Cure Cancer' based on what I had learned and experienced during my journey to optimum health. The book was published and released during 2013 to coincide with the Run, to emphasise the positive message of hope, health and happiness. In the book, I share the story of my journey with cancer and the knowledge I gained about the healing properties of living foods and essential exercise based on my own experience, so that others may have the opportunity to make informed conscious choices themselves.

During 2012 while in training for RunRAW2013, we used our years of running and nutritional experience to design a strategy that would enable us to run a marathon every day for a year without injury or energy depletion. We knew it was possible to be fueled sufficiently with a raw vegan diet for the body to be recovering while running, and that getting sufficient sleep would complete the rejuvenation process in order for us to continue running consecutive marathons. We also knew we would have to keep monitoring our physical fitness and nutritional intake as we progressed each day so that we could change the strategy accordingly. Because we were committed to running a marathon every day, 366 consecutive marathons all the way around Australia, it was crucial that we stay in a state of optimal health both physically and mentally, and to get sufficient sleep for optimal recovery and rejuvenation, since there would be no rest days until we finished.

Our running experience comes from many years of recreational running as well as having both participated in many international marathons and ultra runs around the world, as listed below.

International Marathons:

Royal Victoria Canada (both x 4); Vancouver Canada (Alan x 2, Janette x 1);
Comox Valley Canada (both x 3); Country Roads Canada (both x 2);
Log Train Trail Canada (both x 1);
Seattle USA (both x 1); Philadelphia USA (both x 1); Hawaii USA (both x 1);
Big Sur USA (both x 1);
Paris France (both x 1); Burgundy Wine France (both x 1); Alsace Wine France (both x1); Antwerp Belgium (both x 1); Firenze Italy (Janette x 1);
Hamilton Millennium New Zealand (both x 1); Buller Gorge NZ (both x 1);
Marysville Australia (both x 1); Great Ocean Road Australia (both x 1).

Ultra Marathons:

Burning Boot 60 km Canada (both x 1);
Kneeknacker 50 km Trail Canada (Alan x 2, Janette x 3);
Woodstock Fruit Festival Marathon & 50 km Ultra USA (both x 1);
Great Ocean Road Marathon & Ultra Australia (both x 1).

… and then, there was the Ultra Endurance Event:

To celebrate the year 2000 and my 50th year, we ran the length of New Zealand together, covering 2182 km running 50 marathons in 50 consecutive days. I wrote the following account which was published in 'Marathon & Beyond' Magazine, Vol 5 Issue January 2001

'Running the length of New Zealand to Celebrate the Dawning of a New Millennium'
"When we sailed away from New Zealand in our 40-yacht 25 years ago with our two little children, we never anticipated that we'd eventually return to run the length of the island nation as a way of bidding farewell to the twentieth century while welcoming the twenty-first. As parents in the early 1970s, we searched for an alternative lifestyle and an ideal environment in which our little family could grow. In that idealistic quest, we sailed into the unknown dream world of sea gypsies, water wanderers and wayward travelers through the swollen sea of life. A decade of cruising through a dozen countries while experiencing numerous cultural happenings created a family firmly bonded by a keen sense of adventure. It was this commitment to enjoying each other while living life to the full that hatched the idea in 1997 of meeting again in New Zealand to celebrate the dawning of the new millennium in the year 2000. Over the years we had become avid runners, so it was natural that our new quest involve long distance running. We began to plan the challenge with the same detail we'd used over the years to set sail for new and exotic ports of call. Alan (then aged 54) and I (then aged 50) would run the length of New Zealand some 50 marathons in 50 days, while our then adult children, would help with the planning, organizing and support. It was exhilarating to launch into yet another adventure as a family. Our years of traveling had taught us that good health, attainable through consistent physical exercise and sensible nutrition, was of great importance for any challenge

we might set for ourselves. To run 50 marathons in as many days we figured the training would involve consistent long slow distance running, which would mean getting up early every morning and going for at least an hour's run, concentrating on keeping the pace at approximately six minutes per kilometre. Over the three years of training we would build up the distance run every day to include a 42 km run once a week while slowing the pace to roughly 7.3 minutes per kilometre.

It would be just as important to get the nutrition portion of the equation right. We had always believed that a balanced diet of natural foods and plenty of water is required to maintain a healthy body. Our training diet consisted of fresh fruit and veggies, whole grains, brown rice and pasta, soy products, some fresh fish, pure grapefruit juice and water. We did not eat any junk food or fast food, no red meat or dairy products, no salt and no tea or coffee. We also did not use any forms of drugs, such as painkillers, anti inflammatories and the like. Neither did we use sports drinks. We cannot overemphasize the importance of pure water intake in such an athletic venture toward remaining properly hydrated.

We were able to secure several sponsors for what we were calling 'NZ2000KmRun' including a naturally balanced energy bar and gel. We practiced eating it with a banana and a fresh fruit smoothie before beginning each run and had the energy gel at the end of each run. We made it a practice to always warm up with a 1 km walk and to cool down with a two kilometre walk at the end as a way of preventing injuries from overtaxed cold muscles. Immediately following each run, we stretched for 20 to 30 minutes, using mostly yoga stretches and, when our feet were weary, we would first soak them in ice water to bring down any swelling, then in warm water with Epsom salts afterward. We were also fortunate to be sponsored with 400 litres of pure grapefruit juice which we drank throughout the run. Other sponsorship included mobile telephones essential for communications between us and our support crew, a road bike and 5 pair of running shoes each, 3 pair of which we alternated during the Run, all of which we wore out.

We realised that running a marathon a day for 50 days to cover the 2000-plus kilometres from Cape Reinga in the north to Bluff in the south of New Zealand, would create a fair amount of interest throughout the country (and in fact worldwide primarily through our website), so we decided to seize the opportunity to do some charitable fundraising. As we had two friends who had been disabled as a result of car accidents, we had a personal interest in a good cause. We approached Paralympics

NZ with the idea and suggested any funds raised should go toward helping athletes with disabilities achieve their sporting goals and, ultimately, to compete in the Sydney 2000 Paralympic Games. Upon our arrival in New Zealand from France early in November 1999, Paralympics NZ took over organizing press releases to the news media and set up a website to encourage fundraising. We entered our daily diary notes throughout the run which were posted on the site.

Our son (then 28) who had agreed to be our support crew throughout the Run joined us from Scotland and our daughter (then 30, married and at the time expecting our first grandchild), would monitor the e-mail address from San Francisco where she lived and join us for the last two weeks of the Run. The first thing we did was buy a suitable support vehicle, a solid diesel truck converted to a mobile home that slept 3 and was guaranteed reliable to go the distance. Our son would be our driver, going ahead to stage water and food stops every 10 kilometres. He would also check out the next day's run on the bike after we had finished for the day, which meant that he would bike twice the distance that we would run every day. He pushed us out the door at 5:30 every morning, watered and fed us, and was always there with words of encouragement. He was our life support, and we couldn't have done it without him.

On December 17, 1999, we stood below the lighthouse at Cape Reinga at the northern tip of New Zealand and briefly looked out towards the Pacific Ocean which, 25 years before, had carried us with the wind in our sails away on our first adventure together. Now we were embarking on another voyage of discovery, this time over land with the soil beneath our feet as we ran the length of our country - Aotearoa as it is known to all New Zealanders. It was an emotional moment as the light flashed its last revolution when dawn broke, and we began to run. The trail around the coastland and down to 90 Mile Beach provided a rugged but beautiful start. Our son drove onto the beach and was waiting with water, suntan lotion and camcorder. Two days of sun, sand and diminishing horizons running on 90 Mile Beach was an unforgettable experience. Never before had we run 42.2km in a straight line! Once onto the roads, we settled into a daily routine of 5:30am starts, water and food breaks every 10 km, applying suntan lotion on a regular basis and changing clothes and shoes as necessary, depending on the weather. For the first five days we had various shifts of pain and 'niggles'. We would run along saying "right knee niggle", "left ankle pain", "right shoulder ache" and so on, comparing complaints as we progressed. The camber of the road played a big part in contributing to what we hoped would not become chronic injuries, as we had been training in Canada and Europe on the left side of the road and had to change to the right for oncoming traffic in New Zealand. We changed sides whenever it was safe to do so, on long straights and whenever there was a wide enough shoulder. We also tried to stay on the outside of country roads for better visibility by motorists.

After five days and five consecutive marathons, we were truly into 'unknown territory'. We'd never been beyond that point in training. We continued on, gripped with apprehension, but found, apart from when we encountered adverse weather conditions, that we could hold our own. The weather played a huge role in how much energy we depleted during each run and the time it took to cover the distance each day. Our average daily running time was 5:15 hours, but actual time on the road, including stops, ranged from 5:45 to 8:15 hours. When we had especially heavy rain, strong headwinds or extreme temperatures, we merely changed gear (that is, as in momentum and clothes). When it rained we used vaseline liberally on our toes and areas subject to chafing, so despite several days of constant rain, which meant running in soggy socks for several hours, we did not suffer any blisters, chafing or foot problems (apart from developing toes that looked like pink prunes).

After ten days on the run we realised that as long as we stayed at a constant pace, we would not sustain any major injuries. However, we always knew that rough ground could cause a twisted ankle and that the danger of road running with traffic was ever present. The terrain ranged from flat straights (such as 90 Mile Beach and the Canterbury Plains) to steep hills (such as the Parapara Mountain Range and Dunedin's Steepest Street in the World). We found that flat running caused more aches and pains than running hills because of the constant pounding and minimal range of motion of muscles. Generally, the rollinghills of New Zealand provided the best all-around terrain for running as well as the most interesting scenery.

We have never found running boring because there is always something to look at and something to think or talk about. After 30 years of marriage where we had always worked and played together, you'd think there wouldn't be much left to say. But every day there was something new to discover; a different birdsong, native trees, animal antics in the fields, house design ideas and garden landscapes.

At the end of each day's run, we set up camp in the truck. Sometimes we'd be close enough to a town where we could park in a campground overnight and return the following morning to the point where we'd stopped the previous day. Other days we would drive to family or friends who lived nearby. But often we would simply park where we ended our run: on the side of the road, under a tree or beside a river. Frequently we were treated to local hospitality, including offers of hot baths, laundry and shared meals. After a rough day of cold rain and wind, a free night in a warm motel or a heartwarming room in a country home was very welcome.

The greatest highlights of the run were undoubtedly when we were joined on the road by athletes with disabilities. Throughout New Zealand, Paralympics NZ kept the Regional Para Federation Groups informed of our schedule and in each area it was arranged for athletes and supporters to join us along the way. Having these wonderful people along put many things in perspective for us. The pain in our legs seemed to disappear when we were running alongside someone who was paralyzed or had no legs. We were honoured to run with new friends who had cerebral palsy, spina bifida, and disabilities ranging from visual impairment to tetraplegia. We enjoyed the company of paralympian medalists and youngsters aspiring to reach those heights. Their courage and determination inspired us to continue our commitment to finish the challenge we had set for ourselves. Another highlight was running the Hamilton Millennium Marathon, held on January 1, 2000. The race constituted our sixteenth marathon in our sequence. We pushed a wheelchair with a donation box around the course and collected $800 from runners and spectators. More than 2500 participants came from over the world, including several athletes with disabilities. Of all the marathons we have run worldwide, this was the most inspiring. We were later thrilled to learn that the marathon organisers had pledged $5000 toward our fund-raising effort.

Around the thirty seventh day we went through a tough period, which we attributed to a growing lack of restorative sleep and quality rest periods. At the time we had a lot of media coverage, which involved interviews for newspapers, radio and television as well as fund-raising campaigns where we pushed the donations wheelchair around towns after finishing each day's run. We now refer to this down period as "hitting the wall" because if we were to relate the 50 consecutive marathons to a single marathon, that would have been about the time and place you'd expect to encounter the dreaded 'Wall.' We managed to run through the exhaustion and nausea and come out feeling stronger and fitter than before. As we neared the end and began the countdown from 10 marathons to go to the finish, we experienced feelings of invincibility, of wanting the run to continue and wishing we could turn around and run right back again. (Yes, Forrest Gump is our favourite running movie!) We did, in a rash moment, decide to enter and run the Buller Gorge Marathon, held a week after we were scheduled to finish the NZ2000kmRun. (We figured we must be training toward something and Buller Gorge was a great marathon, Alan did 3:39, I did 4:06 and we raised over $100). However our mortality was reestablished during the last few days of slogging into Southland's cold headwinds, in rain which at times we were sure would turn to snow. We were convinced that the endurance we had built up during the previous 40 marathons helped us run through those days and were thankful we had not experienced those conditions earlier in the run. Although most New Zealanders were disappointed with the summer weather, we considered ourselves fortunate that for most of the run we had near-perfect conditions, with cool, overcast days. As we ran into Bluff on February 5, 2000, emotions ran high, yet we felt sad the run was ending. We even slowed down to make the experience last a little longer.

With the end of the road in sight, our son and daughter joined us and we all ran side by side, holding hands to the finish. It had been a team effort, a challenge we had set out to overcome together and a goal we had achieved as a family. We did it! We had run the length of New Zealand, 2182.2 km, 50 marathons in 50 days!"

The awareness we raised and the funds we attracted through the NZ2000KmRun went towards helping people with disabilities become rehabilitated and reintegrated into the community through the most effective medium of sports, recreation and leisure activities. In October 2000, Alan and I attended the Paralympic Games in Sydney, Australia as guests of the New Zealand Paralympic Team. It was an incredibly inspiring experience and an honour to be in the presence of those incredible athletes who prove every day that if you 'never stop pushing' you can achieve whatever goal you set for yourself.

During the years between the NZ2000kmRun and RunRAW2013, we experienced and learned much about incorporating our conscious way of living with long distance endurance running, as shown with the following comparisons between NZ2000kmRun and RunRAW2013:

Comparisons between NZ2000kmRun & RunRAW2013

	NZ2000kmRun	RunRAW2013
Ages of Alan & Janette	54 & 50	68 & 64
# of Marathon distances	50	365
Total distance run	2182.2 km	15,782 km
Training Time	3 years	3 years
Type of shoes for run	running shoes	Vibram barefoot shoes
Number of shoes for run	3 pair each	16 pair each
Type of Food Consumed	Vegetarian/Vegan	Raw Vegan
Type of Energy Food	'Energy' Bars	dates & bananas
Type of Energy Drinks	boxed juice	fresh juice
Blister prevention	vaseline	Vibram barefoot shoes
Sun screen	chemical based	no sunscreen
Type of Fuel for Vehicles	Petrol	LPG Autogas
Type of Power Energy	electric	Solar

While Running Raw Around Australia we wore Vibram Five Finger (toe shoes designed to assimilate barefoot running) to run as near to barefoot as possible. Running 'barefoot' around Australia was a conscious lifestyle choice to tread lightly on the earth and to eliminate the possibility of injury. The benefits of running barefoot have long been supported by scientific research, coaches and athletes, who believe that a gradual system of training barefoot will strengthen muscles in the foot and lower legs, leading to a better running form through an increased sense of balance and greater agility. Running in Vibram shoes enabled us to experience the freedom and joy of running 'barefoot' while reducing the risk of exposure to obstacles that may cause injury. By running 'barefoot' around Australia in Vibram shoes, we were more in tune with our bodies which deepened our connection with the earth.

In training for RunRAW2013 during 2012, we ran everyday logging approximately one hundred and twenty kilometres per week including one marathon distance. We also participated in several running races, all run in Vibram barefoot shoes:

Warrandyte 8 km Fun Run, Australia (Alan x 1). Third overall of 60 starters and oldest runner.

Sri Chinmoy 15 km, Melbourne, Australia. (Alan x 1. Oldest participant.

Australian Ultra Runners 6 Hour Race (Alan x 1) Thirteenth overall, running 60 km in 6 hours at 66 years of age, finishing 3 km short of the Australian 65-70 record.

Le Semi-Marathon de la Vente des Vins des Hospice, Nuits-Saint-Georges, France. (Janette x 1)

10 km and 21.1 km race, second in Veteran 3 Femmes category for both distances.

Sri Chinmoy 18 km Melbourne Australia. (Alan x 1) First in category, oldest participant.

Sri Chinmoy 30 km Melbourne (both x 1). I finished first, Alan third 60-69 Veterans category.

RunRAW2013 started January 1, 2013, leaving Melbourne heading north following Highway 1 around Australia in a counterclockwise direction. Together we ran at least a marathon distance (42.2 km) with an average of 43 km every day throughout the year (365 days), until we returned to Melbourne via Tasmania. The last marathon (#365) of RunRAW2013 finished at our starting point in Federation Square, Melbourne on 31 December 2013. Then, on January 1, 2014, we ran Marathon #366 along the Yarra River Trail from Melbourne to Warrandyte to set the World Record for the most consecutive marathons Running Raw Around Australia, the only couple over the age of 60, fueled on fruit and veg, wearing barefoot shoes.

Throughout RunRaw2013, while running every marathon every day for 366 days, we used a Garmin GPS Watch to accurately record (via satellite) extensive data on each marathon, including the latitude and longitude of each start and finish, elevation gain, distance run, running time and pace, as well as a graph showing the profile of each marathon and other relative information. We also recorded the distance run with the Garmin GPS device in both support vehicles, and our support crew wrote a separate daily journal entry which verifies our own written daily account of each marathon. Excepts from these written entries were posted through the social network on our Facebook page throughout the Run. All the collective data has been submitted to the Academy of World Records, Guinness World Records and the Australian Records for official recognition.

While Running Raw Around Australia we were also very focused on raising awareness and supporting charities instrumental in making a difference to the health and welfare of people, animals and environmental sustainability within Australia and worldwide. RunRAW2013 was an awareness and fund-raising event for the following charities: Animals Australia, Kids Under Cover, The Gawler Foundation and The Australian Paralympic Committee.

Animals Australia

Animals Australia is a nonprofit charitable organisation financed through community support representing some 40 member societies and thousands of individual supporters. Animals Australia campaigns to protect *all* animals, and is known for its groundbreaking work in investigating and exposing animal cruelty. Animals, like us, are emotional beings. Their desire to be free from suffering is not unlike our own. Yet unlike us, they cannot vote, object, or speak out against violence — making animals among the most exploited, and in need of our protection. In recognising that the raising and killing of animals for food is today the primary cause of animal suffering and that the livestock sector is one of the most unsustainable industries on the planet—and that adopting a vegetarian lifestyle has many health benefits, the WhyVeg.com website was created. WhyVeg.com is an initiative of Animals Australia, Australia's most dynamic national animal protection organisation. In understanding the compelling reasons why people are shifting to a plant-based diet, more people will adopt healthy, compassionate, and cruelty-free lifestyles. Animals Australia believes that we can create a better world for all through promoting kindness to animals. Their goal is to significantly and permanently improve the welfare of all animals in Australia. www.animalsaustralia.org

Kids Under Cover

Established in 1989, Kids Under Cover is a not-for-profit organisation operating in Victoria, Queensland and the ACT. Their vision is for all young people to have the opportunity to reach their full potential. On any one night in Australia, around 105,000 people are homeless. Almost half of these people are under the age of 25 years. 23% of Australia's homeless are children – almost one in four homeless people is under 18. On average, two out of three young people who become homeless while at school will leave school in the same year. Kids Under Cover respond to the needs of young people who are at risk of becoming homeless by offering one or two bedroom, fully demountable studios with bathroom, constructed on the grounds of the family or carer's home. This unique accommodation allows families to stay connected, giving them extra room to live and providing the young person with a secure and stable environment to grow into healthy adulthood. When the studio is no longer needed by the family, it is dismantled and moved to another family in need. Studios last approximately 15 years and can be relocated up to four times. Kids Under Cover also has a Housing Program whereby 14 houses accommodate young people who are currently experiencing homelessness including a strong focus on young mothers and their babies. Young people and their siblings who have lived, or are currently living in Kids Under Cover accommodation, automatically qualify to apply for a Kids Under Cover Scholarship. The scholarships are designed to promote the return to school for individuals who have been absent for extended periods and for those looking to realise their dreams through further education. Through responsive action with a focus on prevention, Kids Under Cover supports young people to be independent with the opportunity to experience family life and pursue educational aspirations. www.kuc.org.au

The Gawler Foundation

The Gawler Foundation was established in 1983 as a nonprofit, non-denominational organisation to provide innovative and integrated support for people affected by cancer and other illnesses. The Foundation's underlying philosophy is that regaining balance in one's life leads to healing. The Gawler Foundation offers a range of lifestyle programs based on nutrition, meditation, positivity and empowerment. Using holistic approaches to healing, the well-being programs foster health promotion, disease prevention and total well-being in body, emotions, mind and spirit. Consistent with the principles of integrated medicine, The Gawler Foundation programs apply a self-help approach designed to improve quality of life. This enables participants to make informed, effective choices and better manage their own healing journeys. The philosophies of The Gawler Foundation are based on the healing experience of Dr Ian Gawler who in 1975, then a young Vet and decathlon athlete, was diagnosed with bone cancer, and as a result, his right leg was amputated. Eleven months later, the cancer returned and his specialist told him he had only two or three weeks to live. Ian then followed an effective self-help program with key principles; good food, positive attitudes, meditation and loving support. He completed a remarkable recovery eighteen months later. Due to his own healing experience, Ian Gawler established Australia's first active Cancer Support Group in 1981. The Gawler Foundation was established in 1983 to further his work. Based in Victoria, Australia at a residential retreat in the Yarra Valley and set on 20 acres at the foot of rolling hills amid natural bushland. The Gawler Foundation Yarra Valley Living Centre accommodating up to 40 guests, offers a place of comfort and nurture for the range of healing and well-being programs offered. www.gawler.org

The Australian Paralympic Committee

The Australian Paralympic Committee (APC) is a not-for-profit organisation and a registered charity, The APC helps Australians with disabilities participate in sport and compete at the Paralympic Games. Participation in sport provides positive social and physical benefits to people with disabilities and plays an important role in changing community perceptions of people with disabilities. The primary goal in creating the APC, was to establish participation at summer and winter Paralympic Games, marketing (sponsorship and fundraising) and public awareness together with a support goal assisting members to develop disability sport within Australia. Current APC Members include: Athletics Australia, Australian Blind Sports Federation, Australian Shooting International Limited, Australian Sport and Recreation Association for Persons with an Intellectual Disability, Basketball Australia,

Australian Sports Organisation for the Disabled, Cycling Australia, Cerebral Palsy-Australian Sport and Recreation Federation, Disabled Winter Sport Australia, Equestrian Australia, Football Federation Australia, Riding for the Disabled Association Australia, Rowing Australia, Swimming Australia, Table Tennis Australia, Tennis Australia, Wheelchair Sports Australia, and Yachting Australia. The Australian Paralympic Committee helps identify potential Paralympians and assists athletes to prepare for competition by providing funding for coaching, equipment and travel in the lead up to the summer and winter Paralympic Games. At the heart of what The Australian Paralympic Committee does are the athletes, who strive to compete at an elite level, upholding the ideals of the Paralympic movement. Australia has participated in the Paralympic Summer Games since the first Games in Rome 1960 and in the Paralympic Winter Games since their inception in 1976. www.paralympic.org.au

These four charities were chosen to be recipients of RunRAW2013 awareness and fundraising because each of them are actively involved in making a difference to the lives and well-being of people and animals through kindness and compassion. Due to the dedicated work of these charities, many children and animals, people with disabilities and people with ill health are receiving support and care for their well being. We were proud to be associated with these Charities and to raise awareness and funds to help them in their endeavours to help others.

Running Raw Around Australia also gave us the opportunity to experience a very personal journey. Although we started out with the feeling that we (as a species), and we (personally) were Running Out of Time to make a difference, it *gave* us time to reflect on our own lives and how we can continue to inspire and motivate others in the future. Running around this Sacred Land, meeting the people and the animals, experiencing the kindness, compassion and support from so many, and understanding that *this* is our natural way of being, it was in so many ways, a Journey of Discovery.

This journey was not only an incredible physical, mental and spiritual experience for us personally, but also one that we were able to share with countless people around Australia and Worldwide. We ran a marathon every day for a year and a day, to share a positive message at a time when people are sick and tired of being sick and tired. A time when people are looking for an answer, when people are looking for inspiration and motivation to take control of their own health, a time when people are genuinely concerned about their environment and their children's future. We went the distance, but we were not alone. By the time we had been running for half a year and were halfway round the country, mainstream TV, radio, newspapers and journalists worldwide were wanting to cover the story....because it was a feel good story, and now is a time when people want to hear a feel good story. By the time we finished Marathon #366, there were over 17,000 people worldwide who had been following the Run on our Facebook page, countless others through Running Raw Around Australia website. They were with us all the way, one step at a time, one marathon a day, going the distance on their own Journey of Discovery. Here is that feel good story:

RUNNING RAW AROUND AUSTRALIA
Route and Schedule

Melbourne - Canberra	January 1 - 22
Canberra - Sydney	January 24 - February 2
Sydney - Brisbane	February 4 - 25
Brisbane -Townsville	February 27 - March 30
Townsville - Darwin	May 22 - 28
Darwin - Katherine	June 3 - 4
Katherine - Fitzroy Crossing	June 5 - July 2
Fitzroy Crossing - Broome	July 3 - 11
Broome - Perth	July 13 - September 3
Perth - Albany	September 5 - 18
Albany - Esperance	September 19 - Oct 1
Esperance - Ceduna	October 2 - November 1
Ceduna - Adelaide	November 2 - 20
Adelaide - Geelong	November 22 - December 7
Geelong - Melbourne	December 8 - 11
Melbourne	December 11 - 14
Spirit of Tasmania Ferry	December 14
Melbourne - Tasmania	
via Devonport, Launceston, Hobart	December 15 - 21
Tasmania Hobart - Devonport	December 21 - 30
Spirit of Tasmania Ferry, Melbourne	
Finish Run at Federation Square	December 31
World Record Breaking Run -	Marathon # 366
Melbourne - Warrandyte	
Along the Yarra River Trail	January 1, 2014

January 2013

MARATHONS #1-31

...And they're off!!! A great turn out this morning at Federation Square, Melbourne- thanks everyone who came to see them off. Janette and Alan were looking fresh and ready for their inspirational adventure!-Eileen, RunRAW2013 PR Person

Marathon #1.

January 1, 2013. Federation Square, CBD Melbourne to Berwick on Hwy 1. We arrived at Federation Square to start the Run and there were over 70 well wishers gathered to send us off, thanks guys! Great media coverage from TV Ch 7, 9, 10 & ABC. Our PR & Media person Eileen set us off at 8:30am with a group of over 30 runners, including Ping one of our Support Team, while the other Support Crew, Tabitha, Maureen, and Graeme drove the vehicles ahead for our first stop. Had other media interviews along the road throughout the day, making it a very long day on the road running on concrete all the way to Berwick. We ate fresh fruit all day and had a salad for dinner after we finished. Camped on the grass verge beside the road where we finished and met a few locals who came by to greet us. Met by Graeme's friend Carol who invited us to her place for showers and laundry, which she returned to us in the morning before 6am, all dried and folded, thanks Carol. What an amazing day, seemed like we were never going to get there! It sure felt like we were Running Out of Time! If every day is like this, we'll need more hours in the day! Temp 15-26 degrees. Distance 42.2 km. Pace 7.47. Running Time 5hrs 43min. Time on the Road 11 hours.

Comments from Facebook/RunningRawAroundAustralia2013:

- *You're absolutely awesome. I keep my fingers crossed for you two.* - **Natalia**
- *I'll be watching you all year! Best of luck every step of the long journey! You are inspiring.* -

Jessica
- *Nice work Alan and Janette.-***Sally**
- *Wowee Zowee. -* **Gladys**
- *Best wishes from Canada - I will be watching -* **Parvati**
- *WOW, best of luck! hope to see you in WA! -* **Willeke**
- *Best of luck- you're awesome. Love the spirit -* **Melanie x**
- *Good luck! -* **Susan**
- *GO Alan and Janette!!! You two are truly amazing!! Best of luck to you both -* **Rhonda X0**
- *Best wishes from Stockholm. -* **Stuart**
- *Sorry we couldn't be there guys, but thinking of you! Go strong. -* **Vegan Smythe**
- *Keep going! Running Raw -* **Marco**

Marathon #2.

January 2, 2013. Berwick to Longwarry. Away at 6am. Legs and feet all good. Fast 12 km to first stop for TV interview for the Today Tonight Show. Also did Radio interviews for ABC Darwin and Perth while on the run and 1 hour of photos for the Leader newspaper. Still on concrete most of the way but todays run easier than yesterday. Ate fruit all day, a big bowl of cherries on finishing and salad for dinner. Thanks for the offer of showers and the donation from Bill and Isabel. Distance 42.27 km. Pace 7.47. Running time 5hr 28min. Time on Road 10 hrs.

Marathon #3.

January 3, 2013. Longwarry to Trafalgar. Away at 5:15am, legs and feet still feeling good, ran 12 km to first stop. Lovely sunrise and rolling hills through countryside. Did radio interview at 7:30am for ABC Canberra. Hilly most of the day, had trouble finding our way through Warragul without going on the freeway, eventually took a country road over the hills and far away!

It was a very hot, slow finish, 36 degrees. Camped in a secluded spot away from the road and ate a whole durian! Distance 42.32 km. Running time 5hrs 41min. Time on Road 10 hrs.

Marathon #4.

January 4, 2013. Trafalgar to Traralgon. Away 5am onto the freeway, we met Trev the local police who gave us permission to run on the wide emergency lane so we don't have to take long detours on the narrow country roads around here. Great sunrise. One car in four tooting and waving. First stop at 12 km ran in heat with no shade 12-39 km and had to make a detour to get water. The radiant heat from the road was burning our faces, the road was melting and so were we! Maureen found a shady spot for us to stop after running in the heat for 17 km and we devoured a whole watermelon each! We finished in 42 degree heat, next 361 have got to be easier! To night we're staying in Park Avenue Tourist Park, Traralgon compliments of Helen and Tom, many thanks. It's 9:30pm and cooling down to 35 degrees so we can use the wifi which melted down on us today! Max Temp 42.3 degrees. Distance 42.2 km. Running time 5hr 39min. Time on Road 10hr. For those in the area, we'll be running from Traralgon on Hwy 1 (Princes Hwy towards Sale, see you on the road!

Marathon #5.

January 5, 2013. Traralgon to 10 km west of Sale. Drove to where we had finished yesterday and started running at 5:30am. Very warm 24 degrees at sunrise. First stop with Tabitha at 13 km while Maureen and Ping went shopping for more fruit! Second stop at 21 km, running with a strong following wind. Alan developed a slight pain above his left knee which got worse until he could barely run. Slow 10 km to finish with his knee pain easing but quads very tight. Finished at 42.41 km and drove down side road to the local airport where the girls had set up camp for the night in the car park. Airport officials offered for us to use the facilities and fridge during the night, thanks! Alan icing his knee while we had a delicious salad for dinner. Food intake for the day each 1 grapefruit, 3 bananas, green smoothie with 10 bananas, bunch grapes, 3 oranges, bowl cherries, half watermelon, chia pudding with extra bananas and salad. Temp 36.5 degrees. Pace 8.12 Running Time 5hr 48min. Time on Road 9.5 hrs.

Marathon #6.

January 6, 2013. West Sale Airport to Providence Ponds Nature Reserve, 30 km short of

Bairnsdale today. A distance 42.63 km running time 5 hrs 56mins in a cool 27 degrees with only 4 corners all day. Slight inflammation on Alan's knee, nothing a little ice and arnica wont take care of. Running fuel intake each: 4 bananas, 1 grapefruit, 1 kg cherries, 1/2kg grapes, 10 oranges, 3 mangoes, 1 avocado, 4 kiwifruit, huge mixed vege salad and banana chia pudding, yum! An emotional finish to the Run met by Remeeka from Kids Under Cover and family.

Marathon #7.

January 7, 2013. Providence Ponds 32 km east of Sale to Nicholson River Camp Ground through Bairnsdale. Slept in! Away at 6:15am. Alan's knee much better but Janette feeling sick and tired! Bit soon for that! Tabitha phoned us to say the ute was not running well so phoned RACV for roadside assistance. They sent a mechanic and both caught up with us at the local garage. Seems the new LPG tank was empty and it had not changed over to the main tanks, so we'll have to keep both full. Filled up and all going well. Long straight roads all day only three corners till we reached Bairnsdale, which also has a very long main street through the town. Finished the run at Nicholson River Campground and set up in a complimentary site, thanks for that and the great hot showers. Maureen and Ping went shopping for more fruit and veg. Food intake each 3 bananas, 4 oranges, 4 nectarines, half watermelon, green smoothie with 10 bananas, 2 bowls chia pudding with extra bananas, 2 glasses fresh carrot & beetroot juice, 1 avocado, large salad, zucchini noodles with botanical cuisine tomato sauce. Distance 42.29 km. Pace 8.34. Running Time 6hr 02min. Time on the Road 10hr.

Marathon #8.

January 8, 2013. Nicholson to Lake Tyers State Forest 10 km past Lakes Entrance. Nice scenery over the Nicholson River and through Lakes Entrance. Up in the hills now, thanks Warrandtye for the hill training! Tomorrow's Run to Orbost. Cooler day 29 degrees. Running time 6hrs 11min. Time on road 9 hrs. Pace 8.46min per km. Distance 42.29 km.

Marathon #9.

January 9, 2013. Lake Tyers Forest to 2 km past Orbost Cool dark start at 4:45am. Rolling hills with a cool wind behind us, a runner's dream. Day 9 and the best day's run so far. Temp 19 degrees. Distance 42.23 km. Running time 6hrs 14min. Time on road 8hrs 30min. Pace 8.51.

Marathon #10.

January 10, 2013. 2 km past Orbost to 30 km before Cam River. We're one thirty- sixth of the way there! Orbost over Mt Raymond to Cabbage Tree Creek, parked overnight in forest. Hills, hills and more hills, cool start 4:45am. Phone interview with ABC East Gippsland Radio on the run. Thanks to those who stopped us on the road and gave donations and Lester who gave us local road info for tomorrow. Thanks to all the motorists for the toots and waves. Best days run yet. Today's food (fuel) intake: grapefruit, 4 bananas, banana chia pudding, brazil nuts, large banana & orange smoothie, rock-melon, large veg juice, 6 nectarines, 6 dates, 1 avocado, large mixed veg salad with stuffed mushrooms & red peppers. Tomorrow's run to halfway between Cann River and Wingan River. Temp 23 degrees. Distance 42.4 km Running time 6hrs 15min Time on road 9hrs.

Marathon #11.

January 11, 2013. 30 km from Cam River to Wingan River. More steep hills from Orbost to Wingan River. Camped on roadside where we met lovely raw vegan couple Carina and Patrick who are traveling around in their van. Conducted phone interview with German newspaper in the afternoon. Distance 42.16 km. Running time 6hrs 32min. Time on road 10 hours. Today's food intake: 1 grapefruit, grapes, banana pudding, smoothie, melon, nectarines, tomatoes, 1.5 avocados, dates, brazil nuts, large salad of tomato, cucumber, avocado and greens with tahini/citrus dressing.

Marathon #12.

January 12, 2013. Wingan River to NSW/Victorian border. On the road at 5AM, lovely sunrise at 6am. We met a swagman on a bicycle with his little dog who had ridden down from Brisbane en route to Melbourne to get away from the heat. Also met the lovely, hospitable Marianne in Genoa who gave us lemons and apples. Best run so far! Felt so good at 42.2km that we decided to run on to the border making 46.43 km for the day. Running time 6 hrs 43 mins. Time on road 9.5 hours. Today's food intake: grapefruit, apple, grapes, 3 avocados, dates, smoothie, melon, almonds, brazil nuts, more grapes, nectarines, zucchini spaghetti with creamy tomato sauce and salad.

Marathon #13.
January 13, 2013. Vic/NSW Border to 5 km south of Eden. Away at 5AM. Left the van in Victoria and ran across the border into NSW in the dark. Very narrow shoulder on the road and all hills! Camped at sea level at Twofold Bay, just before Eden. Great hot showers and did some laundry at Discovery Holiday Park on the beach. Sadly, it rained all afternoon and evening… Running time 6 hours 40 mins. Time on road 9 hours. Today's food intake: apple, lemon juice, 3 oranges, dates, nectarines, big smoothie, soaked almonds, large green salad. Distance 42.35 km.

Marathon #14.
January 14, 2013. 5 km south of Eden to 10 km before Bega. Away in the dark as always. Very hilly, passed thru Eden, nice coastal views. Tough last 12 km running on very stony shoulder. Stopped at a roadside campsite with a beautiful view. Running time 7hrs 4mins. Time on road 12 hours (due to being photographed by media for three hours!) Today's food intake: 3 bananas, large bowl of steel cut oats with figs and almonds, half watermelon, spinach smoothie, cashew and brazil nuts, 6 nectarines, 1 rock-melon, dates, avocado, fruit salad. Distance 43.00km.

Marathon #15.
January 15, 2013. 10 km before Bega to Quaama. Away at 5:15. It was just getting light. Lots more hills! Ran thru Bega, NSW. Very narrow shoulder and rough asphalt. Hot and windy all day. Flies very bad in eyes, ears, nose, mouth, may have to dig out mosquito net masks soon… Nice quiet camp beside St Saviour's Church in Quaama. No road noise tonight! Today's food intake: Bananas, steel cut oats with figs and almonds and fresh-made almond milk, dates,

green smoothie with banana, apple, spinach, 1 watermelon, 4 yellow nectarines, avocado, more dates, 2 large salads with tomato. Distance 43.00km.

Marathon #16.

January 16, 2013. Quaama to Island View Holiday Park, Narooma. Great run down the hills to the sea! Ran from the quaint town of Quaama to just before Narooma. Met a Japanese cyclist on the way who had cycled down from Darwin en route to Adelaide and a couple on a motorbike with a sidecar who gave us a $30 donation. Many thanks to Jason, manager of Islandview Beach Resort for giving us a free night despite being super full! Super great facilities at a gorgeous beachside location! After dinner we all walked to the beach 5 mins from our camp and had a swim. Beautiful view of Montague Island from Handkerchief Beach. Today's food intake: oranges, dried figs, green smoothie, bananas, 6 nectarines, 1/2 watermelon, avocado, sun-dried tomatoes, olives, green salad. Distance 42.70km.

Marathon #17.

January 17, 2013. Narooma to 30 km south of Batemans Bay. Alarm didn't go off this morn, so had a late start. LOL! Away at 6AM with a cool sea breeze. Beautiful coast and inlets. One of our easier days. Felt good at finish. Ran from Island View Holiday Resort (thanks again Jason) to just south of Moruya. Today's food intake: 3 bananas, figs, 3 glasses of banana/greens/date smoothie, half watermelon, veg juice, cashews, olives, 2 large salads, fruit salad. Distance 43.97km.

Marathon #18.

January 18, 2013. Moruya-Batemans Bay to Nelligen. We were expecting a hot day today (40 degrees) so got an early start to beat the heat. Only ran 3 km before our water was boiling, almost too hot to drink. Heat from the road was searing, it was like being in an oven. Steep hills. REALLY hot, the day peaked at 44 degrees, but luckily, we found a really lovely campsite for the night on the banks of the Clyde River in Nelligen. Lovely gent and his mum offered us their place on the river for the night and went to get water for us. Many thanks! Went for a swim in the salty water which cooled our core temperatures beautifully! The river location was too good to resist for the night, but was not quite 42.2 km, so after a quick dip, we ran around the wee town of Nelligen to make up the kilometres. Today's food intake: 1 grapefruit, 4 bananas, grapes and more bananas, green smoothie and leftover salad, tahini, yellow zucchini, olives, figs, half watermelon, oranges, large juice of beetroot, apple and orange, rock-melon, fresh coconut juice with vanilla bean, zucchini spaghetti, green salad, pineapple. Distance 42.28km.

Marathon #19.

January 19, 2013. Nelligen to 6 km before Braidwood. Away at 4:45, but the Garmin watch wasn't charged overnight, so it stopped at 9 km. Put it on the charger for the next leg, and took it for the last two legs, but our stats for the day were stuffed up Still ran 42.2 km though. Ran in light rain most of the day. The Clyde was so steep we could smell the brakes of the traffic coming downhill and the clutches of the traffic going uphill. Very dangerous with little or no shoulder all the way up. What shoulder there was, was very rocky! Time on road 11 hours. Stopped for the night in another gravel pit (the Universe knows how we love those) 6.5 km east of Braidwood. Today's food intake: 1 grapefruit, 4 bananas, left over zucchini spaghetti, 7 nectarines, brazil nuts, 8 nectarines, 1.5 avocados, sun dried tomatoes and tahini. Distance 42.20km.

Marathon #20.

January 20, 2013. 6 km before Braidwood to 10 km east of Bungendore. Away at 4:55. Ran thru Braidwood in the dark while the town was sleeping. Smooth shoulder on the road. Met two young men going home from a party who offered us a rum and coke! Also talked to a highway patrol officer from Sydney and asked his advice on negotiating Sydney traffic. After seeing how steep the Clyde was, we decided on a different route out of Canberra going through Goulburn and Shell Harbour and into Sydney through Sutherland. New schedule being posted on the website soon. Today we finished crossing the Great Dividing Range at 851 metres above sea level. Ran through where bushfire had burnt 3-4 days ago and met Dave and Cat Prentice, who gave us a generous donation. Many thanks! Today's food intake: 1 grapefruit, 4 bananas, mangoes, avocados, nuts, large banana cinnamon smoothie, drinking coconut, nectarines, rock-melon, large green juice (kale, spinach, orange), and more avocado, watermelon. Distance 42.92km.

Marathon #21.

January 21, 2013. 10 km east of Bungendore to Canberra. Away at 4:45 on smooth roads through the wee town of Bungendore. Found wounded kangaroo on the road in the first 15 km. Called wildlife people who came to see her but the poor girl's leg had been broken by a collision with a vehicle and she had to be euthanised. At least she wasn't alone in her final minutes. Thank you Diane from WIRES for coming to the rescue (so to speak). PLEASE slow down on country roads, people, especially at dusk and nighttime! We ran through Queanbeyan and into Canberra in 30+ degree heat. We stopped for the night in Fyshwick. Many thanks to Anne from the Canberra South Motor Park for our complimentary night! In the afternoon, the folks from Gas Energy Australia came and took photos of us with the vehicles. Our Subaru station wagon was converted to gas and is now dual fuel. The Ford Falcon is a dedicated gas vehicle with two fuel tanks that will be driving right through the Northern Territory and WA on only LPG Autogas. Today's food intake: 1 grapefruit, 4 bananas, left over salad, avocado, soaked figs, banana and watermelon smoothie, brazil nuts, 6-7 nectarines. Post run: 1 avocado with 2 dates, large salad of lettuce, carrot, beetroot, olives, fresh and sun-dried tomatoes, fresh corn. Distance 42.27km.

Marathon #22.

January 22, 2013. Canberra. Running around Canberra along the lake trails and up to Parliament House. Very quiet on the streets with Parliament on holidays, but don't worry, we'll keep running the country! Fun to meet up with Melbourne couple on the run and found we'd been in same races with last year. On our own for the run (no support crew) so food intake was plenty of water and dates with 1 pineapple at 17 km and 1 avocado at finish. Great turn out at Sweet Bones Vegan Restaurant for our talk and delicious raw vegan 3 course dinner, green smoothie, zucchini noodles with tomato sauce and banana chia pudding. Thanks Jyoti, Emily & Russell. Great to meet everyone and thanks so much for your support. Temp 30 degrees. Distant 43.04 km, Running Time 6hrs 56min.

Marathon # 23.
January 23, 2013. Watson, Canberra. Running around (in circles!) near Canberra, through the northern suburbs lovely tree lined streets and a few kangaroos in the bush on Mt Majuro. Temp 28 degrees. Running time 5hrs 53min Pace 8.21 Distance 42.25 km. Heading out of Canberra tomorrow and being joined by new crew Graeme en route. Finally downloaded all videos and photos taken since start of Run tonight! Good night folks!

Marathon #24.
January 24, 2013. From Watson, Canberra ACT to Arthur Stanley Gurney VC Remembrance Rest Stop at George Lake, NSW. Away from campground 5:15am eating 1 grapefruit and 2 bananas onto Federal Hwy. still dark. Huge wide bike lane mostly concrete all the way. Ran a fast 13 km to the first stop, ate 6 oranges then ran very fast pace (fastest 10 km since leaving Melbourne) to 26 km, start of George Lake with wind farm on the hills 100 windmills. Thanks to the passing tourist who gave a donation. Ate 4 bananas and 2 peaches. Ran along edge of dry lake for 10 km where our friend Graeme was waiting having flown in from Melbourne and driven the ute and caravan on to meet us with Maureen and Ping for the third stop. All had a sit-down salad lunch, great to have our dear friends all together with us. Great rest stop just 2 km on so the Team parked and got set up for the night while we ran on and back the last 4 km for the day's run. Temp 29 degrees. Distance 42.21 km. Running time 5hr 49min. Pace 8.16. Will be setting up official Garmin stats in the next couple of days. Now the question is, which Vibrams shall we wear tomorrow?

Comments from Facebook/RunningRawAroundAustralia2013:
- *Great work guys!* - **Roy**

- *I love this couple such an inspirational story and gives hope to so many people everywhere that it's never to late to live and do the things you want.* - **Tara**
- *That is a lot of vibrams. Clearly your preferred footwear? Are you not eating any proteins?* - **Nikki Greens Nikki, lotsa greens!**
- *All plant foods have proteins in them.* - **Nalin**
- *Jeanette, are the food amounts you are listing for both of you together, or each? A raw vegan diet provides plenty of protein. Great going Alan and Janette... you guys are an inspiration!* - **Vee**
- *Legends* - **Maryanne**
- *Wow. It still doesn't seem like enough food for all that work. I hope you are both watching the scales. Cheering you on.* - **Nikki Xx**
- *Awesome work and its great to here about your food intake. Stay safe.* - **John**
- *Looking fantastic guys!* - **Remeeka**
- *Inspiring! All the best.* - **Patty xx**
- *Truly amazing.* - **Lisa**
- *You are both so inspiring!!!! Absolutely amazing!* - **Robyn** *Xxx*
- *How long do a pair of vibrams last?* - **Lee**
- *Nice collection of shoes you got there.* - **Minsk**
- *A pair of vibrams last for at least 500 miles in my experience.* - **Steve**
- *I vote for the pinky-red ones.* - **Alana**
- *...and I thought i had a Vibram obsession! You guys are so incredible!* - **Fiona**
- *You are both such an inspiration. Great work.* - **Taylor**
- *Keep up the great work - amazing inspiration.* - **Rachel**

Marathon #25.

January 25, 2013. George Lake to Goulburn South. Away 5:15AM running alongside misty lake. Flat concrete cycle lane. Crossed Great Divide 740 meters. First break at 13 km ate bowl of fruit salad. Graeme and Ping off to Goulburn to have the SuperRoo checked and do fruit shopping. Maureen at next stop 25 km with nectarines and peaches. Stopped to talk with two brothers who are walking from Melbourne to India to experience life through nature. Shared fruit with them and ran on into the mounting heat. Third stop at 32 km ate whole melon and nectarines. Temp 36 degrees with 6 km to go, very tiring, but perked up when we got to the campground in Goulburn for cold showers and another delicious dinner of 2 salads and fruit chia pudding, thanks to Maureen and Ping. Catching up on laundry and updating the website - check out the Events page if you're in Sydney for our charity dinner evening on 2 Feb and run to the Opera House with us on 3 February. Distance 43.66 km. Running time 6hr 15min. Pace 8.36. See you on the road!

Marathon #26.
Goulburn South to Marulan. Australia Day 26 Jan 2013. Where's everybody going? Don't they know it's a holiday? We were out on the Hume Hwy with thousands of cars and trucks racing past in both directions. Is that why everyone is asking how we're coping with the traffic? Well, we can now say that it was incredibly draining, especially the last 10 km. So, can everyone please stay home on the holidays? Thanks! Departed Watson Campground 5:15am arrived Marulan Rest Area off road on Old Hume Hwy 3pm, no more road noise! Cool breeze behind us most of the day, temp to 29 degrees. Distance 42.2 km. Running Time 6hr 7min. Pace 8.41. Food intake (each) 1 grapefruit, 3 bananas, 5 peaches & nectarines 1 avocado with olives & brazil nuts, half water melon, 10 dates, very large and delicious salad, and almond smoothie. Alan & Graeme installed new solar panel on caravan roof before spectacular lightning and thunder storm. Shut everything down including the computer (reason why this post is a day late) and watched the show. Nature provided a better show than any fireworks display for Australia Day!

Marathon #27.
January 27, 2013. Marulan to Burrawang. Lightening storm brought heavy rain throughout the night which continued this morning. Depart 5am in dark, light rain, temp 19 degrees. Rain increased to very heavy after 40 min, we were wet through and getting cold by the first stop. Changed to dry clothes but kept wet Vibrams on, no blisters. Alan developed painful

shin splint on right leg, iced the swelling at 3pm and 5pm. Rain eased and rest of run very pleasant after turning off the Hume Hwy onto Irriwarra Hwy, so peaceful with no traffic noise. Through farmland reminiscent of the English countryside. Farms with English names and village of Sutton Forest had great little fruit and veg market - thanks to Jim for the gifts of produce! Through Moss Vale and on to lovely spot to camp of the road. Temp 23 degrees. Distance 42.29 km. Running Time 6hrs 10min. Pace 8.45. Food intake (each) 1 grapefruit, 4 bananas, 6 peaches, banana watermelon smoothie, 5 mangoes, green smoothie, half avocado, large salad and zucchini noodles with tomato sauce.

Marathon #28.
January 28, 2013. Burrawang to Dapto on Lake Irrawarra. Heavy rain all night, delayed start at 5:30 waiting for rain to ease, gave up and ran out into it, through Robertson (where we saw the New Idea) and on to first stop at 12 km top of Macquarie Pass. Fantastic nonstop fast run downhill (10% grade) thru the Pass in heavy rain. Beautiful thru misty rainforest and sheer rock face on edge of road. No road shoulder, running on rumble strip with severe drop-off or ditch on edge. 12 km from top to bottom of Pass. Hairpin corners so tight, trucks have to back up to get around. Several cars had gone over the edge (in the past) and lay rusting in the forest below.Good thing it was a holiday today, so little traffic and no trucks. All the motorists were very considerate as they passed us, they could see that we had nowhere to go but run on the rumble strip. Talk about being caught between a rock and a hard place! Second stop at 25 km bottom of Pass. Graeme waiting with the ute & caravan having navigated the Pass downhill with no dramas. On, on into the heavy rain and head winds increasing to 35 km just past Albion Park. Maureen & Ping waiting for us. Short stop as we were drenched and needed to finish with 6 km to go and rain and wind increasing. On to Dapto with a brief run along the freeway, finished at 42.3 km in residential area, so we all drove 2 km away to park at Lake Illawarra for the night. Will drive back in the morning to start where we finished today. Weather is forecast to increase severity, rain and wind, throughout the night and easing during tomorrow. Spin off from cyclone Oswald so we'll be on the lookout for flooding and

high tides when we hit the ocean road. Temp 22 degrees. Distance 42.3 km. Running Time 6hr 31min. Pace 8.40 Food intake each: 1 grapefruit, 8 bananas, green smoothie, 10 peaches, 1 avocado, 10 dates, 2 large salads.

Comments from Facebook/RunningRawAroundAustralia2013:
- *I love this mountain!! The terror of many a childhood holiday.* - **Amanda**
- *Hi guys really inspiring running. Do you guys take any supplements or vitamins each day? It doesn't seem like enough calories as I estimated it to be about 2600 calories. When you factor in the running effect of burning about 4800 calories this leaves you with a net negative 2200 calories. How do you do it?* - **John**
- *When you eat raw food you get all the vital vitamins, nutrients and phytonutrients the body needs which means you don't have to eat as much. All the protein needed is in there too.* - **Tisha**
- *Well done guys.* - **Matthew**
- *Inspirational you two.* - **Madeleine**
- *I was thinking of the two of you as i ran through Warrandyte this morning.* - **Jo**
- *Well done!* - **Stuart**
- *Quite a challenge, my friends.* - **Carolyn**
- *Hey Everyone, We're still here and still running. Had a couple of interesting days being blown into Sydney, fringe benefits of Cyclone Oswald. Internet connections not good and we've been doing long days due to the weather, so priorities have been to eat and sleep.* - **J&A, Run RAW 2013**

Marathon 29.
January 29, 2013. Dapto, Lake Illawarra to Stanwell Park. Rock'nRoll all night with hatches battened down as the tail end of Cyclone Oswald came through, very heavy rain from 4pm to 5am and strong winds, but the caravan kept it's wheels on the ground. Departed at 5:30am after Graeme drove us back to the finish-start point. Slow going all day with head wind and rain clearing later in the day. Through Wollongong early in the morning as people just opening

shops. Some approached us and said they "Thought they recognised us," they had seen some of the TV coverage. They also said, "What you're doing is so inspiring and your message gives us all hope." Yay! So happy that it's working! Beautiful scenery along the coast road and crossed the amazing Sea Bridge (suspended above the sea) had an interesting hollow sound under our steps. Waves from Oswald crashing on the rocks below. Evidence of flooding and trees down on the roadside along the way. Camped beside the beach at Stanwell Park after running close to 48 km for Janette as she did some extra 'running around.' Temp 20-26 degrees. Garmin Distance 44.27 km. Pace 9.40. Total Km to date 1236.21. Food intake each 1 grapefruit, 3 bananas, large green smoothie with bananas, peaches & oranges, watermelon, rock-melon, 1 avocado with olives, 2 large salads.

Marathon #30.

January 30, 2013. Stanwell Park to Ramsgate Beach. Great sunset last night with spray drifting across from the surf crashing on the beach. Booming sound of surf rolling in all night, thanks Oswald! Away at 5:30am up the hill at dawn, misty sunrise over the ocean with cool breeze. Onto Hwy 1 for 22 km, built-up getting closer to Sydney. Several people stopped to talk at 3rd break including people and dogs from Assistance Dogs who help people with disabilities. Kids at the Taren Point school all excited and ran with us as we came in to our last break outside the school. Over the Capt. Cook Bridge, beautiful scene of boats in the bay, through suburb streets to Ramsgate beach and the Campground. Temp 18 - 27 degrees. Long day with extra km finding our way, Janette did 48 km again. Garmin distance 44.54 km. Running Time 8hr 47min. Pace 11.50. Food intake each 1 grapefruit 5 bananas, green smoothie with bananas, pineapple, peaches, 3 mangoes, watermelon, 2 large salads.

Marathon #31.

January 31, 2013. Ramsgate Beach around Botany Bay. Awoke to the sound of jet planes at Sydney airport, just over the Bay. Away at 6:30 running along the beach around Botany Bay, sunrise over Sydney City. Thanks to Brad & Irene at Kogarah Bay who gave a donation and hopefully will come to our speaking dinner event tomorrow. Back along the beach trail through Brighton Le Sands to the Airport into strong head wind, sand blowing everywhere. Back through the suburb streets to finish at the campground. Temp 19 - 32 degrees. Graeme installed the wiring for the new solar panel today while we were running. Food intake each 1 grapefruit, 10 bananas, grapes, watermelon, 1 avocado, 2 large salads. Distance 42.27km

Comments from Facebook/RunningRawAroundAustralia2013:

- *Amazing what you are doing. Stay strong!-Andrew Mmmm watermelon!* - **Marty**
- *So inspiring!* - **Brighde**
- *Welcome to Sydney!* - **Lennie**
- *Awesome!* - **Juliet**
- *Yes, this is VERY inspiring and amazing and you look so happy! more power to you both!* - **Patty** *Thanks for sharing Patty, was wanting to know how they were going. Keep doing what you do guys great stuff.* - **Raelene xxx**
- *The watermelon looks amazing* - **Sharon**
- *1 month in!!! YAY! Great work guys...each day see's me looking for your latest post! You rock.-Jan Welcome to Sydney, looking forward to meeting you tonight at the Brighton Le Sands RSL fundraiser, you are a truly inspirational couple.* - **Denise**
- *The best foods for runners.* - **Gunter**

February 2013.
MARATHONS #32-59

Marathon #32. February 1, 2013. Ramsgate Beach around Botany Bay, over Taren Point Bridge to Cronulla and back, up to Brighton Le Sands and back through back streets as the beach trail is too windy, getting sand blasted! Weather changing rapidly to thunder storm and strong head winds, finished just in time! Cold stormy day on the beach. Distance 43 km 88. Running time 6hr 22 min. Pace 8.42. Food intake each 1 grapefruit, 2 mangoes, 1 pineapple, green salad, bunch grapes, 2 passionfruit, 1 rock melon. Looking forward to the Raw Dinner and speaking event tonight, will report on that tomorrow! If you're in Sydney, come out and join us run thru Hyde Park to the Opera House, meet at the Pool of Reflections in Hyde Park at 7:30am for a leisurely 2 km run to the Opera House. Don't miss the sunrise - See you there!

Marathon #33.
February 2, 2013. Ramsgate Beach to Turramurra through CBD Sydney. Great raw vegan charity evening last night, thanks to Kym and others who made it possible and thanks to everyone who came out on such a stormy night! Up at 4:30am and away by 5:30am into torrential rain and strong head winds. Water on roads up to ankles in parts, made for a slow run into Sydney to meet up with our stalwart friends who braved the weather to come out and run with us from Hyde Park to the Opera House. A sad goodbye to our dear friends and enthusiastic support crew from Melbourne, Ping, Maureen and little Lucy. We will miss you, thank you for being there for us. Also thanks to Craig for bringing our mail and the box of yummy raw foods from botanical cuisine. A warm welcome to Francine who blew in with the storm yesterday to join us on the road to Darwin. Graeme is staying on with us for another week while we find someone else to come on board to Darwin. Wet and windy run over the

Sydney Harbour Bridge, thanks to Bob for the guided tour through the Rocks to the Bridge and to Brett & Ryan for escorting us over. Continued on thru Nth Sydney suburbs in steady rain to finish at a quiet park in Turramurra. Temp 14-17 degrees. Distance 44.46. Running time 7hr 26min. Pace 10.02. Total Km to date 1411.36 km. Off to bed for an early night with wind howling in the rigging...

Marathon #34.

February 3, 2013. Turramurra to Mt White. An amazing run today after 9hrs sleep, quiet spot off the Hwy, but still in Sydney suburbs after first stop at 12 km. Raining and cool. Finally out into the bush and rain forests after 20 km. Incredible 5 km run downhill to the Hawkesbury River. Sheer rock cliff on one side and steep drop-off into rainforest on the other. Beautifully sculptured rocks, red, pink and white, reminiscent of the Red & White Terraces at Tarawera NZ, I swear I could smell the sulphur! Many motorbikes and cyclists on the road early, sharing the sycopath. Oops, cycle path! On our last legs, oops, the last leg, climbing up Mt White we came across Robert, out for a Sunday stroll in his wheelchair. A retired Paralympian out there just pushing on. Spent some time on the road together swapping Paralympic stories then called Francine to drive back and pick Robert up and take him to the train in Gosford. See you on the road, Robert, "Never Stop Pushing!" We ran on to the top of Mt White to finish at 42.73 km. Temp 18-26 degrees. Running time 6hr 36 m in. Total Km 1454.09. Food intake 1 grapefruit 14 bananas, 8 oranges, 1 pineapple green smoothie, large salad and shared a jar of botanical cuisine classic cheese with the crew, thanks for the treat Omid!

Marathon #35.

February 4, 2013. Mt White to Forresters Beach. Depart in the dark on Hwy 83 Pacific Hwy. Dawn breaking with birdsong. Beautiful 12 km run downhill through misty rain forest to first break and green smoothie. Another steep downhill run into Gosford for the second break at 27 km. Onto the Central Coast Hwy to third stop at 37 km. Francine had done the food shopping and had a ripe red pawpaw for us, the best we've had since arriving in Australia! (Also the cheapest, oh yay, bring it on!) Running along and heard someone call out "Go

Raw!", met up with Glen who was driving past, he and his wife Michele have been following us on Facebook, great to see you on the road. Finished at Forresters Beach to set up camp for the night. So great to get the legs into the rolling surf. Distance 43 km. Running time 6hr 47min. Pace 9.27. Total Km 1497.09. Food intake each 1 grapefruit, 12 bananas, green smoothie with pineapple passion fruit banana and cos lettuce, 1 pawpaw, Pad Thai salad with zucchini, beetroot, carrot noodles and orange lime ginger coconut sauce made by Raw Chef Francine, Yum! Graeme off to visit friends Deb & Gerry and Sammy who visited us yesterday at Mt White. Great to meet you and thanks for doing our laundry and the offer of showers and real bed for the night, the sea was too inviting and we're off to sleep to the sound of surf rolling in. Goodnight folks.

Marathon #36.
February 5, 2013. Foresters Beach to Catherine's Hill Bay. Depart in dark 5:15am on Central Coast Hwy. Colourful sunrise over The Entrance and the bridge over the lake. Big Daddy Pelican sitting on lamp post on bridge counting the cars going underneath! Over causeway through massive mangroves, roadworks everywhere, but otherwise the road was clear with wide shoulders. Finished the run on the Pacific Hwy and drove down to the beach to set up camp for the night and to go in for a swim! Temp 20-29 degrees. Distance 42.22 km Running time 5hrs 44 min. Pace 8.09.

Marathon #37.
February 6, 2013. Catherine Hill Beach to Tomago Motor Camp (10 km north of Newcastle) Daybreak start with Graeme driving us up to the Hwy to start where we finished last night 3 km up from the beach. Good run on Hwy with wide cycle lane through Newcastle suburbs and down to the beach at Sandgate with 6 km to go to finish at Tomago. Temp 20-27 degrees. Distance 42.49 km Running time 6hr 20 min. Pace 8.56. Total km 1581.80. Food intake: banana kiwifruit orange passionfruit smoothie, quarter watermelon, banana vanilla lemon date pudding, 1 avocado, large green salad, zucchini noodles and tomato sauce with botanical cuisine Walnut Bolognese YUM!

Marathon #38.

February 7, 2013. Tomago to 4 km from North Arm Cove on Pacific Hwy 1. Stayed in motor camp and had the luxury of a warm shower before we left this morning. Away at 5:30am in the dark on Hwy, concrete cycle path mostly flat all day with strong headwind. Got hot very quickly with heat coming off the road and the glare from the concrete. Many large trucks on the road, draft from trucks passing hard to run into. Two trucks passing one behind the other generate about 60 km wind that almost knocks us off our feet! We now understand the question we've often had, "How is the traffic noise?" answer; "very tiring!" Needed more breaks as the day went on and felt quiet exhausted when we finished at a quiet spot in the forest about 1 km off the highway. Temp 18-30 degrees. Distance 42.93 km. Running time 6hr 33min. Time on road (with breaks) 10 hrs. Pace 9.09. Total Km 1624.73. Food intake each 1 grapefruit, 10 bananas, 1 pawpaw, 4 peaches, green smoothie, 3 fresh orange juice, 1 avocado, 1 vege juice (carrot, beet, apple, kale, ginger).

Marathon #39.

February 8, 2013. Nth Arm Cove to 10 km past of Bulahdelah. Out on the road at 5:30am running along slip road beside the Hwy for 5 km. In serious mosquito country, swarming all over us if we slow down or stop, they're big enough to pick us up and carry us away! Running through Myers Lake area must be a huge breeding ground. Back onto Hwy and the trucks blow the mosquitos away, back onto concrete cycle path, will have done 80 km of constant running on concrete so far by the end of today. Not effecting our feet so much as the glare from the (white) concrete in our faces. Undulating hills and some roadworks in rising heat along with the noise of the traffic making it tiring. No towns for 36 km until coming into Bulahdelah. New crew Brad arrived and took over from Graeme driving the last 10 km to finish at a truck stop alongside the road, it's going to be a noisy night with the trucks going by. Said goodbye to Graeme, so grateful for his help and support, we are blessed to have such a good friend, thanks Graeme. Temp 17-35 degrees. Distance 44.51 km. Running time 6hr 04min Pace 8.11. Total km 1669.24. Food intake each: 1 grapefruit, 10 bananas, 8 oranges, green smoothie, 1 pineapple, grapes, mango & passionfruit, 4 nectarines, 1 avocado, veg juice (beet, carrot, apple, kale, ginger, celery, lettuce), mixed veg dish with botanical cuisine Pepperberry Sauce.

Marathon #40.

Wahoo! February 9, 2013. 10 km past Buladelah to Fordfail. 5am start on Hwy 1 back to the concrete and headwinds, but less trucks because it's Saturday! Found a tiny bird on the edge of the road, winded by the updraft from a truck. Picked him up and he looked at me then closed his eyes. I held him to the first stop and kept talking to him until I was able to place him amongst the bushes off the road. He opened his eyes, looked around, hopped off my hand, took a few steps, turned and looked at me and said, "peep" then flew up into a tree. Fly safe little one. It's hard to see those who don't make it, we move them to the trees or grass whenever possible. Gorgeous camp spot last night beside the river serenaded by Francine on the violin, magic! Temp 20-33 degrees. Distance 42.7 km. Running time 6hrs17min. Pace 8.50.

Marathon #41.

February 10, 2013. Fordfail to Moorland on Hwy 1. Start 5:15am in dark, oh yay, asphalt cycle path, a relief after 100 km of concrete. Garmin had not charged during the night so did first leg without, setting the vehicle odometers to track the distance. Met with Mike & Vicky who stopped on their way to a triathlon in Forster. They had read about us in the New Idea mag and were following us on FB, so exciting to meet up. They drove on to meet up with Brad and Francine and sign our book to document that we were running on that stretch of road. Thanks for stopping and for the donation guys! Garmin charged and back on the job from 14 km. Faster run on tar seal while Francine did a food shop, thanks to the local fruit & vege market in Taree for the free produce! Brad got fuel and checked the ute and caravan then drove on to catch us for the third break just past Manning River. On to finish in small village of Moorland. Temp 20-32 degrees. Distance 43.79 km Running time 5hr 59min. Total km 1755.73. Food intake each 1 orange, 10 bananas, quarter rock melon, 2 nectarines, 6 lychees, fruit smoothie, half watermelon, vege juice (carrot, apple, cucumber, beetroot, silver beet, celery), and dinner; pumpkin & zucchini noodles with botanical cuisine Mushroom and Black Olive Sauce.

Marathon #42.

A momentous occasion! February 11, 2013. Moorland to Oxley Junction above Port Macquarie. Dark and cloudy start at 5:15am accompanied by Francine for 3 km, when she turned around and returned to camp while we ran on 12 km to first stop. Mostly concrete cycle path, very humid which zapped energy quickly so had to stock up well at each break. All on Hwy 1 but not so much traffic, was today a holiday? Finished at Oxley Junction (turnoff to Port Macquarie) Temp 21-32 degrees. Humidity 91%. Distance 42.45 km Running time 6hr17m Pace 8.53.Total km 1798.18. Food intake each 1 grapefruit, 10 bananas, fruit smoothie (apple, banana, nectarines), quarter watermelon & honeydew melon, green smoothie (banana, kale & ginger), 1 avocado, tomato & basil salad & mixed green salad. Drove down to Port Macquarie and lovely to meet up with Jen, thanks for the delicious fresh tomatoes and basil from your garden which we had for dinner by Shelley Beach. Interview with local Port Macquarie newspaper, watch for the article.Thanks to Pete & Teresa who stopped by and gave us a donation. Quick swim and bed as a dark and stormy night approaches....

Marathon #43.

February 12, 2013. Oxley Turnoff to Port Macquarie to Kempsey. Francine drove us back from the beach to start at 5:30am. Humid with thunder and lightening. Easy running mostly flat and asphalt. Green smoothies at first 2 breaks (bananas, pineapple, kale, spinach, peaches) Heavy rain showers during third leg, completely drenched but felt good as it was so humid. Caught up with Francine & Brad who was fixing a car for a young man who turned out to be a magician (not for fixing cars though). So he offered to do a little show for us in return for his car being fixed. Fun show in a truck stop somewhere on the Pacific Hwy! Nice river crossing and finished in Kempsey, nice quiet park under the trees. Interview with journalist from Kempsey newspaper. Temp 21-30 degrees. Distance 42.27 km. Running Time 6hr 15min. Pace 8.52. Total Km 1840.45. Food intake each: 2 green smoothies, 10 bananas, grapes, 4 nectarines, 1 avocado, half watermelon, fruit salad.

Marathon #44.

February 13, 2013. Kempsey to Paddy's Rest on the Hwy. Departed 5:15am with Francine joining us through the town for a 7 km run. Kempsey get our vote as the cleanest, greenest, quietest, friendliest town so far. Not even a cigarette butt on the ground! Daybreak revealed flat green farmland, ran through quaint village of Fredericton where Alan met up with one of his relations, next stop Jurassic Park! Francine picked up some locally grown watermelon from roadside, $5 a piece! Took a long break midway to catch up with media interviews and instal new shelf in the ute for ripening fruit. Quick run to finish at roadside rest stop. Temp 21-27 degrees. Distance 42.33 km. Running time 5hr 59min. Pace 8.29. Total km 1882.78. Food intake each 1 grapefruit, 10 bananas, half watermelon, fruit salad, 1 papaya, 3 peaches, 1 avocado, raw lettuce tacos with ginger lime coleslaw, garam masala tomato curry, guacamole.

Marathon #45.

February 14, 2013. Paddy's Rest to Uranga. It was a dark and stormy night, and the crew said to the runners, "Get going, these marathons aren't going to run themselves!" So, we departed in the dark 5:15am accompanied by crew Francine for the first 3 km before she turned sand disappeared into the dark and stormy morning. Continued into the dawn of Valentine's Day on the road. First break did phone interview with CNN Atlanta for CNN London, for our UK & US followers. On, on along the Hwy, stopped at roadside produce stall with locally grown bananas and persimmons, first of the season, yum! Cut down off the Hwy through forest road to Uranga, quiet after the Hwy traffic noise. Almost finished when it became dark and stormy again and the clouds burst with a torrential downpour, drenching us to the skin for the last 5 km. Finished at campground in time for another phone interview for German news, then into hot shower, oh yeah! Temp 21-24 degrees. Distance 44.68 km. Running time 6hr 30min. Pace 8.44. Total km 1927.46.

Marathon #46.

February 15, 2013. Urunga to Moonee Beach (through Coffs Harbour) What an amazing day! Departed 5:15am in the dark, joined by Francine for the first 3 km before she turned back. The truckies must be wondering what's going on, there's three of us now, out there in our flashy neon jackets! Warm early morning shower to send us on our way as dawn broke, ran 15 km to first break, where we stopped for a couple of hours to try uploading the Garmin data, but still not working. Sorry folks, it will be next week now before we get the full data online. Lost the first 15.33 km from today's data in the process. Meanwhile, back on the road with 15 km to Coffs Harbour and folks to meet. Wonderful lunch break at The Happy Frog Organic Produce & Restaurant in Coffs, complimentary salads and juice, with gift bag of fruit, thank you so much Kim. Met up with Brenda & Richard, Vivienne, Tania & Paul, Janna and friends of 36 years ago from Rabaul, PNG, Alison & Bill, how fun was that! Thank you all for your gifts of fruit and friendship. Another 15km through roadworks to finish at Moonee Beach thanks to Russell at the Sapphire Motel for the recommendation, and for the refill of water on our way. Temp 20-29 degrees. Distance 44.66 km Running time 6hr 44min. Pace 9.31. Total Km 1973.22. Food intake each 1 grapefruit, 10 bananas, half watermelon, vege juice, fruit smoothie, mixed salad, 1 avocado, fruit salad.

Marathon #47.

February 16, 2013. Moonee Beach to Half Way Creek (half way between Coffs Harbour and Grafton) Departed at 5:15am in the rain with Francine doing 6 km. Ran first 14 km along new (not yet open) hwy, as no-one working today Sat. Interesting to see the stages of construction and equipment, had the whole road to ourselves away from the traffic. First break at 15 km, next leg rolling hills, wide shoulders on the road and more rain showers. Stopped by the police who wanted to have a chat since he'd seen us on the road several times in the last few days. Snr Constable Wal Broom of NSW Police pulled into our third break stop with lights flashing, jumps out of the car and says he's going to attract some attention for us! He told us that if we ever need help or more water to just flag him down. Thanks for keeping the roads safe Wal. Passed through the 2013 km mark on top of Dirty Creek Hill 110 metres and finished at

Half Way Creek Truck Rest Stop with the best $2 showers. Francine made a great sign so we could take a photo, we were joined by Janna who arrived with durian to celebrate. Temp 19-23 degrees. Distance 42.3 km. Running Time 6hr 6 min. Pace 8.40. Total km 2015.52. Food intake each 1 grapefruit, 10 bananas, 6 peaches, 6 lichees, 2 plums, half durian, 1 avocado, green smoothie (silver beet, pineapple, apple, avocado).

Marathon #48.

February 17, 2013Half Way Creek to Ulmarra. Well, today was a day to remember! A rainy night in the truck stop surrounded by big rigs and kangaroos! Departed in the dark 5:15am with Francine doing her 6 km morning run. Ran 14 km through farmland and forest in the rain to first stop. Second leg to Grafton still raining most of the way. Noticed the rivers have a slick of oil on top of the water and there is a pungent smell in the air from the flooding in the area a few weeks ago. This part of the Hwy was closed for over a week during the floods. Continued on to Ulmarra with only 5 km to finish when Janette was struck in the legs by a flying missile thrown from a car, which turned out to be an icecream in a cup from MacDonalds. Hit full force (with around 60 km per hour impact) just above the knee on the right leg, bounced onto the left leg before exploding all over both. Janette doubled over with the pain of the impact, both of us in shock with the realisation of what had happened. A young mother in a following car witnessed the action and pulled over to see if we were okay, thank you Sarah. Limped over the road to the Ulmarra Post shop and was given some ice, stopped there to ice both legs. So kindness overcame stupidity, thanks to both. Finished the Run just past Ulmarra. Temp 20-27 degrees. Distance 42.47 km. Running Time 6hr 11min. Pace 8.44. Drove to Lawrence to stay the night with friends Narelle and Robert. Treated to a delicious raw meal prepared with much love by Narelle. Robert showed us his garden and picked tropical fruits fresh for the meal. Janette soaked in a hot bath with Epsom salts to relieve the leg pain, showers for everyone else and laundry done. Delightful evening with delightful friends, then a quiet sleep in a real bed, what luxury! Thank you Narelle & Robert for your wonderful hospitality, much appreciated. Food intake each 1 grapefruit, 10 bananas, melon smoothie, green smoothie, 6 nectarines, 2 large salads, mango, banana & passionfruit.

Marathon #49.

February 18, 2013. Ulmarra to Mororo Truck Rest Stop. Drove from Narelle & Robert's place back to the spot we had finished yesterday to start at 5:30am, just getting light, roads very wet from rain all night. Running along between sugar cane plantations still water logged from the flood brought by the last Cyclone, worst flood in 60yrs. Remnants of the flood are rubbish everywhere, oily slick on the water and in the river, dead frogs, lizards and turtles on the road, branches, leaves and other organic matter over the road, and a very pungent smell, combination of rotting flesh, sulphur and tar. We were getting drenched with grit filled water being sprayed up over us from the trucks going through the surface water on the road. Flat all the way, grit in our waterlogged shoes causing rubbing on the toes and ankles. Janette's right leg causing some discomfort but still able to run at normal speed, until slowing on the last 4 km. Stopped for break at McLean where the river was particularly polluted, oil visible on the water birds. Ran on, stopped by photographer James Pitman of photo events.net.au who took pics of us on the road. Finished at a Truck Stop on the Hwy near Mororo. Temp 21-25 degrees. Distance 42.64 km. Running time 6hr 03min. Pace 8.31. Total Km 2100. Food intake each 1 grapefruit, 10 bananas, 1 fruit smoothie, 1 green smoothie, 6 peaches, half pawpaw, zucchini noodles with tomato sauce.

Marathon #50.

(Oh yeah!) February 19, 2013. Mororo to Broadwater Depart from Rest Stop at 5:15am, our little caravan surrounded by big rigs, trucks coming in during the night. Into the dark and rain, feet in surface water, heads down to keep caps on when trucks spray us with gritty water as they pass. Discovered when it got light that the Garmin watch hadn't started. Finally got going after a few km, then the phone stopped working, got to first break and Francine's phone had shut down too. Everything is waterlogged. Janette's legs now sporting large blue and green bruises compliments of MacDonalds (product and resulting attitude), but otherwise no after effects. Worse pain from two ant bites received during compulsory squat! Meanwhile Francine unloads oranges into a puddle as the bottom falls out of the box, followed by Fran(tic) scrambling to retrieve said oranges in the pouring rain accompanied by profound statements about the nature of existence! Photographer from local newspaper caught up with us on the road and took pics in the pouring rain. Ran past Little Italy where the first Italians established a settlement in 1880. Took photo of Janette with David, remembering the Florence Marathon. Finished the run at Broadwater Stopover Tourist Park where Tina & Bart made our day by providing a spot for us. Thanks for your support! Spent the rest of the afternoon trying to get the Garmin stats sorted to no avail. Thinking of getting a refund on today, will do it again tomorrow and see if we can improve our performance! Weather report for more rain and wind, that will make a change! Temp 20-23 degrees. Adjusted Distance 44.45 km. Running time 5hr 52min. Total Km 2147.08. Food intake each 1 grapefruit, 10 bananas, 6 peaches, 2 fruit smoothies (banana, pineapple, orange) & (rock-melon, peach, blueberry), half pawpaw, 1 avocado, cabbage leaf wraps with seed spread, tomatoes and mixed veg salad.

February 19, 2013

WOW! Eileen here, Janette and Alan are really braving it out up there, water logged shoes and rubbing toes today, but they always find a smile, they are true 'silver lining' people. TODAY they have completed 50 Marathons in 50 Days which equals their NZ record!!!! CONGRATULATIONS YOU TWO! Please share this amazing feat (and their amazing feet!) with everyone you know, please ask them to give generously to this campaign (through the website) let's make all their seemingly impossible (to the rest of us!) hard work worthwhile! A wonderful note arrived on here this morning from Kaje, A & J's son and thanks for your wonderful support last night everyone, great sharing in celebration of this milestone! Eileen

"Just over 13 years ago my Mum and Dad did an amazing thing. They ran – one foot after the other – the length of New Zealand - from Cape Reinga to Bluff. Over 50 marathons in 50 consecutive days! That is: running a marathon every day for seven weeks!...And today they have done exactly that again, only this time they still have another 45 weeks of consecutive daily marathons to complete their goal of running around Australia! 365 marathons in 365 consecutive days… each. They are in their 60s. While you are pondering on that, take some time to think how hard a task they have set for themselves. Most of us would consider completing 'one marathon alone' a huge achievement in one's

lifetime...and it is. A few of us may get 'hooked' and train hard to complete a few marathons… and a mere handful would complete more than say, a handful!

For my parents, this is more than just an amazing personal undertaking, an amazing journey to see every inch of the road that encircles their country. They believe in treading lightly on this earth, in kindness and helping others. They want to bring awareness to all they meet that anyone can set goals – however small or humble – and set out to achieve them. They want people to be inspired to make conscious decisions about their own path, their health, the health of others and the health of the planet.

They are supporting four worthy charities who could benefit from your attention and your donation. One answering the cry against youth homelessness; one supporting those with terminal and chronic diseases; one valuing our determined Paralympian athletes and hopefuls; one striving to prevent endemic cruelty to animals.This is how you can help my parents, Janette and Alan, achieve their goal:

- Follow their progress on their website and Facebook page. Share their dream and discuss with others. Check their schedule and go out to give them a word of encouragement as they pass your gate. Ask your local MP or media outlet to get involved.
- Pick a charity (link below) that resonates with you and encourage others to join you in supporting or donating to that cause. These charities exist because of issues that really are there - and they seek your generosity to help improve the lives of those you may never otherwise have been able to touch so kindly.
- Be inspired and inspire others to achieve their dreams.

Congratulations, Mum and Dad - enjoy each new day… somewhere out there on the road!"

"Friends are as companions on a journey, who ought to aid each other to persevere in the road to a happier life" ~ Pythagoras

From Kaje

Marathon #51.

February 20, 2013. Broadwater to Lennox Head. Someone heard about what we're doing, running a marathon a day for 365 days around Australia, and commented that we won't be doing any PBs (Personal Bests). Well, folks today was THE day, the day we achieved our own PB ultra endurance running 51 consecutive marathons and a distance of 2187.37 km, breaking our own record set February 5, 2000, of 50 consecutive marathons and 2182.2km. So, for the record, every day for the next 314 we'll be doing a PB, just like everyone else who does their personal best in everything. So on this wonderous day, we departed in the dark and torrential rain, into headwinds and surface water, taking 4' waves from the trucks to a standing ovation from the clapping frogs in the floodwaters beside the road. Heads down into the driving rain and howling wind we felt like we were going nowhere, and at times going backwards, but eventually we made it to the first stop for a rejuvenating fruit smoothie and a change of clothes. Second leg much of the same, clothes drenched within seconds and shoes holding water. Second break in Ballina, greeted by Maxine with gifts fresh from her garden and orchard, as well as a generous donation, thank you so much for your support and kindness. We enjoyed the delightful cherry tomatoes for dinner. Had photographs taken for the Northern Star newspaper, then on towards Lennox on the coast road as the wind and rain increased. Joined by Belinda and Dante on the road and later by Anthony who ran with us to finish at Lake Ainsworth just north of Lennox Head. Thanks for the company, it made all the difference at the end of a very wet and windy day. Distance 42.34km.

Marathon #52.

February 21, 2013. Lennox Head to Yelgun Rest Stop (near Brunswick Head) Awoke 4am to the heaviest rain we have had so far. Put on wet clothes and shoes from yesterday and head out the door 5:15am, soaked to skin within seconds. Running on Coast Road to Byron Bay, not much traffic so a relief not to have the trucks spraying us with surface water. Ran 20km without a break into Byron and stopped at the produce market. Had a large smoothie (orange, banana, peach, silver beet) then went to market for fresh passionfruit and dragonfruit. Interview and photos with Sharon from Echonetdaily, then ran out of Byron in torrential rain onto freeway. Very soggy run to finish at Hwy Rest Stop. Temp 20-26 degrees. Distance 47.42 km Running time 6hr 44min. Elevation 52 metres. Total km 2234.84. Food intake each 1 grapefruit, 15 bananas, 1 avocado, large fruit smoothie, raw lasagna (zucchini, fresh cherry tomato sauce, botanical cuisine nut cheese, thanks to Raw Chefs Francine and Brad!

Comments from Facebook/RunningRawAroundAustralia2013:

- *You guys amaze me every day!* - **Katharina**
- *Awesome!!* - **Lisa**
- *Wow, you guys are unstoppable!* - **Nalin**
- *Love what you guys are doing. Safe travels.* - **John**
- *Kept going.* - **Melanie**
- *So sorry guys! You deserve better weather!!* - **Sieghilde**
- *This is amazing! I cannot believe you consume enough calories to provide the necessary energy.* - **Frederick**
- *Amazing! Keep it up guys!* - **Stephan**
- *Hopping into wet clothes!* - **Tania**
- *Saw you heading out of Byron Bay along Ewingsdale Rd. Really wanted to stop and say hello, but nowhere safe to pull over along that stretch, especially in the wet. You are legends for keeping it up in this weather!* - **Jannine**
- *Doing great guys!* - **Anita**
- *You guys are RAWSOME! Truly Inspirational.* - **Regina**
- *Amazing effort you guys are an inspiration! Peace and love to you two wonderful people!* - **Rawsomely Good**
- *That's dedication, not many people have!!* - **Irma**
- *It's a VERY humid day up here, I just ran with them and was drenched in sweat in 1 km!* - **Eileen**

Marathon #53.

February 22, 2013. Yelgun Rest Stop to Currumbin. Torrential rain all night, surface water all over the Rest Stop. Left in the dark and rain 5:30am onto Hwy and into the truck wash again, strong tail wind pushing us along, clothes and shoes wet through, drenched to the skin in minutes. (So here's a question; if you're not wearing any clothes, can you get drenched to the skin? Might have to try that tomorrow as we're literally running out of dry clothes!) First two legs 14 km each to the turn off to Tropical Fruit World. Drove up to TFW where we were greeted by Kelly who showed us all around and treated us to some delicious fruit tasting and gave us gifts of mangoes, dragon fruit, starfruit, avocado, miracle fruit, macadamia nuts and the biggest jackfruit! Thank you so much Kelly, Jason and Tropical Fruit World at Duranbah Drove back to the spot where we came off the Hwy and started running again AND it started raining again! Continued on the Hwy coming into Tweed Heads which became a Freeway, no pedestrians allowed, so climbed over the barrier onto road works area and ran along the new road for a couple of km until we came to a 15' fence, fully locked and completely closed off. Instant decision, up and over the chain link fence (easy with Garmin toe shoes!), looked back to read the sign on the fence: "No Entry-Under Camera Surveillance!" A hearty wave and we were off! Down to Kirra Beach and onto the beach path, huge waves rolling in, salt in the air and sand in the face! Finally arrived at Currumbin, a long day, but a fruitful one! Temp 21-23 degrees. Distance 46.81 km. Running time 6hrs 37min. Pace 8.30. Food intake each 1 grapefruit, 15 bananas, fruit smoothie (orange, banana, silver beet, passionfruit) half rock melon, fruit smoothie (banana, nectarine, kiwifruit, grapes, plum, silver beet), 1 avocado, fruit salad (dragon fruit, kiwifruit, papaya, passionfruit, peaches, nectarines, mango, macadamia nut, basil)

Marathon #54.

February 23, 2013. Currumbin to Helensvale Howling wind and rain storm, lightening show all night. Parked right above the estuary with a view of Surfers in the distance. Off in the morning 5:30am in the light, we're on Queensland time now. Stopped at 10 km to meet up with our friend Michaela who is joining us as Support Crew. Many thanks to Brad for jumping on board to help out for the past 15 days, how blessed were we to have met in Sydney, keep in touch Rain cleared and sun came out for a hot sunny day running along the beach trail amongst hundreds of other runners, then through Surfers Paradise along the Esplanade amongst the crowds looking at the amazing sand sculptures. Across the bridge to stop at the marina for 2nd break. Michaela and Francine had been joined by Eileen (our intrepid PR/

Media Person Extraordinaire) who has flown in from Melbourne. Left the girls to organise shopping, laundry and dinner menu and ran on in the heat, such a change from yesterday's weather. Finished at Helensvale where they had set up camp for the night at the Gold Coast Holiday Park had given us a complimentary site, thanks for your support! Francine & Michaela were luxuriating in the pool while Eileen was creating a delicious raw dinner in the caravan, having done our laundry at her friend's place nearby, thanks, so much appreciated, we didn't have many dry clothes left with all the rain we've had in the last few days! Had a quick soak in the pool before dinner, then a shower and bed, a great day! Temp 20-29 degrees. Distance 43.53km. Running time 6hrs 10min. Pace 8.30. Food intake 1 grapefruit, 15 bananas, fruit smoothie, half watermelon, zucchini carrot noodles with carrot fennel pate compliments botanical cuisine and Super Raw Chef Eileen

Marathon #55.

February 24, 2013. Helensvale to Springwood (20 km South Brisbane) Today's Run dedicated to our dear friend Barrie and to her family who are Celebrating her Life today. Fly free dear one.

Set off 5:30am in very heavy rain for first 30 min, enough to get thoroughly drenched again! Intermittent showers all day with 110% humidity, otherwise an easy run along the Surfers Paradise to Brisbane Cycle Path (84 km mostly alongside the Hwy) with the girls driving on the Old Hwy. Passed a group of cyclists and wheelchair racers getting ready to race, wheelchairs have evolved to amazing low slung hand pedal machines since we last saw them in 2000. Road closed for the race just after we went through so the girls were diverted into the suburbs and we all eventually met up for the first break at 14 km. Continued on and met up with Eileen joining us for a run on the next two legs. Finished in Springwood where Eileen prepared delicious dinner and the girls made dessert, what a Team! Temp 27-28 degrees. Distance 42.45 km. Running Time 6hr 26min. Pace 9.06.Total Km 2367.63. Food intake each 1 grapefruit 15 bananas fruit smoothie, 1 dragonfruit, half pawpaw, 1 avocado, large green salad, pumpkin fettuccine with botanical cuisine Olive Pate.

February 26, 2013

NEWSPLASH! If we had the power to control all this wild weather, we'd be able to control the news too! Unfortunately, due to the flooding situation up in Qld, Sunrise are having to divert their crew tomorrow, which we totally understand. They plan to do a live cross from the Sunshine Coast, but we'll keep you posted! Fortunately, our story goes on....and on.... and....on!

Rain, rain and more rain! Watching the drips on the visor of my cap collect and run together before pouring off in a stream in front of me. Momentum puts my face in the waterfall, splashing into my eyes, running down my cheeks and dripping off the end of my nose. I watch as the sleeve of my shirt becomes moist with raindrops, rapidly changing to be completely wet, clinging to the top of my arm, flapping back and forth underneath. My shirt is drenched, the water seeping through to my skin. I feel the rivulets running down and soaking my shorts, the wet material clinging to my legs. On, on, my feet continue to pound the pavement, sloshing through ankle deep water, the socks are soaked, the shoes holding water, splash, squelch, slap, my toes feel like pulp. Water, water everywhere, rushing past my feet in a storm-water drain, splashing towards me from the wheels of the oncoming cars and being drenched by a wall of water as a truck passes. On, on, my feet continue to pound the pavement, splash, squelch, slap, splash, squelch, slap. On, on, the road goes ever on. Rain, rain and more rain; 41, 42, 43 km, at last we stop. Standing in a puddle, peeling of the wet clothes, another day, another marathon, running in the rain.

Hi all, Eileen here-media wrangler and occasional raw chef. I am normally luxuriating in my office near Melbourne writing stories and taking long lunches (I wish!), but last week, thought it was time I got on the road to find out what it was really like to be with these two legends! I've now seen first hand what they are doing- and make no mistake, it is HARD! I have never met two individuals (not to mention the hardy crew!) with such fortitude and commitment. I've done a number of endurance events in my life, but I'm used to getting geared up, doing the race, and basking in the afterglow. For these guys, every day is another mountain to climb and they just keep getting up and climbing it, day after day. 58 days on the trot today. Amazing. Forget the afterglow, they have a glow, ALL THE TIME! For those who have concerns, I can unreservedly assure you that they look fantastic and they eat amazingly well: they eat A LOT of food! They stop every 10-15 k ms to refuel briefly and as soon as they stop each afternoon, they eat constantly for about 2 hours! I am not only reassured that they will absolutely reach their goal, I am so INSPIRED by their commitment. They are running in conditions most people would refuse to (um, I may have been a tad 'un keen' when it was 34deg, hosing down and the road was covered in water, but could hear Janette telling me to 'Harden Up!" so I got cranking!).

Hi Everyone, We've had some very busy and long days in and since Brisbane and just haven't had a chance to update daily, BUT we're still on the road, we're still running and we're still getting all your supportive comments, so thanks for your patience. We'll be back online with all the updates tomorrow, which will be Marathon #60, we'll be a sixth of the way, yay!

Marathon #56.

February 25, 2013. Springwood to Gordon Park via Brisbane CBD Departed in pouring rain at 5:30am running along Logan Rd into Brisbane CBD to Southbank to meet up with media. Interview with Channel 10 in rain by the flooding river. (Aired at 5pm and late news) Turned off the Garmin and drove to Gordon Park where we were staying for next 2 nights. Caught bus back to CBD and turned Garmin back on to finish the Run around the city. Ran along the river walkways, out to Kangaroo Point and through the Botanical Gardens, all in the pouring rain. Garmin off, bus back to Gordon Park with 10 km to go to finish, ran around the neighbourhood, splashing through puddles on the trail with the local kids and dogs. Temp 27 degrees. Distance 42.51 km. Running Time 6hr 17min. Pace 8.52.Total Km 2410.14. Lovely evening out and excellent salad with Brisbane Raw Vegans at the Forest Vegan Cafe. Thanks Bren for the delicious raw desserts afterwards and for having us invade your home!

Marathon #57.

February 26, 2013. Brisbane in the Rain. Stayed the night in 'a real bed' in Gordon Park (big thanks to Bren) and ran back to CBD to cover the distance we had driven yesterday. Still pouring rain through flooded Victoria Park, into city streets amongst people rushing through the puddles in their office suits and brightly coloured gumboots, umbrellas blown inside out! Met up with Phil from Kids Under Cover to receive more $$$ gift vouchers from Coles (Thanks Coles) then to 'In Training' to pick up more Vibram shoes sponsored by Barefoot Inc (Thanks Vibram Barefoot Inc). Ran along the flooding river trail, through the Botanical Gardens and CBD. Turned off the Garmin and jumped on a bus back to Gordon Park, Garmin back on to continue the run. Stopped with 5 km to go so we could go and speak at a local ROTARY meeting, (Thanks for the donations). Finished the run after returning to Gordon Park, 5 km in the dark by the light of the moon in misty rain. Finished 11pm. Temp 27 degrees. Distance 42.41 km. Running Time 6hr 49min. Pace 8.16. Total Km 2452.55.

Marathon #58.

February 2, 2013. Brisbane (Gordon Park) to Caboolture Up early to meet up with the Sunrise Show crew, but postponed till tomorrow, so waited for our friend Sarah to join us. Departed 8am, three of us running in the rain and surface water on the Hwy while Francine & Michaela navigate with the vehicles through the wet chaos getting out of Brisbane. Stopped on Hwy by Police asking if we were okay and warning us that the Hwy would become the Motorway where pedestrians are not allowed, but said it would be okay if we were really careful and stayed in single file as there was no other road to go on. So, off again against the traffic, lots of toots from motorists and truckies. Stopped again by Police about 10 km further on to tell us that there was a slip road ahead that we could use. Thx to both Police Patrols for your concern and help. Finished the run in Caboolture at Satrah's house. Temp 26-28 degrees. Distance 43.08 km. Running Time 5hrs 46min (keeping up with Sarah!) Pace 8.02. Total Km 2495.63. Shared a delicious meal of 3 salads made by Chef Michaela in Sarah's huge kitchen (by comparison to the caravan!) Delivery of a beautiful basket of organic fruit and veg from Kylie of Organics at Redcliff Jetty Market (Thanks so much) and thanks to local Soft Tissue Therapist Sue Black from Bowette in Kurwongbah, who kindly gave Alan remedial massage therapy (Thanks, much appreciated, Janette's turn next time!)

Marathon #59.

February 28, 2013. Caboolture to Mooloola. Up early to do the Sunrise show live from outside Sarah's house. Departed with Francine joining us for 6 km then on into the rain. Stopped to talk with David & Janeth from Caboolture who came out to find us after seeing us on the Sunrise Show, lovely to meet you. Running along in the rain through the lush green countryside and up through the beautiful Glass Mountains. Met up with fruity friends Anne and Cappi, and the sun came out! Great to see you again and thanks for the mangos and sunshine!

Comments from Facebook/RunningRawAroundAustralia2013:

- *Two Raw Vegan Superstars, and Two Beautiful People. Great to catch up with you today on the Sunshine Coast. Best Wishes for the rest of your adventures. You both Rock!* - **Anne & Cappi** ♥♥♥
- *In a time where people complain about taking the stairs or having to walk 5 minutes from a car park to their intended destination, you really put things into perspective. Just saw your feature on Sunrise, and I have to say I'm thoroughly impressed and inspired, by both the charitable and physical aspect of this initiative. Your dedication is phenomenal & I only hope that I could do something of this nature with as much passion. Just wanted to wish you guys all the best, good luck and happy runnings.* - **Sydney fan x**

March 2013

MARATHONS #60-90

Marathon #60. March 1, 2013. Mooloolah to Eumundi. Rained all night. Rose drove us back up the hill 3+km to the spot where we'd finished last night, where Sarah was waiting to run with us for the day again. She ran ahead handing out flyers and telling everyone she met about RunRAW2013, arranged for the kids in school to come out and cheer us on, stopped the local politicians to talk to us, asked the shopkeepers to come out and cheer! Great to have her energy with us and to help spread the word, thx Sarah. Rose rode on her bike with us for part of the way and was also joined by her friend James, great to have you both along for the ride! Rained in showers throughout the run. Finished in Eumundi at Rose's friend Kathy's house, to spend the night in comfortable beds and have dinner at a real dining table! Thanks Kathy for sharing your home in your absence! Dear friends of 43 years Tony & Barbara (from NZ & PNG days) who live 30mins away came up to visit for the evening, great to catch up again, you haven't changed a bit! (Well, maybe your beard Tony!) Thanks for the delicious tomatoes and greens from your garden which went into the salad that Rose made. Francine opened up the enormous jackfruit that we'd been given by Tropical Fruit World and we all ate heartily, as the rain continued to come down, turning the tropical garden into a steaming jungle. A great way to end Marathon #60 and two months on the road. Puts us one-sixteenth of the way. Yay! Temp 25-30 degrees. Distance 42.27 km. Running time 6hr 23min. Pace 9.03.

Marathon 61.
March 2, 2013. Eumundi to Gympie. Another wet day out on the Bruce Hwy. Evidence of the recent flooding and road closures, running through surface water all day. Francine & Michaela visited Eumundi Market and solved their rain problems while Rose did the first two stops for us. Thanks Rose, see you next time you join us on the road. Tourist info before Gympie

advised us to continue through to the other side of the town to stay above high water as more flooding expected. Wet mud everywhere as we passed Gympie in torrential downpour for last 3 hours and set up camp on the other side compliments of Gympie Caravan Park, thanks. Laundry and showers were very welcome! Temp 23 degrees. Distance 43.08. Running Time 6hr 22min. Pace 8.52. Total Km 2623.32.

Marathon #62.

March 3, 2013. 7 km south of Gympie to 7 km south of Maryborough. Heavy rain most of the way, heads down, plodding along, one step after the other...lots of signs of past flooding, surface water and mud everywhere. Less traffic as it is Sunday, and most trucks stopped. Finished near Glenwood outside the local Fire Station. Wet and wild Michaela had beautiful fruit ready for us. Temp 21-24 degrees. Distance 44.49km. Running time 6hr 23min. Pace 8.36. Total km 2667.81.

Marathon #63.

March 4, 2013. 20 km south Maryborough to Junction Hwy 1 and Maryborough Truck Stop. Depart 5.15am daybreak, NO RAIN! Cloudy and some sun. Ran good pace for first 14 km to break, greeted with great smoothie; banana, starfruit, orange and dragonfruit. Second leg the same, smoothie made with banana and jackfruit. Continued through rolling hills, lush green scenery, through pine forests, sugarcane plantations and farmland. Francine met us with pineapple at 37 km while Michaela drove on to set up camp at a truck stop as all the camping grounds were flooded. Girls drove to Maryborough to do laundry and shopping while we finished the run. Temp 20-26 degrees. Distance 42.24km. Running time 6hr 11min. Pace 8.47. Total Km 2710.05.

Marathon #64.

March 5, 2013. Sth Maryborough to 21 km south of Childers. Away from Truck Stop 5:15am, warm, sunrise in a watery sky, wind behind us. Francine joined us for 3 km before returning and we ran on, both feeling very strong. Ran 17 km to first stop, not many places to pull over with the vehicles, virtually no verge on the edge of the road. Girls had a delicious fruit smoothie ready then on we went again for another 14 km. Flood damage everywhere, rivers high and mud where the flood waters had receded. Finished at Truck Stop with covered table and seats, where we shared a watermelon with a little sugar glider who came to visit. Second day with cloud cover but without rain. Temp 24-29 degrees. Distance 42.32 km. Running time 5hr 58min. Pace 8.27. Total Km 2752.37.

Marathon #65.

March 6, 2013. 21 km south Childers to 25 km north of Childers on Bruce Hwy. Away 5:15am warm clear morning. Francine with us for 3 km running and Michaela taking videos. Ran 17 km to first stop, great green smoothie ready for us. Continued for another 14 km through sugar cane plantations and gum trees, looking for koalas but didn't see any. Into Childers township, girls shopping and Michaela taking some more video footage. Stopped by several locals who had seen us on TV. Became very hot and humid for last leg. Finished at truck stop in the bush. Had telephone interview for Take 5 Magazine while sitting on a log in the bush, good to sit down after being on the road all day. Temp 24-29 degrees. Distance 45.82km Running Time 6hr 52min Pace 9.00. Total Km 2798.19.

Phew! Thank goodness for that! Standing on the side of the road as a large truck goes past, got it on good authority from our local 'Blue' that the truckies "won't hit a good looking Sheila like you!" Now was that hit, or hit on? Well, at least that's one less thing to worry about then! Now here's how the story goes....We're running along the road heading out of Childers, past the local pub. Suddenly 'Blue' comes rushing across the road towards us, his white hair and wispy white beard flying. "Hey," he calls, "are you the old buggers running around Australia?" We laugh and reply, "Yes that's us." He says, "Hold it right there while I get a picture" and pulls out a phone from his pocket. We keep running towards him as he fumbles with the phone muttering, "Don't know how to use this new-fangled thing." He realises that we're not going to stop, so he starts running backwards, still trying to figure out the phone. We watch as he navigates on the side of the road, retro running into the traffic. "Got it" he yells and snaps a couple of shots of us. He stops and puts out his hand. "I was just having a beer over at the pub when my friends said, "There go those old buggers running around Australia," so I had to come and get a photo! How old are you?" he asks. We tell him, 67 and 63. "Wow" he says, "Don't you think you're a bit old for that sort of shit?" We laugh again and reply, "No, actually we're getting younger every step." He says, "Well, I'm 60 and I'm knackered from running 30 yards!" We laugh again. "Are you doing this for some charities?" he asks. "Yes," we reply and tell him about the four charities. "Well, good on you mates" and digging in his pocket he hands us a note. "Hope you make it," he says, heading back down the road, "I need to have another beer!"

Marathon #66.

March 7, 2013. 25 km north of Childers to 10 km past Gin Gin on the Bruce Hwy 1...and now for a little drama! Late start 6am after a lovely night camped in the bush, beautiful starry sky during the night. Had only been running about a km when Janette tripped over concealed stick off road and landed heavily on shoulder and ribs. Couldn't breath for a few seconds as the air in lungs completely expelled on impact. Continued running very slowly but had extreme pain in the ribs with each step, so phoned the girls to come with the vehicles to the 5 km mark. Strapped the rib cage and chest area after rubbing comfrey salve on the skin. Ate a whole pineapple for the bromeliad enzyme which acts as an anti-inflammatory and pain reduction then continued on at a slow pace, with more breaks through sugar cane plantations on either side of the road. Ran through Gin Gin thinking that could be just what I need to dull the pain!! Finished the run at 5pm, very long and painful day. Will be interesting to see how quickly everything heals while on the run. Note: Alan also injured his ribs with a fall 3 weeks ago and was healed within 10 days. Francine picked us up and drove us back to the Gin Gin Showgrounds Campground where Michaela had set up camp in a complimentary site and laundry. Very welcome hot shower, complete with cane toads watching on! Dinner - delicious salad cabbage leaf wraps with botanical cuisine Kale & Basil Pesto. Temp 24-28 degrees. Distance 42.35 km. Running time 6hr 27min. Pace 9.09.   Total Km 2840.54.

Comments from Facebook/RunningRawAroundAustralia2013

- *Well Done Team Rawsome...* - **Lee**
- *I hope you have a quick recovery* - **Margot**

- *I ran Port Macquarie half marathon today, struggled. Every day u guys inspire me to keep on trying. Thank you.* - **Janelle x**
- *keep up the great work Well done!!* - **Sylvia**
- *Heal well and swiftly, Janette.* - **Kel**
- *Thank you for the pineapple lesson. Hope you heal quickly Janette* - **Dan**
- *You guys are so amazing!* - **Amanda**
- *Wishing you a speedy recovery. I did the same thing a few months back, but I only tripped over my own feet. Took about a week for me to heal. Thinking of you* - **Michele x**
- *Wishing u a speedy recovery. U are both so inspiring* - **Kylie**
- *Please get better soon you are what you eat they say. Pineapples are tough on the outside sweet inside, may you be the same* - **Milt**
- *So sorry about your accident, I hope you heal quickly.* - **Annemaree**
- *Hope you get better real soon!* - **Lisa**
- *Kia kaha ehoa ma, stay strong my friend* - **Barbara**
- *Tell us when u go thru Esk! My family will greet n help if need be.* - **Collin**
- *Sorry to hear of the fall for Janette* - **Brenda**

Marathon #67.

March 8, 2013. 10 km past Gin Gin to Woora National Park 6am start with Michaela driving us on to where we finished last night and doing some video footage of us on the road. Janette running quicker today but still in pain, just settled into a steady pace where the pain level is stable. Narrow shoulder on edge of road, rolling hills and road works on last leg. Girls finding it difficult to get a place to stop for the night, meanwhile we see a local farmer and ask if we can park in his driveway. He replies. "I would say yes, but it's not my driveway!" However, he tells us to go another half km through the roadworks to a road that goes into the National Park that would be ideal for the night. We finish the run in the middle of the road works and call the girls to drive back. The traffic controller on the road calls her partner at the other end to direct the girls back, thanks Bronwyn. While we're waiting for the girls to arrive, we're attacked by thousands of sandflies, Bronwyn says she's been amongst them all day jumping around to keep them away. The girls arrive, Alan takes over driving the ute and caravan up the dirt track while Michaela and Janette walk, and eventually have to run to the caravan as the sandflies are swarming us. We all dive into the caravan and suddenly the sandflies are gone. Great quiet spot to camp in the bush away from the road. Temp 24-28 degrees. Distance 43.31 km. Running time 6hr 28min. Pace 8.56. Average 42.344 km. Total Km 2882.89.

Marathon #68.

March 9, 2013. Woora National Park to 5 km of Miriam Vale - The Day of the Sandflies! Quiet night, managed to keep the little critters out of the van, but they were waiting for us at dawn! First 14 km was extremely miserable, biting us on the legs, face and arms. Put on net masks and long sleeve shirts at the first stop then only had to keep them off our legs. Extremely hot and humid and felt like we were suffocating under the nets. Tried various oils but nothing scared them off. Swarming us every step. Exhausting running, Janette lost the plot and tripped with 2 km to finish, down on the rocky road in a screaming heap, knees and elbow gashed. "How come I have all the luck?" Michaela picked us up and drove to the complimentary campsite at the Star Roadhouse & Caravan Park, thanks Debbie. Under the hot shower to ease the bites and road rash. Tomorrow has got to be a better day! Temp 22-29 degrees. Distance 42.41 km. Running time 6hr 21min. Pace 8.59. Total Km 2925.30.

Francine's account of The Day of the Sandflies - (Or The Resurgence of Jurassic Park) Janette and Alan up at the crack of dawn to run down the rocky road to the highway. As dawn broke they were befriended by a plague of sandflies, who found their legs, arms, face and back to be quite the delicacy. Michaela and Francine, blissfully unaware of the sandfly onslaught as we hung around the caravan before heading out to meet J & A at the first stop. Francine directs Michaela at the bottom of the hill and is suddenly under siege from 1000 sandflies. Doing what would to otherwise unaware passing motorists look like some kind of tribal dancing, Francine manages to kick her way back across the road to the safety of the Subaru. Find J & A looking like they are playing karate chop with their hats. Alan exclaims, "that was the worst morning of my life!" Second stop, and J & A are worse for wear though Alan touts the benefits of his stylish mosquito net/beekeeping hat as a method of protection against facial onslaught. Janette too decides to adopt mosquito net hat technology. Francine meets

J & A for third stop, then carries on to organize night in caravan park in Miriam Vale. Michaela collects J & A only to find an injured and bloody Janette after yet another fall. Just another traumatic day on the road. Michaela and I have taken refuge in the caravan to escape the blood sucking sand flies that are absolutely annihilating us!!! Poor Janette and Alan are covered in bites and currently look like the cast of Arabian Nights as they run along the side of the highway! This is a veritable plague!! Give me mosquitoes anyway... Did I just say that? Francine

Hi folks, just letting you know that we're okay, covered in bites from an epic 42.4km run accompanied by millions of sandflies! Will update with more details tomorrow. Had dinner and a hot shower and now we're all heading for bed because we're all dog-tired. Goodnight.

Marathon #69.

March 10, 2013. Miriam Vale to Bernaraby Truck Stop. Michaela drove us back to yesterdays finish spot to start at 5.30am. NO sandflies! Janette's knees working okay but slightly more pain in the ribs after yesterday's fall, so another slow day coming up. The roadworks crew escorted us through the site, holding the traffic at both ends. One of them gave us all the change in his pocket for a donation saying, "You guys are film stars, I saw you on TV!" Ran long legs of 14, 12 and 15 km with 3 km to finish as there was nowhere for the vehicles to pull over with the road works. Girls had set up camp in Truck Stop which we all rated as 5-star because it had toilets and rubbish bins and was far enough away from the road for the traffic noise. Beside the Boyne River which showed signs of previous massive flooding, had warning signs to watch for crocodiles, but no warning about the Goliath Mosquitoes, who arrived in swarms when it got dark! Not to worry, we're old hands now with pesky critter attacks, best method is turn out the lights and go to sleep! Temp 23-29 degrees. Distance 42.9 km. Running Time 6hr 18min. Pace 8.59. Total Km 2968.20.

Marathon #70.

March 11, 2013. A significant number and past 3000 km today! Bernaraby to Gladstone Nth. Michaela drove us back to yesterday's finish spot to start at 5:20am. Both feeling a bit slow today, must be the after effects from the sandflies. Painted ourselves with calamine lotion to stop the itching. Janette's knees painful for first few km and ribs still the same level of pain with every step. Running through more roadworks until the turnoff to Gladstone. We had been warned by locals not to continue on the Hwy bypass because of the roadworks, so diverted through Gladstone an extra 6 km. Quiet and picturesque road into Gladstone, but there the scenery changed, very industrial through the town and out the Nth side. Finished the run after several km of roadworks in a roadside gravel pit 15 km north of Gladstone. Had sponge bath in gravel pit amongst dingo prints! Temp 23 degrees. Distance 42.96 km. Running time 6hr 47min. Pace 9.28. Total Km 3011.16.

Marathon #71

March 12, 2013 Nth Gladstone to Marmor. Off at dawn, Janette still in pain, slow 12 km through industrial area, running alongside the railway line with trains carrying coal to the power station, some over 1 km long with 4 engines and 300 carriages, going back and forth, empty and full all day long. Spent 3hrs on phone with Garmin at first break with some success, now have data up to Feb 28, will upload in the next few days. Back on the road through flatlands, looks like Africa but no giraffes or lions! Very long day, finished just before dark. The girls had set up camp next to a park with picnic tables so had delicious salad dinner outside until the mosquitoes arrived and chased us into the caravan. Temp 23-30 degrees. Distance 43.54 km. Running time 6Shrs 8min. Total Km 3054.70.

Marathon #72.

March 13, 2013. Marmor to Rockhampton. Another long day on the road alongside the train line and through roadworks. Very rough and rocky tarseal. Ran extra km to get into Rockhampton. Temp 23-32 degrees. Distance 45.94 Km. Running Time 6.46 Pace 8.51. Total Km 3096.64. Food Intake: grapefruit, bananas, oranges, mandarines, green smoothie, salad.

Marathon #73.

March 14, 2013. Rockhampton to Yaamba Depart 5:30 running through outskirts of Rockhampton, over bridge river still in flood, and past lovely gardens and large shopping centres, out to first stop at 13 km. Girls drove on to second stop and left Janna there while they went shopping for week's food and supplies. We ran on through suburbs and into the countryside to second stop opposite farmhouse near The Caves. Had a visit from Beau, Brielle, Buddy & Rosie, thanks for the veges and donation and doggy cuddles! Thanks also to Henry from up the road who stopped and offered showers! Pity we were only halfway through the run! Ran on through bush and mild hills to third stop at 38 km where we demolished 10 oranges each before finishing the last 6 km past Yaamba Truck Stop. Michaela drove to pick us up and back to the truck stop for the best $3 shower and yummy salad. Found out from the servo that there is no LPG for the next 200 km so Alan disconnected the ute from the caravan and drove back to Rocky, he said the 42 km seemed like a very long way driving it! Truck stop filled up with campers, trucks and trailers spending the night. Temp 26-33 degrees. Distance 42.35km. Running time 6hr 27min. Pace 9.09. Total Km 3188.99.

Marathon #74.

March 15, 2013. Yaamba to Kunwarara Good cool start, Michaela drove us to 3.3 km where we finished last night. Ran first 1-2km before turning the Garmin on (!) Too bad we can't bank the extra kms! Ran 13 km to first stop, first hour with mosquitoes swarming us. Spent 2hrs getting Garmin data uploaded and updated, then on for another 11 km and had 10 oranges and 4 bananas. On through very nice scenery, flat plains with lush grass and flood water still lying in fields like lakes. Stopped at the last fruit stall till after Mackay. Plenty of variety and locally grown produce all overseen by a very friendly bird who landed on Michaela's shoulder and went to sleep! Bought pineapples for $1.50 each and was given free ripe bananas! Ran on a final 10 km, stopped part way to take photos with banner for 3213 km. Rough road past magnesia quarry and tough running. Girls had found a great campsite off the road and presented us with durian, that made us feel much better! Temp 21-29 degrees. Distance 43.46 km. Running Time 6hr 33min. 125 Total Km 3232.46.

Marathon #75.
Kunwarara to Gravel Pit 20 km north of Marlborough. Depart at 5:30am with Raelene & Gavin from Rocky Road Runners who came to join us on the Run for the day. Set off at 7min pace, good company and time went very fast as we chatted on the way. Thanks for joining us on the road guys! Met a couple of truck drivers stopped on the way and told them what we're doing and why and gave them a flyer about RunRAW2013. They said all the truckies were trying to figure out what we were doing on the road every day and that they will call each other when they see us to let them know. Temp 21-33 degrees. Finished by 2pm. Distance 42.31 km. Running time 5hr 54min. Pace 8.21. Total Km 3274.77.

Marathon #76.
March 17, 2013. Gravel Pit to Waverley Creek Rest Stop. Early start 5am in the dark with stars still out. Nice daybreak to the sound of emus calling, kangaroos and emus in the mist watching us through the long grass. Found old abandoned service station at 11 km for first stop. Michaela and Francine stayed to do some video footage while we ran on through the mosquitos. Edge of road very rough with pyramid shaped stones everywhere just waiting to get us under the toes, instep and heels. Did some fancy footwork to avoid them and plenty of fancy comments when we hit them! Janette's ribs complaining as she twisted while trying to avoid the stones, knees almost healed and not jarring any more. At least there's not so much traffic on the road as it's Sunday. Michaela went ahead with the caravan to set up at Rest Stop while Francine stayed with us for the last stops. Very hot with heat radiating off the road, registered 38 degrees in the vehicle at the last break. Last leg took a lot of focus to keep going especially for the extra 2 km, but we could hear Francine calling out to us in her thick Russian accent "You can do it!" so we kept going, sweat dripping on the road, water hot in our bottles and the road ahead looking like a mirage of water with the heat waves rising. Finally staggered in to the best Rest Stop since we started the Run. Free camping, toilets, water, picnic tables and shade trees far enough off the road to cut down the traffic noise. Cooled down with a bucket of cold water while Michaela made a great meal of cabbage wraps which we ate outside until the sun went down and the mosquitoes chased us into the caravan. Temp 21-36 degrees.

Distance 43.56 km. Running time 6hr 23min. Pace 8,41. Total Km 3318.33.

Marathon #77.

March 18, 2013. Waverley Creek to Clairview Beach. Off in dark at 5.15am. Beautiful sunrise, red sky with trees silhouetted on skyline, perfect 'Out of Australia' scene. Early morning chorus of birdsong and sounds of animals waking, I'm sure I heard a lion! Very warm and no breeze. First stop 14 km had large banana smoothie then on through a changing landscape of flatlands with long grass, pools of water with blue lilies and tall thin trees, to rolling hills with dense bush. Feeling the rough stones underfoot while running on the edge. Realised after 7 km that the Garmin watch had not started so used the vehicle odometer to adjust distance run on road. Only a few km from the coast but not seeing it until finally finished at Clairview Beach Holiday Park on a complimentary site right on the beach with showers and laundry! Thanks for your hospitality and support! Straight down to the water to plunge in and found the girls sitting on the edge. "Do you want to know the good news or the bad news?" they asked. Looking out at the beach and rolling waves we couldn't see what could be bad. "Great beach but there are crocodiles in the water!" Francine said pointing out to what looked like logs surfacing on the waves. Not to be deterred, we walked down to the edge and watched for a while as the animals occasionally surfaced out past the breakers, then decided it would be safe enough if we stayed by the edge behind the rocks. So we lay down in the warm water, keeping an eye on the waves and wondering if we could get up quick enough to outrun the critters! Clearly they were not interested in us as they stayed just out of sight. Wonderful feeling to soak in the saltwater after the Run. Well, the good news is that those critters were not crocodiles, but dugongs! (manatees), very docile delightful marine mammals that look like elephant seals without the tusks. Could have gone out and swum with them had we known! Apparently there is a pod of around 100 of them that live in the waters off Clairview. (Note to self: Coming back to this spot when we have more time to stay). Francine made a delicious salad and banana and pineapple pudding for dinner. Temp 21-31 degrees. Distance 42.61 km. Running time 6hr 27min. Pace 9.11. Total Km 3360.94.

Marathon #78.

March 19, 2013. Clairview to 10 km south of Ilbilby. Stormy night (Cyclone Tim off coast) Departed in dark and rain with Leona & Andy whom we met at the campground last night. They ran with us 4 km up the Clairview Road to the Bruce Hwy, thanks for joining us, it was great to have your company. Continued on accompanied by very large mosquitoes in drizzling rain, cool showers on and off all day with a following wind, welcome change to the heat of the last few days. Banana and pineapple smoothie at first two stops. Landscape changed from bush to sugarcane plantations. Ate 6 oranges each at last break then on to finish in an old gravel pit at exactly 42.2 km.

Marathon #79.

March 20, 2013. Depart at daybreak 5;30am. More rough rocky roads with narrow edges. Rolling hills with Brahman cattle and sugar cane plantations. Cool following wind with constant showers throughout the run. Seemed very easy running today, fastest day for many weeks. Finished 5 km short of Serina. Michaela and Francine doing recordings for the RunRAW videos - stay tuned! Michaela drove ahead to find great complimentary campsite at Tropicana Caravan Park in Serina, thanks for your hospitality and support Sierra and Olga. Great showers and laundry, keeping up with the wet clothes. More rain and wind forecast for the next week, but it's better to run in than the heat so we're not complaining! Distance 42.30 km. Running time 5hr 47min. Total Km 3445.48...off to bed.....

Marathon #80.

Oh Yay! March 21, 2013. Serina to Mackay Started at 5:15 after Michaela drove us 7 km south to where we had finished yesterday. Light showers alternating with heavy rain all day running past huge sugar cane plantations with own narrow gauge railways. Ran easy first 13 km to first break, then 12 km to second break. Michaela and Francine drove on to Mackay to do the shopping while we continued the 20 km to finish, taking dates and water on the way. Stopped at fruit & vege stall entering Mackay to eat bananas, then continued on to finish past Mackay township. Drove the ute and caravan back to Premier Campground where Bev gave us a complimentary site. Thank you for your hospitality and support! Went into the pool to soak our feet and legs in the cool water then had a hot shower, wonderful! Temp 19-27 degrees. Distance 43.78km. Running time 6hr 43min. Total Km 3489.26.

Congratulations! By reaching MacKay, you have officially passed the halfway point on your route to Darwin!!...and to put the size of this country in perspective to those others following your journey - be amazed as they run this already colossal distance of 80 non-stop marathons, four and a half more times in order to finish their circumnavigation of Australia...Keep on plodding! Kaje xx

Marathon #81.

March 22, 2013. Mackay to Mt Ossa Very warm night 27 degrees. Michaela drove us Nth to our finish point from yesterday, raining and hilly most of the morning, then into flatlands amongst the sugar plantations. At one of the breaks, a lady came out of her house where the caravan was parked to ask if everything was okay and was there anything she could do for us. Francine told her about RunRAW2013 and that we were there for a break on todays run. She kindly gave us a donation, thank you. Very hot and humid between second and third breaks (10 km), ran out of water so stopped to wait until girls arrived, felt dehydrated very quickly. Ate 5 oranges each and recovered within 20 mins. Ran the last 6 km in heavy rain storm which was cooling. Finished at exactly 42.54km at Mt Ossa Rural Store where we were offered showers, thank you so much! Parked across the road for the night as another heavy rain storm surrounded the caravan and tent with water! Temp 27-33 degrees. Running Time 6hr 14min. Pace 8.46. Total km 3531.80.

Marathon #82.

March 23, 2013. Started in the dark, rain all night, wet road but better surface and wide shoulder. Truck coming from behind blew a tyre, sounded like a rifle shot. Driver stopped to inspect then carried on. We often see the remains of tyres on the side of the road, wouldn't be good to be there when they explode. Both feeling weary today as a result of being dehydrated yesterday and not much sleep last night. Battled on between heavy rain showers and steaming humidity, but with 2.5 km to go Janette lost the plot and fell asleep at the wheel! It only takes a split second to go from upright to horizontal with the legs still going but the brain shut down. It's not the falling asleep or the falling down that gets you, it's the waking up a split second before hitting the ground and knowing there's nothing you can do before the impact brings everything back to reality...and then the pain screams at you as the first impact cracks another rib, you bounce onto your elbow and shoulder with the second impact and slide to a halt on the palms of your hands. The sound of someone screaming brings your brain back to full clarity and you realise the scream is yours, and you know this is really going to ruin the act. What to do? You pick yourself up, brush yourself off and start all over again! Got to the caravan and cleaned up, had a salad and fruit and a 45min nap, which got us through the next 16 km. Finished in Bloomingdale where Michaela had set up camp on the grass behind the Community Hall, the sun came out to give us a lovely twilight and sunset before the mozzies arrived. Early to bed for a long recovery sleep. Distance 42.13 km. Total Km 3574.11.

Marathon #83.

March 24, 2013. Bloomingdale to Proserpine. Had a good nights sleep and departed in the dark at 5am, both feeling back on track. Long straights on the road through sugar plantations all day, very humid again. Very few trucks, but many motorbikes on the road, out for a Sunday ride. Ran extra km to finish at Gunna Go Caravan Park 6 km past Proserpine, thank you for the complimentary site, Clive. Found the girls cooling down in the pool and joined them, then had hot showers, did the laundry and had delicious dinner of cabbage rolls stuffed with salad and botanical cuisine sauce. Another early night and good sleep, after the locals went home from the bar and the cane toads finished their conference outside and a brown snake departed the toilet block! Love the wildlife in this area! Temp 24-29 degrees. Distance 44.77 km. Running time 6hr 28min. Total Km 3618.88.

Marathon #84.

March 25, 2013. Proserpine to 12 km south of Bowen. Departed in the dark at 5:15am, Janette picking up speed already. Ran through the last of the sugar plantations into rough scrub and flatlands. Warm but not so humid, with following wind to keep cool. Lots of tiny frogs on the roadside, helped a bright green one go away from the road and into a pond. Thought about how well they stay hydrated. Carried more water and called the girls for more when we ran out before getting to the break stops. Did 18 km the first leg as there was nowhere for the vehicles to pull over, then 12 km and last 2 legs of 6 km each. Found a spot to camp by a babbling brook with a live resident turtle looking like ET as he swam upstream. Temp 22-32 degrees. Distance 42.46 km. Running time 6hr 04min. Total Km 3661.34.

Marathon #85.

March 26, 2013. 12 km south of Bowen to Guthalungra Departed in the dark 5am after another good night's sleep, stars still out in a clear sky. Dawn broke over a flat landscape heralded by the raucous sound of kookaburras laughing. Didn't think we looked that funny, but obviously they did! Running towards Bowen saw an amazing phenomenon of spiderwebs completely covering a line of trees like a net. Millions of spiders in the webs, apparently this happens after floods. We ran around the airport to continue on Bruce Hwy towards Townsville, while the girls left the caravan for our first break and drove into Bowen for a look around. Continued on with humidity rising, hard going on rough rocky road. Francine brought water and oranges, a small shower broke the humidity and a cool breeze picked up so it was easier to run the last 7 km. Finished at 43.37 km and Francine picked us up to drive on to where the girls had set up camp for the night in a very large gravel pit on what remains of the old road between the Hwy and the railway line, the only place to park the vehicles off the road.

Marathon #86.

March 27, 2013. Gutalungra to 13 km south of Inkerman. Michaela drove us back to where we finished last night and we started at 5:15am in the moonlight. Lovely daybreak as the moon set, enjoyable 14 km run to great picnic area for first break, great smoothie to get us on the way. Nowhere along the road to stop the vehicles so Francine came back in Subie with water and oranges so we could go the extra distance with only 12 km to finish. Split it up into two 6 km runs because of the heat and humidity. Francine found a good camping spot at exactly 42.42km. Great salad for dinner compliments of Chef Francine. Temp 22-34 degrees. Running time 6hr 05min. Pace 8.37. Total Km 3752.13. (Hey, we're still ahead of the Facebook 'Likes'!)

Marathon #87.

March 28, 2013. Sth Inkermann to Ayr. Departed at 5:15am Beautiful day break with the moon setting for first hour. First break at 14km, 2nd at 13km and 3rd at 15 km, long hot running day with a few stops on the way to make phone calls in the shade of the sugar cane. Finished 4.5km past Ayr. Francine picked us up and drove back to Burdekin Cascade Caravan Park in Ayr, thanks for your hospitality and support! Lovely campground and friendly folks. Temp 23-35 degrees. Distance 42.25km (Forgot to turn Garmin watch off when driving back so Garmin data registers 4.5km extra) Running time 6hr 35min. Pace 8.25. Total Km 3794.38.

Marathon #88.

March 29, 2013. Ayr to Giru Eco Park. Driven 4.5km north to where we finished last night, started as the full moon was setting. Running through very tall sugar cane plantations, all ready to harvest. All being irrigated by flooding. Hot and humid, we've figured out that the sugar cane creates it's own climate as we noticed the humidity drop when we are not amongst it. Finished near Giru at the Eco Park set against the bush covered hills, very beautiful and quiet spot beside a lake, owned and run by a friendly family who gave us the site for free, thank you for your hospitality and support. Big mob of resident wallabies all standing around amongst the campers. Temp 22-33 degrees. Distance 42.27 km. Total Km 3836.65.

Marathon #89.

March 30, 2013. Giru Eco Caravan Park to Townsville. Drove 2 km north of the park where we finished last night and started at 5:30pm in the dark. Got into the ute at one of the stops to turn the caravan around, turned the Garmin watch off and forgot to turn it back on when we started running, so no data for 4 km from that break to next just past the Wildlife Sanctuary 17 km from Townsville. Continued in to Townsville, joined by Anthony and Cameron from Townsville Road Runners 10 km from finish who had run out to meet us and run in with us.

Great to have the company as chatting while running made the time and distance go quicker. Ran extra 4 km to Anthony's house so the Garmin data would register 42.22 km. Michaela and Francine drove the vehicles to Anthony's where we will stay for the weekend, then they packed up their things to leave a few hours later, staying with friends at a campground in Townsville overnight before they leave for Cairns. We chatted with Anthony for a while then got prepared for a long day getting everything organized for the long haul over to Darwin. Temp 22-34 degrees. Total Km 3878.87.

Marathon #90.

Easter Sunday, March 31, 2013. Townsville. Start at 5am from Anthony's house joined by Anthony and Cameron, met up with other Townsville Road Runners and ran trails along the river then back to Anthony's at 7am. Made a green smoothie and then drove to The Strand Park on Townsville waterfront to meet with media and other runners. Did some photo shoots then ran up and down The Strand with Wayne (running barefoot) who had come to meet us. Continued to run The Strand meeting up with several other runners and some people who recognised us from being on TV. Met up with Michaela and Francine at the Rock Pool on the Strand for a sad goodbye. Thanks for everything girls, we really appreciate how you took care of us and wish you all the best on your quests. Turned off the Garmin and drove to Coles to put in the produce order for pick up tomorrow then started the Garmin to run another few km before heading back to the Strand for more media interviews and photo shoots. Townsville folks arrived for the Meet, Greet & Eat in the park, also joined by John & Marleen who will be with us as support crew from Townsville to Mount Isa. Lovely to meet everyone and thank you all for your support and donations. Finished the last 6 km with Anthony and Cameron along The Strand under the lights to the Casino amongst many people taking a stroll in the warm evening (27 degrees) A very long and full day, but enjoyable to meet everyone in Townsville, we'll be back! Distance 42.51 Total Km 3921.38. We're a quarter of the way there and heading west tomorrow.

Hi everyone, Eileen here. Alan and Janette have turned left! They've now run over 4000 km and are presently between Charters Towers and Hughenden on the Flinders Hwy- over 40 deg for the last

10 km today-autumn anyone? Internet is a bit of a challenge at present but they'll update when they can. Meanwhile, we're gearing up for their 100th marathon next week, a world record-how amazing is that!!!! They're entering a really tough phase now so keep that support coming!

April 2013

MARATHONS #91-120

Hi everyone, we're back online after a great Easter weekend in Townsville. Thanks so much to Anthony and Cameron of the Townsville Road Runners who ran out to greet us on Good Friday and ran with us into Townsville. Anthony kindly offered for us to camp at his place and Cam did a great job of installing a new water tank into the ute for us. Both ran with us every morning, showing us the wonderful trails along the river where we saw lots of turtles. Also ran along The Strand in the city with Wayne and later in the evening to see all the lights along the waterfront. We made lasting friendships and enjoyed being in Townsville, which is a delightful town. Had a very busy 3 days getting organized for the next leg west, had to fit the runs in between doing shopping and other jobs. We're currently camped in the bush alongside the railway track and half km from the road, (Flinders Hwy) on our way towards Mount Isa. Will update the blogs for Marathons #88 to #92 tomorrow as we need to catch up on sleep now. Hope everyone had a lovely Easter.

Camped in a field of long grass amidst termite mounds, feels like we've found Avebury! We're near Dingo Creek somewhere between Balfes Creek and Homestead on the Flinders Hwy and we've got internet! Yay, so here goes with the updates since Townsville:

Marathon #91.
April 1, 2013. Townsville and 25 km west on Flinders Hwy. River run with Anthony and Cameron at 5am, fast 15 km loop with a stop to watch the sunrise and the turtles at the rivers edge. Back to Anthony's place, Cam installed the new water tank in the ute while we got everything else organized. John and Marleen (our new Kiwi Crew) arrived and drove to Coles to pick up the produce order then helped to stow everything when they arrived back. Thanks to Richard, the Produce Manager at Coles for going to the market this morning especially to get the freshest produce for us. Everything looked great and should last us to Mount Isa.

All packed and ready to roll at 12:30, said goodbye and thx to Anthony and Cam for all their help and friendship and for showing us around the running trails of Townsville. Drove out to the start of the Flinders Hwy (where we had passed coming in to Townsville on Sat) and started running at 1pm, heading west with the sun and wind at our backs. Ran quite fast in 36 degree heat, stopped along the way to get water from a house, thanks Lance for the ice cold spring water. Marleen drove ahead in the Subaru to find a spot for a break, John driving ute and caravan. Great spot on a side road where Cam joined us and ran with us for the next 3 km as the sunset. We said goodbye and he turned around to run back as we continued into the dusk. Finished last 7 km in the dark. John and Marleen had camp set up off the road beside the railway line. Late dinner and late to bed but good to be back on the road. Temp 26-34 degrees. Distance 42.28km Total Km 3963.66

Marathon #92.

April 2, 2013. 25 km west of Townsville to side road near Woldston. Depart at 5:20am in the dark with less than 6 hours sleep two nights in a row, feeling a bit weary. Ran 14 km for first and second legs, feeling the heat and lack of sleep so ate a whole watermelon and some dates. Finished at a secluded spot in the bush off the road, but found that it was the night shunting area for the trains! Temp 21-34 degrees. Distance 42.25 km. Total Km 3975.91.

Marathon #93.

April 3, 2013. Woldston to Macrossan River. Away by the moon at 5:15am Very remote, only saw two houses all day. Good running but slow. Anthony drove out to meet us at 15 km, delivering the botanical cuisine package and mail, thanks for the special delivery Anthony! Our keen Kiwi Crew John & Marleen very organised and busy with projects around the vehicles and caravan. Good cloud cover for the last 10 km made for a cool finish. John had set up camp beside the river and run out to meet us. We had 3 km to go so he drove on and ran back again together to finish today's run. Passed an amazing flood marker showing the biggest flood of 21 mtrs, good thing we planned not to be here in the rainy season! Forgot to stop the Garmin watch (again) as we drove back to camp, so Garmin data registered 45.42 km, but actual distance run 42.42km. Temp 25-28 degrees. Good cold showers and dinner of zucchini noodles and delicious tomato sauce made with botanical cuisine Walnut Bolognese, yum! Went over the 4000 km mark today with a Total Km of 4018.33.

Marathon #94.
April 4, 2013. Macrossan River to Black Jack near Balfes Creek. Depart in the dark 5am, very quiet on the road except for several 4 trailer road (truck) trains. John drove ahead to Charters Towers to do shopping for new battery and parts for new solar system that he will be installing in the Subaru and Marleen drove to the next stop. Went into a small roadside grocery store to refill water bottles and several people getting out of their cars recognised us from the article in the Townsville Bulletin - "Good on youse guys," they said and gave us a donation, thanks guys. Continued running to Marleen's stop, got very hot 38 degrees. Last 10 km was slow going, John had found a great campsite and ran out to meet us, so it was great to have him with us to finish. Temp 20-38 degrees. Distance 42.24 km Total Km 4060.57.

Marathon #95.
April 5, 2013. Black Jack to Termite Land off Hwy. Start 5:15am in dark, no moon so running with the torch (flashlight). Early trains lighting up the landscape and passing with an eerie sound. After about 5 km, Alan discovered he had not started the Garmin watch, so called John to make sure the ute odometer was zeroed off before starting so we could adjust the distance later. Stopped at the Balfes Hotel, Janette talking to the pet Brahman cow and ostrich (not emu), while Alan talked to the pub owner. When Alan told him we were running around Australia, he said, "I've got an old car out back you can have cheap!" Alan said we were about to set a few records and the pub owner replied, "Oh, that's those black round things with a whole in the middle!" Janette went in to find Alan and the owner said, "Well, are you going to buy anything or did you just come in for a yarn, 'cos I've got a cigarette outside waiting for me if you want to join me out there." We said thanks, but we had to run! Weather a bit cooler today so running easier, temp 19-29 degrees. John ran out to meet us again and finished together at a great campsite amongst the termite mounds. Distance 42.44 km (adjusted distance from

Garmin 37.64 km and from ute 4.8 km) Total distance Km 4103.01.

Marathon #96.
April 6, 2013. Termite Land to 3 km past Pentland. Start 5:15am in dark, very quiet Saturday morning, no traffic so running down middle of the road for several hours until two truck trains (4 trailers) passed each other right where we were (we had moved off the road). Easy 14 km first leg and still very quiet for second leg of 12 km. Ran through Homestead with a population of 100, a school and general store which is closing next week, time has passed by this sleepy town and so shall we. The traffic increased a little and without exception every motorist waved, tooted and/or gave us the thumbs up as they passed us. With only a few km to go a car pulled over and the driver asked if we were running for charity as they had seen us earlier when they went to Townsville for shopping and now here we were still on the road. We told them about the Run and the charities and they gave us a donation, even though (as they pointed out) they were cattle farmers. Finished 3 km past Pentland at 42.33 km. John picked us up and drove back to Pentland Caravan Park where he had set up camp in a complimentary site, thank you for your hospitality and support. Temp 19-29 degrees. Total Km 4145.34

Marathon #97.
April 7, 2013. 3 km past Pentland to 9 km east of Torrens Creek. Marleen drove us out to the spot we had finished last night, started in the dark and light rain 5:15am. Long straight roads uphill all day with cool breeze. Running up through the Burra Ranges and into White Mountain National Park to the top of The Great Dividing Range at 500 metres. Big bush fire had recently been through the area leaving a scorched and eerie landscape. John very busy installing the solar system in the Subaru, Marleen had the laundry hanging out at the second stop, what a crew! The last 17 km was one long straight stretching out into the distance in both directions, a taste of things to come! John found a good roadside place to camp at exactly 42.25 km. Temp 19-28 degrees. Total Km 4177.57.

Marathon #98.

April 8, 2013. 9 km east of Torrens Creek to Little Emu Creek. Departed at 5:15am in the dark, cool morning. What to say about being on the road today - 2 corners in 42 kilometres! One neat and tidy little town, population 20, 1 pub and petrol station, train station (1 passenger train per week). Running alongside train track all day, a few very long freight trains - carrying cement, chemicals and cattle. Ran down middle of the road most of the day, road very rough with sharp stones, hard on our shoes. Thirty road (truck) trains with up to 4 trailers, 40 cars, 20 caravans. Cows wandering along the train track and edge of road. That's it! Finished at a great spot beside the railway track at Little Emu Creek. Temp 19-28 degrees. Distance 43.23km. Total Km 4220.80. John finished the solar system in the Subaru, now has solar panels on roof connected to battery inside car that is powering tow fridges also in car. Thanks John, it works great and now we have more room in the caravan! Made a special dessert for John and Marleen as it is their twenty-fifth wedding anniversary today, spending it in the Great Queensland Outback!

Marathon #99.

April 9, 2013. Little Emu Creek to 7 km east of Hughenden. Alan decided to sleep out under the stars last night, but a storm came and blew over his tent with him in it! Hasty retreat to caravan at 3am leaving tent attached to the ute! Started at 5:15am in dark with starry sky, watching the Southern Cross sink in the sky as dawn breaks. Ran through the little hamlet of Prairie (population 30) with huge wind-wheel to pump water. Stopped to talk to a truck train driver and told him about the run. "Thought you must be up to something crazy like that, I've seen you on the road every day since Townsville." We asked him to let the other drivers know and he said he would send out the word, "I've seen your crew out there too, don't worry, we'll all look out for you." The next road train to approach us went right over into the other lane and tooted loudly, driver with thumbs up. Thanks guys. Today on the road it got really interesting, two sweeping corners on one long straight! Kept a good pace today, felt like we were closing in on the big 100! Finished 7 km east of Hughenden, 42.45 km. Temp 19-32 degrees. Total Km 4263.25. Marleen picked us up and drove to the campground where John had set up the caravan, unhitched the ute and gone to town for supplies and fueling the car and we arrived to find him washing the ute. Marleen and Janette drove into town for food but the fresh produce is being delivered tomorrow morning so Marleen will stay behind to stock up. Back to camp, Alan doing laundry and John washing the Subaru. Hot showers all around and delicious chili dinner. Finally got internet access so Janette catching up on the daily posts then off to bed with the rain on the roof and wind in the rigging....it's going to be a big day tomorrow, off to set a few world records....

It was a dark and stormy night, the lightening struck and the thunder crashed and the crew said to the runners, "How are you going to run in this tomorrow?" and the runners said, "One step at a time." So, early in the morning as the town slumbered, the intrepid crew drove the runners back to the last finish point, the wind whistling in the rooftop solar panel and the rain beating on the windscreen...and the crew said to the runners, "Well, better you than me, so off you go." ...and he urged them out into the dark and stormy night....

Marathon #100.

April 10, 2013. 7 km east of Hughenden to 35 km west of Hughenden on Flinders Hwy, Queensland Outback, Australia. Started at 5:15am in the dark, roaring wind and horizontal rain beating on our left side, water filling our ears and wind blowing us sideways. Surface water all over the road and we were drenched to the skin, shoes sodden within seconds. A few trucks past us sending a wall of water onto us and pushing us backwards. We could see the lights of Hughenden in the distance and as we closed in the wind and rain intensified, lightening flashed across the sky creating an eerie display. As dawn broke the town emerged from the mist and we ran into a lake of surface water on the road. Sloshed through the water to take shelter and phoned John to come and get us in the car so we could change into dry clothes. Rain had cleared when he dropped us back to continue running through the town and out onto the long straight road towards Mount Isa. Strong tail wind pushing us along, lightening and thunder in the distance, very desolate land with no grass or bushes, no sign of animals or farmhouses. Ran fast first leg to stop with John, Marleen had stayed back in town to get fresh produce from the Hughenden Grocery Store, as they were getting a delivery first thing and they gave us a box of bananas free, thank you for your support! We continued on, running well until we were drenched again with a sudden downpour of torrential rain that turned to hail! A cool, clear but cloudy last two legs of the run on very rough road with sharp stones and potholes. Having everything thrown at us on our one-hundredth marathon! Finished fast, step for step, side by side, 100 marathons in 100 days, only 265 to go! Emotional finish on the road with John there to take photos, Marathon #100 completed! One hundred consecutive marathons in 100 days, 1 January - 10 April 2013. Total Km 4305.52. Distance 42.27 km. Pace 7.54. Running Time 5hr 34min, our fastest day since the first day out of Melbourne. Average 43.05 km each day (marathon distance is 42.2km) World Records - First Female; (On June 19, 2010, Kalyn Jolivette of Ohio set a new Guinness World Record by running 11 marathons in 11 consecutive days), First Male over 65; First Couple; First Female and First Male Raw Vegan: First Female and First Male to run 100 consecutive marathons in Vibram Barefoot shoes.

Comments from Facebook/RunningRawAroundAustralia2013

- *How amazing, inspiring and exceptional. I hope the tail wind keeps up all the way to Three Ways.* - **Jo**
- *The way you write it is as if one is there with you both - minus your lived experience. Exceptional.* - **Jamie**
- *Real, real HEROS!* - **Peter**
- *Wow, what a challenge, well done. I hope number 200 isn't twice as bad!* - **Margot**
- *I hope you guys write a book.... This is true inspiration, well done on your heroic achievements! The best part...... You are VEGAN!* - **Jazz**
- *Well done! You are amazing people and a true inspiration.* - **Kylie**
- *Unreal amazing achievement you two congratulations.* - **Ingrid**
- *Unbelievable!* - **Jenny**
- *Amazing! So inspirational* - **Megan**
- *Phenomenal...* - **Filip**
- *Such an inspiration - keep up the great work.* - **Rachel**

- *Keep up the great work. There are many of us watching and cheering you on.* - **Doug**
- *Hell yeah barefoot running! Only way to go.* - **Adele**
- *Amazing!!* - **Kelly**
- *You two are a wonderful inspiration! Stay safe!!* - **Jessica**
- *Amazing, a massive congrats to you for achieving this!!!* - **Bart**
- *Our hearts are with you...* - **Colin**
- *Congratulations!* - **Merindi**
- *Congratulations guys! What an amazing achievement! You're an inspiration!* - **Sam**
- *Very inspiration and keep up we Australian are very proud of you xo All the best.* - **Tracey**
- *Gods of running! Hardaznailz the pair of ya!* - **Cameron**
- *You are incredible and this photo is very moving. You are inspiring so many people all over the world* - **Annie xx**
- *We love you Janette & Alan!* - **Marcos**
- *Just amazing.* - **Denise**
- *Absolutely incredible!!* - **Emma**
- *Way to go guys, congratulations. You are heroes.* - **Roch**
- *Way to go u 2, fantastic effort! Congrats on century.* - **Minsk**
- *Go, vegans! Go vegans. Go vegan. GO VEGAN!!!!!!! Imagine how emotional it's gonna be at the end of this triumphant achievement, guys. Already heroic beyond belief. Congratulations. 27.4% of the way. We're with you every step.* - **Peter**
- *Awesome effort Janette and Alan!! Congratulations!!* - **Michelle**
- *Were sending you so much love and energy.* - **Linda**
- *You two are superheroes. I will tell my children about you (when I have them). I hope you are staying strong within your minds, because that is most important. peace and love, I send my best wishes.* - **Kurt**
- *Kale Ya, RAWESOME, good or bad it is an adventure, and look at those kms!!!* -**Odinn**
- *You guys are truly amazing...thank you for inspiring me, I hope you run somewhere near Barossa when u get to SA.... Good luck!* - **Mel**
- *I love how mentally and physically tough you both are. Your support and love for one*

another is incredible to watch and I wish you both success on your journey. Go Vegans. You guys rock. - **Mark**
- Happy Anniversary you two. Not sure what day it is for you, but Terry and I will be celebrating 5 years tomorrow, so it must be 44 or 45 for you I think. Much love - **Tanya**
- Amazing - **Deanne**
- For us runners (in whatever capacity) out there, this is inspirational. Good on ya. - **Sian**
- Thinking of you daily and hope that you are OK after the big storm! - **Brenda**
- Awesome Couple congratulations on no 100! You two are inspirational Keep Safe & Take Care! - **Sylvia**
- Well done - **Rita**
- The both of you are very inspirational to my running. keep up the good running.. peace and good juju always. .- **JuJu Jay**
- Running is all that and more congrats!!! and keep it up. - **Maria**
- Well done !!!..nothing like a several challenges on your 100th marathon just to remind you of your strength to overcome anything. - **Liz**
- I couldn't run that much in my whole life! Good job and congrats - **Avalon**
- Fitness plus - **Kerry**
- Awesome! - **Jen**

"How to run a Marathon 101 - get up at a ridiculous hour, put on wet clothes and shoes and run out the door into dark and stormy morning. Tear along the dotted line until completely perforated, only moving off to side of road when road trains appear on horizon. Hold onto hat and stand aside when road trains pass, continue in straight line for 32km (count three power poles per km) and stop at sign to Marathon Station (42 km off Hwy). Use conveniently placed toilets at rest stop across the road then continue in straight line for 1 km. Turn corner. (Don't get too excited!) Continue in a straight line for remaining 9 km..."

Marathon #101.

April 11, 2013. 35 km west of Hughenden to Stamford Gravel Pit. Rain and wind throughout the night with road (truck) trains parked alongside at 2-3am. John drove us back to yesterday's finish spot to start at 5:15am in the dark, wind and rain. A slower day's run plodding along enjoying the scenery alongside the long straight road, a vast land of tussock grass and scrub; 1 house; 2 dogs running alongside the fence line barking; 20 road trains (most tooted), 20 cars, 2 workers fixing potholes, straight railroad track, 1 passenger and 3 freight trains (all tooted), narrow rough roads, counting power poles. Finished 42.61km. Total Km 4348.13.

Marathon #102.

April 12, 2013. Stamford Gravel Pit to 8.5 km west of Richmond. Blowing a gale and raining when we started in the dark at 5am, many road trains during first hour and one railway train, could see the glow of the lights for 10 minutes before they came into view. Almost straight all the way today except for a left turn through the town of Richmond. Strong following wind and rough rocky road, Alan suffering from BBAS and Janette suffering from BBOS especially when passed by road trains from behind! First and second breaks on the roadside where we could see for miles across the scrubby landscape. John and Marleen went ahead to Richmond, John to set up camp in the campsite and Marleen to pick up more bananas, do the laundry and make juice and dinner. Stopped by family who were passing through and knew about us, took photos and ran through Richmond past the campground and on towards Julia Creek for 8.5km through Dinosaur Country. John drove out to pick us up and back to camp for hot showers and delicious salad for dinner. Marleen made a very decadent fig dessert to celebrate Alan & Janette's forty-fourth wedding anniversary. Forty-four years on the trot, that could well be another world record! What else are you going to do on your anniversary but run another marathon! Temp 19-25 degrees. Distance 42.27 km. Total km 4390.45.

Comment from Facebook/RunningRawAroundAustralia2013:

- Alan and Janette, both are an example of effort, struggle to get what you want no matter what. I hope you manage to complete the rest of the way with the same energy and excitement as when you started this adventure. I send a lot of extra energy and motivation from Spain (Europe), and that nothing will halt on the road, just the end goal. You are already making history. - **David Possé (Madrid, SPAIN)**

Marathon #103.

April 13, 2013. Richmond to Rest Stop 52 km west of Richmond. John drove us out 8 km to where we finished yesterday and we started at 5:30am in the dark. No traffic as we ran in the middle of the road, gradual uphill through dinosaur land. Stopped to look back at the lights of Richmond in the distance. Daybreak brought a clear sunny day. Watched a family of kangaroohoosaurus, 2 adults and 2 youngsters hopping across the road without looking for traffic and up to the railway line where they stopped to watch for trains. Carefully they crossed the railway line, looked back at us as if to say, "uthinktheysaurus" then continued on their way. The road went ever on, undulating uphill in a straight line, on reaching one of the rises we looked back for 20 km and forward for 20 km, and still the road reached into the distance. On either side the power poles stretched in a never ending line, the vast treeless landscape reached the horizon and beyond. As the sun rose higher and the temperature rose with it, the flies came. At first there were just a few, settling on Alan's hat and hitching a ride on his back. After an hour of running into the heat, the fly population increased to where we were both covered with them, mostly coming along for a free ride, but a few flying around our heads, landing on our faces, trying to get into our ears, nose and mouth. Then within half an hour they were swarming, Hundreds of flies buzzing in our ears, crawling on our eyes, nose and mouth. Then it happened. Alan suddenly choked, stopped running and coughed up a fly that had gone into his mouth. "Keep your mouth closed and breathe through your nose," I said, attempting to do the same. "OK," he said, then choked again. Too late, this time he had swallowed it. Continued running hoping to get to the caravan where we could shake them off. Alan choked again, this time it really didn't sound too good. "Not again?" I asked. He recovered and said, "Yep, only this time it went in through my nose and down the back of my throat!" "Oh, that's gross!" "Yeah, they must be desperate is all I can say," he replied. "Ever tried to laugh with your mouth shut?" Finally we made it to the caravan and took refuge with John & Marleen while we had a break. The rest of the run we wore the fly nets under our hats, now that really confused them, but they didn't let up and hung on to us right to the end. That was the day of the flies. Finished 2.5 km past a great rest area with toilets and picnic tables where John had set up camp for the night. John drove out to pick us up and Marleen had made a delicious dinner of zucchini noodles with tomato sauce and beetroot & carrot salad. Temp 18-31 degrees. Distance 42.26 km Total Km 4432.70.

Marathon #104.

April 14, 2013. Rest Area 52 km west of Richmond - Nelia Rd Gravel Pit. Noisy night with trucks pulling in and at midnight John & Marleen discovered their tent was on top of an automatic sprinkler system! John drove us forward to where we finished yesterday, started at 5:15am. Very clear starry morning with orange sunrise. Very quiet, running down the middle of the road most of the day. Discovered all the trees on the landscape are wattle as they are just coming into bloom, will look amazing in another week. We were just leaving after our 2nd break when we heard someone calling out and there on the road was a lady (from Hamburg, Germany) with a touring bike, who is cycling around Australia and had heard about us from the girl in the grocery store in Richmond. She was very excited that she had caught us up and asked many questions especially about what we eat. She decided there and then that she would eat more fruit herself, "Especially bananas to get the energy I need to cycle all day." She signed our guest book, we took photos and filled up her water bottles for her and she gave us a donation for the charities. Such a lovely person and making the most of her 75 years! Got very hot on the road for the rest of the run, but finished well. John picked us up to drive on to the campsite. Temp 18-34 degrees. Distance 42.27km Total Km 4474.97.

Marathon #105.

April 15, 2013. 4.6km from Nelia Rd to 8 km east of Julia Creek. Good nights sleep with no lights or traffic through the night. John drove us back to where we finished yesterday and we started at 5.05am in the dark and starry morning. Stopped to sun gaze at sunrise 6:40am. Very little traffic so ran down middle of road for most of the day. Very straight road, could see forever in both directions. Removed a few roos off the road that had been hit and saw many cattle that had wandered onto the road and not made it. Found an injured goat on the side of the road, he was able to walk but had been bleeding from the nose, must have happened just before we saw him. We herded him back to the fence line so he could find his way through

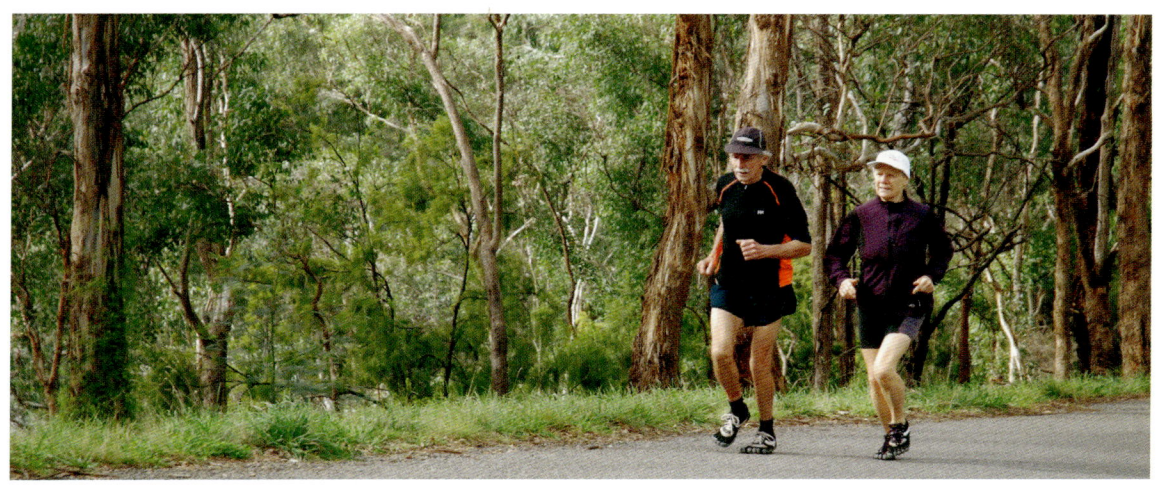

Alan & Janette in training VIC (Photo courtesy Alana Phillips)

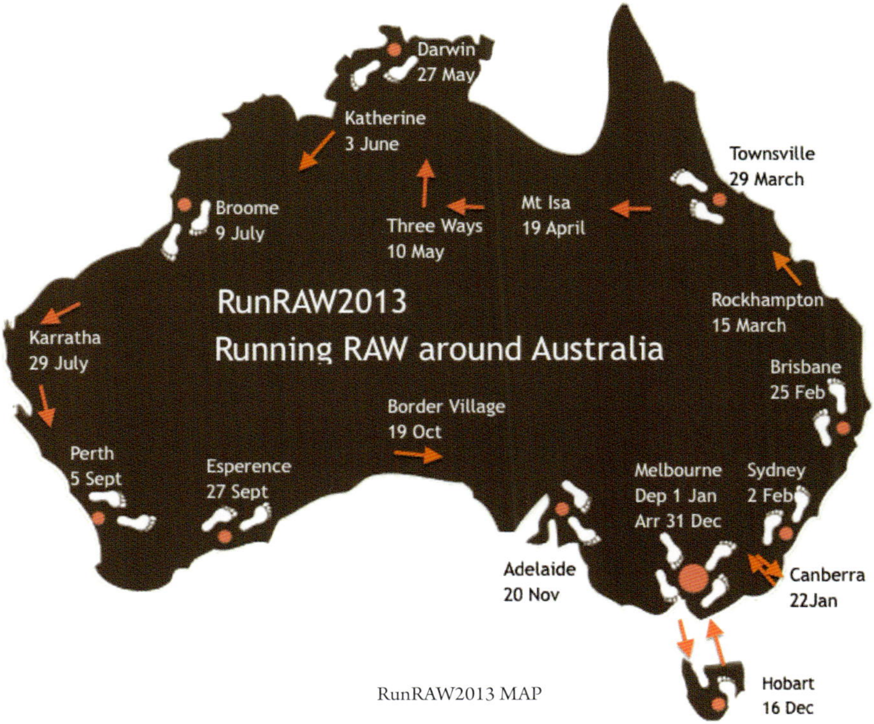

RunRAW2013 MAP

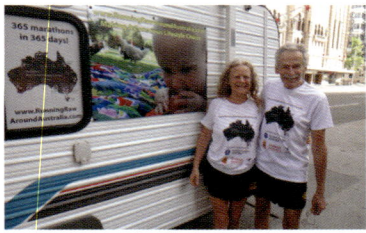

Start day January 1, 2013 Melbourne, VIC.
(Photo courtesy Ping Chan)

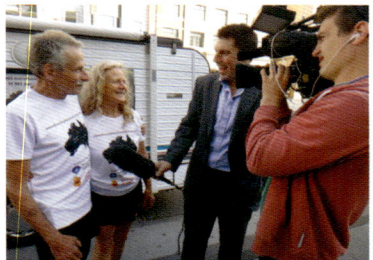

TV Interview Jan 1, 2013
(Photo courtesy Ping Chan)

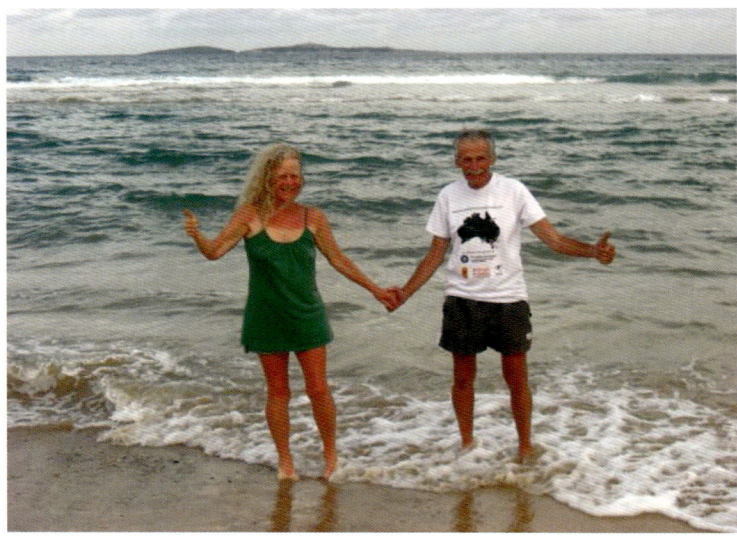

Made it to the Pacific Ocean, VIC (Photo courtesy Ping Chan)

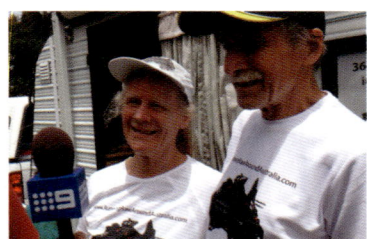

Talking to Ch 9 TV Jan 1, 2013
(Photo courtesy Ping Chan)

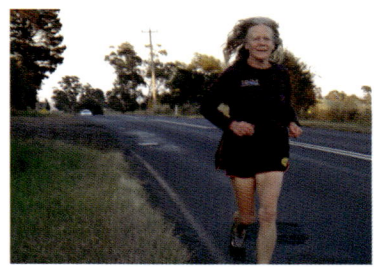

Janette at sunrise VIC.
(Photo courtesy Ping Chan)

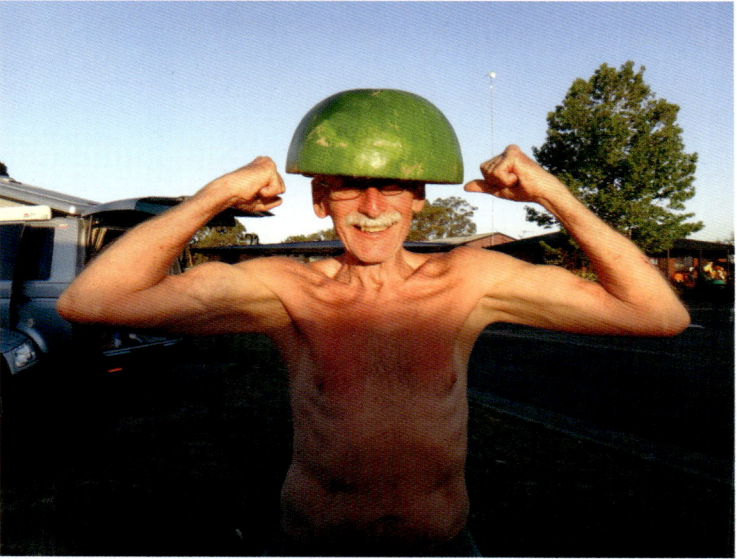

Watermelon muscles (Photo courtesy Ping Chan)

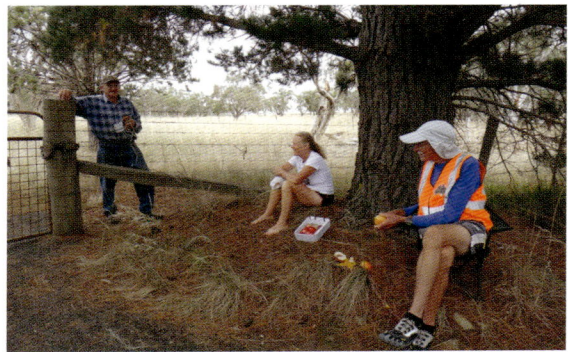
Taking a break with farmer, VIC (Photo courtesy Ping Chan)

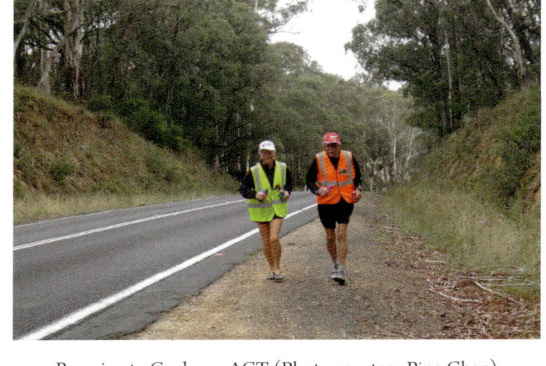
Running to Canberra ACT (Photo courtesy Ping Chan)

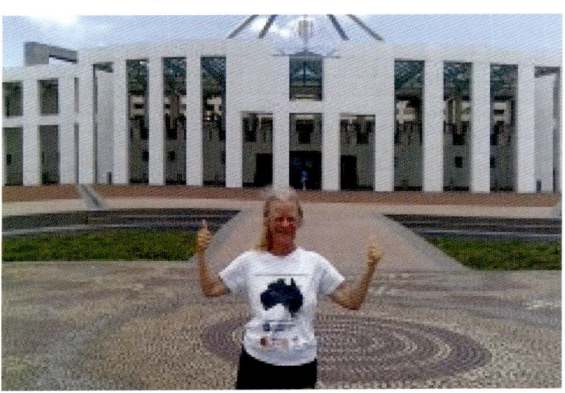
Who is running this country? Canberra ACT.

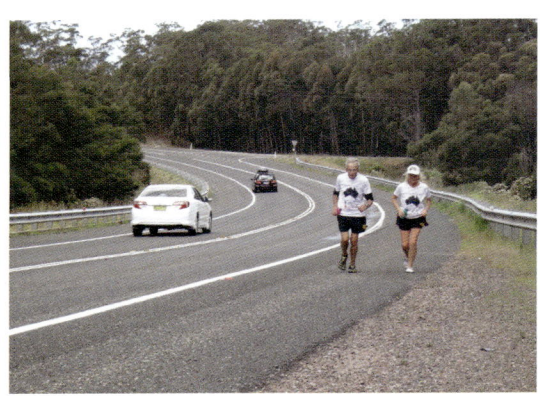
Into NSW
(Photo courtesy Ping Chan)

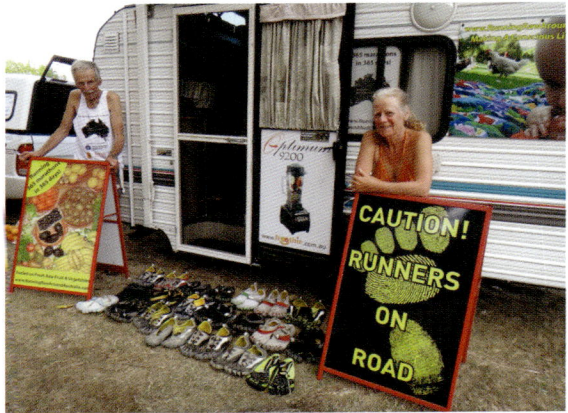
Which Vibram shoes to wear? (Photo courtesy Ping Chan)

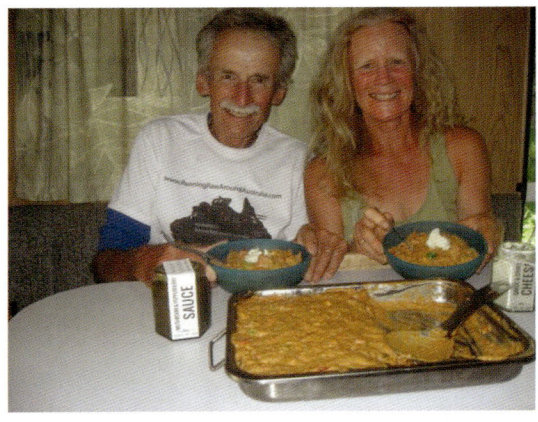
Enjoying dinner. (Photo courtesy Ping Chan)

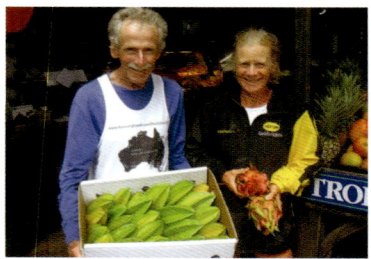
Thanks Tropical Fruit World.
(Photo courtesy Francine Maas)

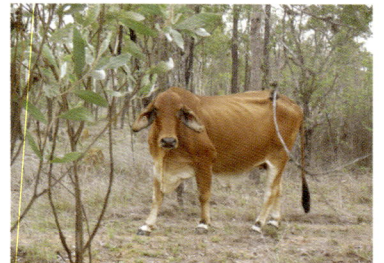
Beautiful Brahman
(Photo courtesy Marleen Kilkelly)

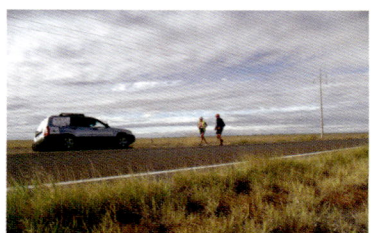
Finish 100 marathons Flinders Hwy, QLD.
(Photo courtesy John Kilkelly)

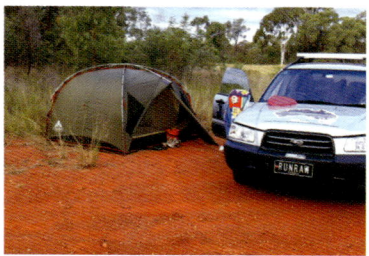
Outback tenting.
(Photo courtesy John Kilkelly)

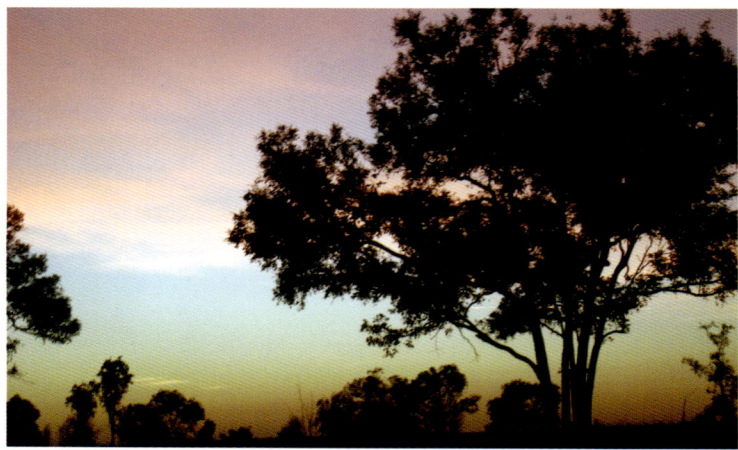
April Sunset, QLD (Photo courtesy Marleen Kilkelly)

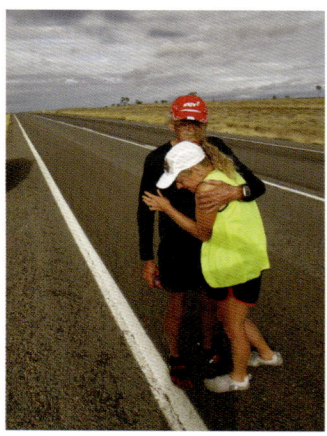
Overwhelmed at 100
(Photo courtesy John Kilkelly)

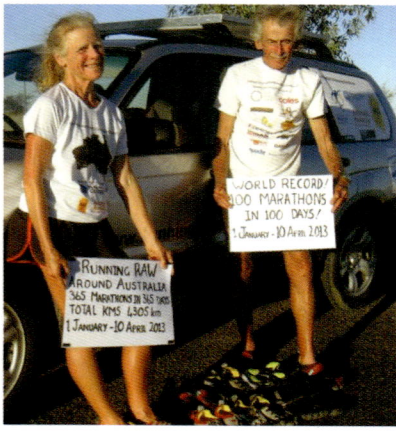
Only 266 to go.
(Photo courtesy Marleen Kilkelly)

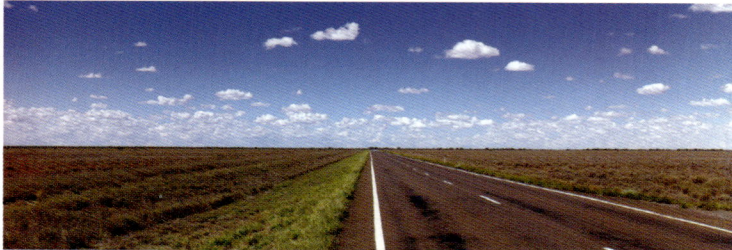
Long straight road, QLD.
(Photo courtesy John Kilkelly)

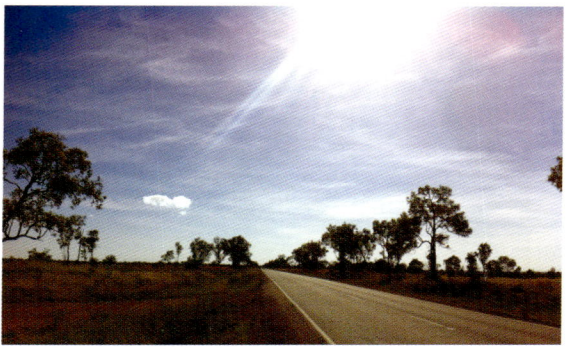
White sunburst, QLD (Photo courtesy John Kilkelly)

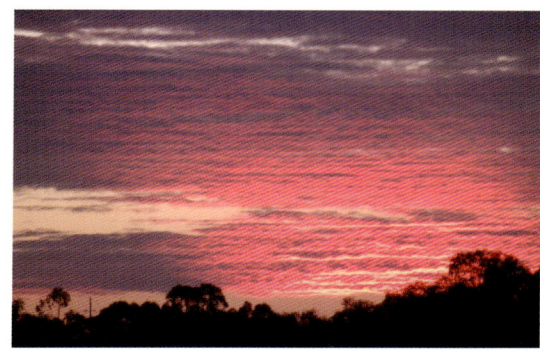
Pink sunset, QLD. (Photo courtesy Marleen Kilkelly)

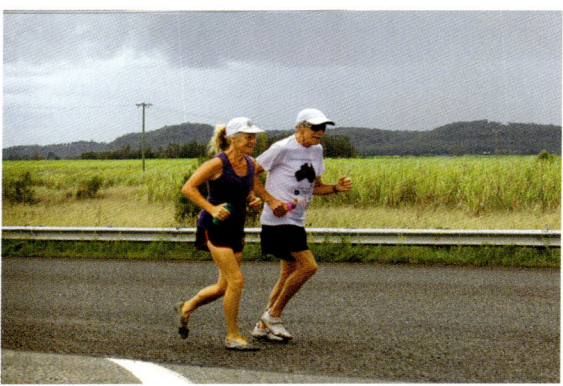
On the road, QLD.

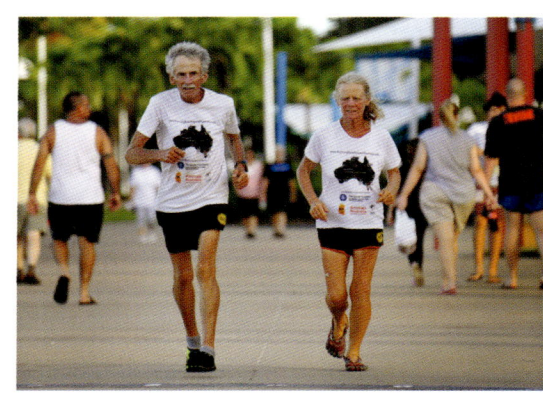
Running through Townsville, QLD

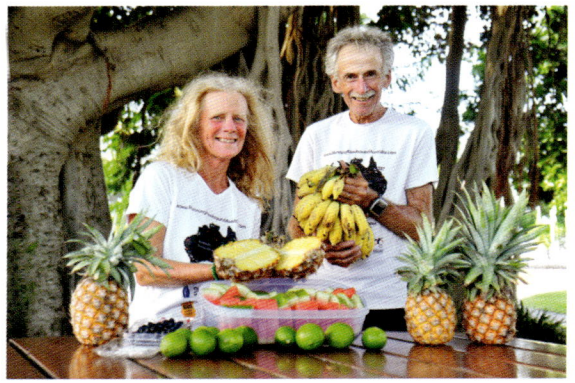
Fueled on fruit

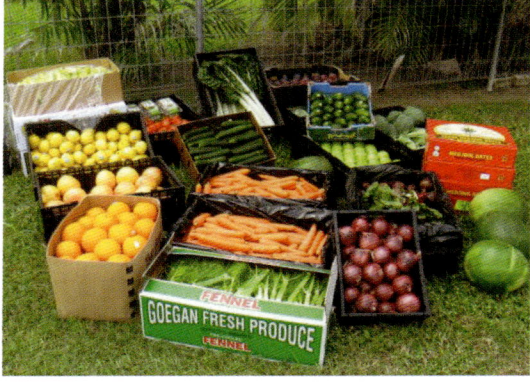
Thanks Coles for Fruit & Veg

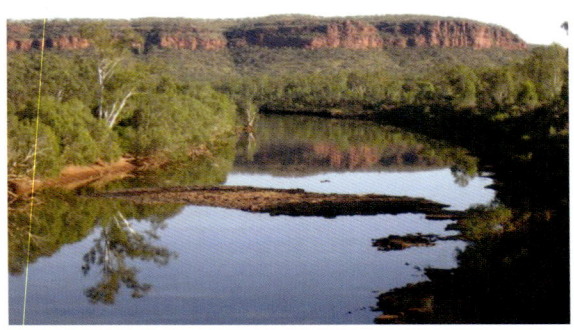
Victoria River NT.

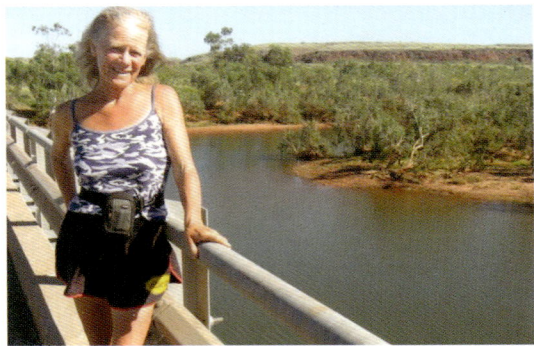
Water in the river, NT.

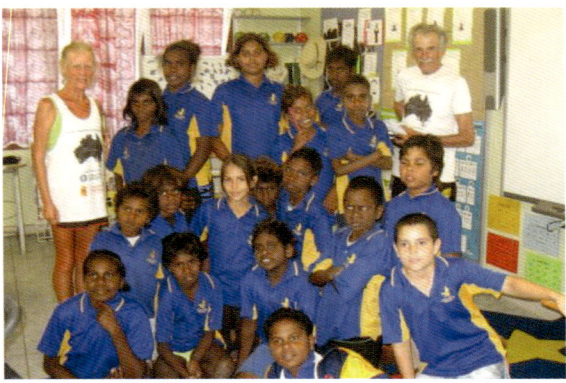
Timber Creek School, NT (Photo courtesy Melissa Kilkelly)

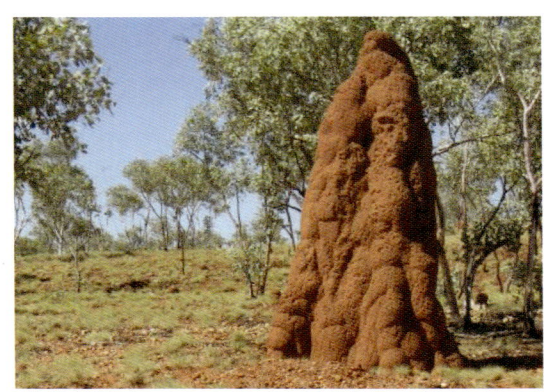
Tall termite mound, NT

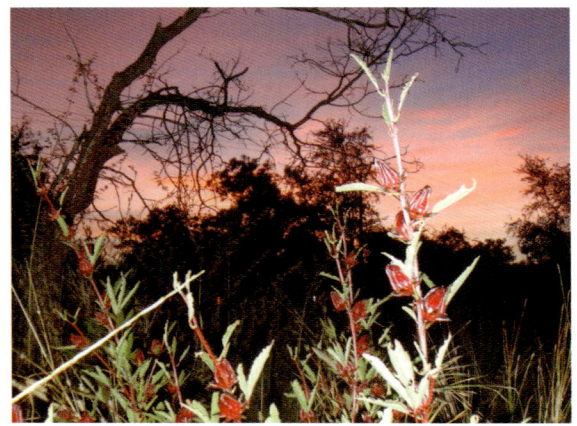
Bush tucker sunset, QLD. (Photo courtesy Narelle Chesworth)

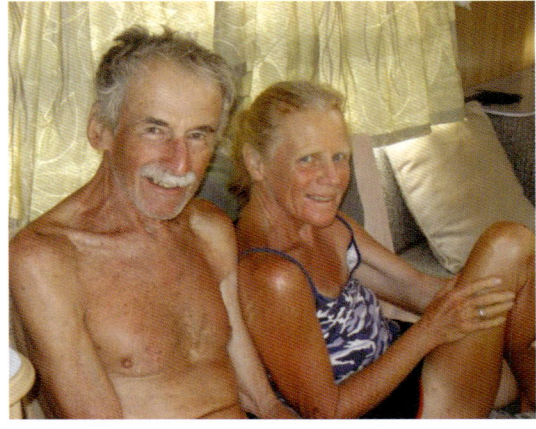
Relaxing (Photo courtesy Narelle Chesworth)

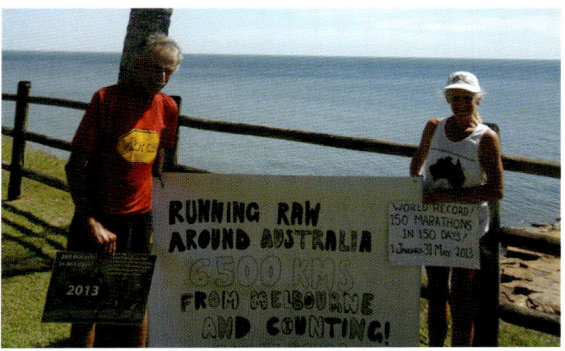
150 marathons/6500km Darwin, NT (Photo courtesy Myke Tran)

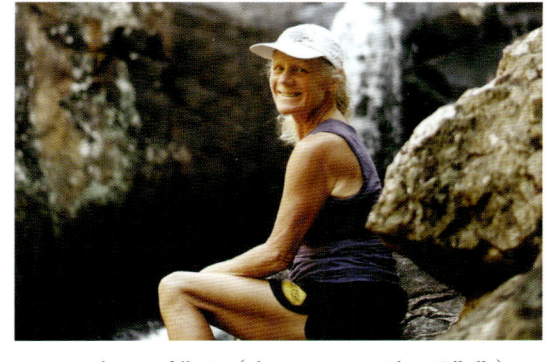
Found a waterfall! NT. (Photo courtesy Melissa Kilkelly)

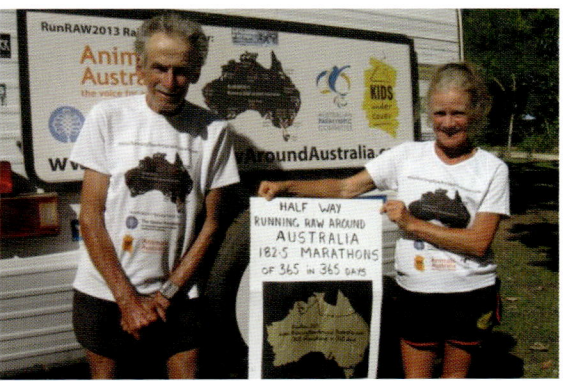
Halfway, WA (Photo courtesy Melissa Kilkelly)

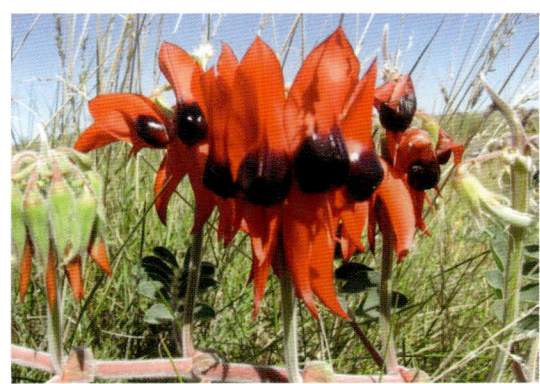
WA wildflower

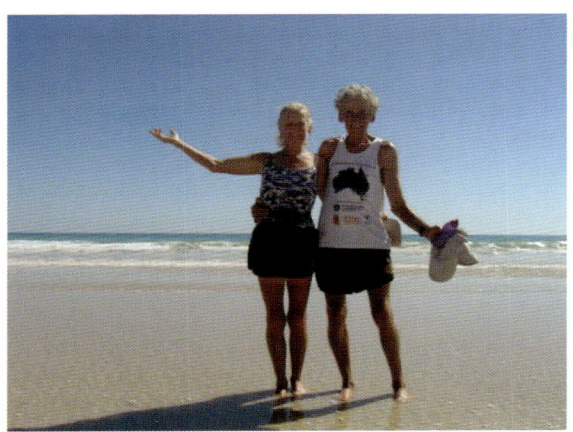
Made it to the Indian Ocean!, WA

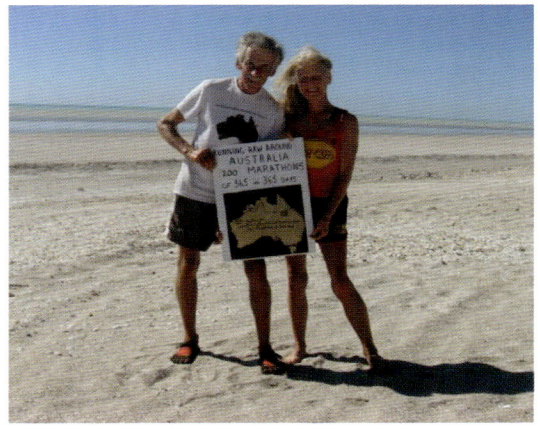
200 Marathons, WA. (Photo courtesy Melissa Kilkelly)

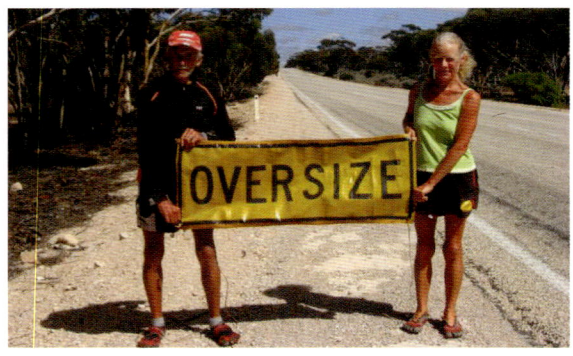
Are we Oversize? (Photo courtesy Melissa Kilkelly)

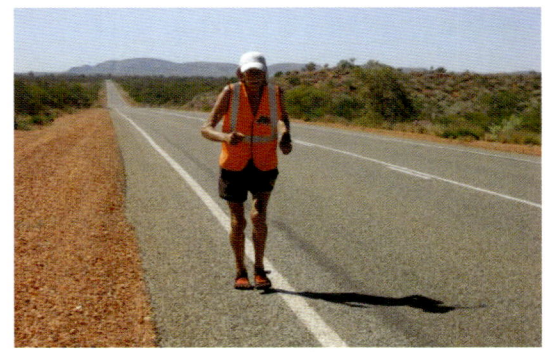
The road goes ever on WA

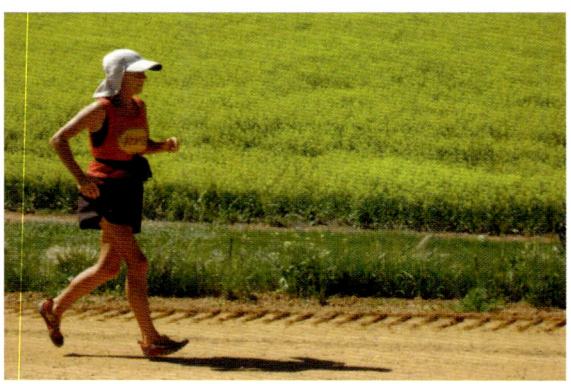
A field of flowers, WA

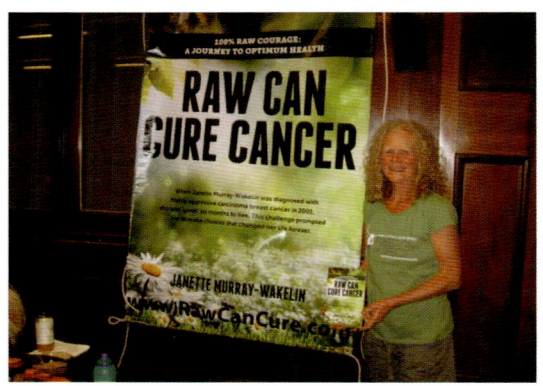
At the Perth event

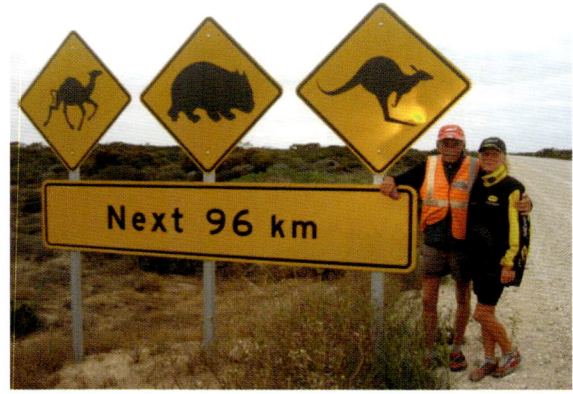
Any sign of animals? (Photo courtesy Narelle Chesworth)

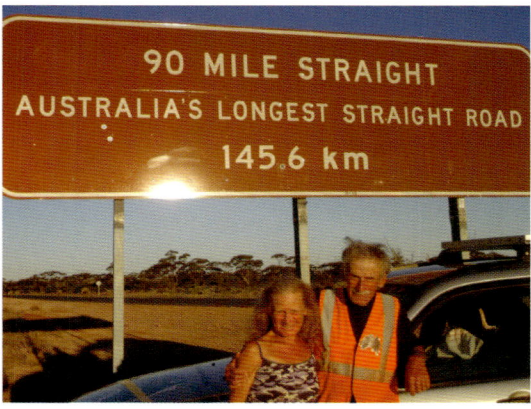
90 mile straight, WA. (Photo courtesy Narelle Chesworth)

to join his herd. Very sad to see so many animals killed or hurt on the road. Got extremely hot for the last 14 km, very hot underfoot, the road was melting and so were we. Checked the temperature of the road surface with a thermometer from our fridge and it went up to 50 degrees, didn't measure any higher! Temp today 18-35 degrees. Glad to be finished at 42.34 km with Marleen there to drive us into Julia Creek where John had set up in the campground. Cold showers and laundry done, Marleen & John went into town to do food shopping and fuel the car. Janette catching up on emails and FB before we leave internet coverage tomorrow. Will be in Cloncurry on Thursday when we'll have coverage again, until then it's time for sleep, after another cold shower as it's 33 degrees at 8pm! Total Km 4517.31.

Marathon #106.

April 16, 2013. Dedicated to all those affected by what has happened at the Boston Marathon today. We have been updated with the news throughout the day and our thoughts have been with all the runners, supporters and spectators as we felt blessed that we were able to continue running our Marathon #106. 8 km east of Julia Creek to Gilliat Channels. John drove us back 10.9 km to where we finished yesterday, started 5:15am in the dark with a starry sky, keeping the Southern Cross on our left and the Big Dipper on our right. Daybreak and a clear sky, big orange sunrise at our back. Ran through Julia Creek township, very quiet and tidy little town, famous for it's Dunnart (endangered cute critter that looks like a little mouse with a fox head). It's nocturnal so of course we didn't see any, but there were many signs about it. The day got very hot, 37.5 degrees with an estimated 48 degree radiant heat from the road, and with the heat came the flies. Thousands of them, hitching a ride on our head, shoulders and back, and buzzing around our face. We put on our head nets and continued on, with our feet overheating on the melting road, a bit hard to stay focussed. John and Marleen were there at the breaks with cold water and foot baths and we put our shoes in the freezer during the break so they were cold to put back on when we left. Not much traffic today, road trains very considerate moving well over when they pass us and tooting and waving. Finished in the middle of nowhere, John picked us up and drove 2.4 km to where he had set up camp. Distance 42.33 km. Total Km 4559.64. Marlene had a delicious early dinner ready and we're all off to bed just after sunset...the sun comes up at 6:40am and the sun goes down at 6:20pm and the flies go to sleep for the night ready to rise again tomorrow...

Marathon #107.

April 17, 2013. Gilliat Channels to Quarry Rd, Flinders Hwy, Qld Outback. John drove us back 2.4 km to where we finished yesterday. Started 5am in the dark, running by the light of the stars in a starry, starry sky. Ran the 2.4km back to caravan and realised that we hadn't started the Garmin watch (again!) We really ought to wake up before we start running so we remember! John has taken on the job of reminding us before we get out of the car. The rest of the run today was the same as yesterday, extremely rough road surface, extreme heat and extreme amount of flies. Only difference was that there was no wind at all. So what do we do to stay upright and moving on days like this? We play the numbers game. Any runner knows how to play, whether you're in a race or just out for a run around Australia, the numbers will come into your head and you can play with them anyway you like. Our numbers game is always about counting and figuring things out. So, today we started by counting our footsteps per km and then figuring out how many steps we would take to run 365 marathons. A marathon is 42.2 km and we estimate that we will take 42.2 million steps (between us) to run a marathon a day for 365 days. Now this is where it gets really interesting! If, during those 365 days we were to fund raise just 1 cent for every step we take, the amount raised would be $422,000. Now that sounds like a reasonable goal to fundraise over the course of a year, and it just so happens that as we passed 4200 kms last week, our Facebook Page reached 42,200 people. If each person reached was to donate just $10, we'd reach $422,000 fundraised. Well, whadyaknow! At our midway break I checked on the Facebook Page and today the count is up to 61,833 people reached, just think where we could go with this! However, at this point of the game, we'd like to thank everyone who is following us on Facebook for your support and encouraging comments, every day we run another marathon (and especially on days like today) it really means a lot to us out here on the road...but this is not really about us running a marathon a day for 365 days around Australia, this is really about sharing a positive message with everyone while raising awareness and fundraising for four very worthy charities. So, we've decided to make our fundraising goal $422,000 and we'd love your help in achieving this. Obviously from the numbers game you can see that if everyone 'Likes' and 'Shares' our Facebook Page more people will be reached and those can do the same, maybe we can reach 42.2 million! Please also share the link to our website, where we have more information about RunRAW2013 as well as details about the four charities AND you can MAKE A DONATION through the website. You can choose to donate to any of the four charities by clicking on the Donations button on the Charity Page, or you can donate to RunRAW2013 and all profits will be divided equally between the four charities. (Many thanks to those who have already done so). We'll keep running those marathons every day and knowing that every step we take, others will be taking steps to help share the positive message and to fundraise for the charities with kindness and compassion. Thank you everyone, we really appreciate your support.

Marathon #108.

April 18, 2013. Quarry Rd to Landsdowne Hwy Junction, 13 km east of Cloncurry. John drove us back to where we finished yesterday and we started in the dark at 5am. Remembered to start the Garmin watch this time! Many road trains this morning, could see the glow of their lights for up to 15 minutes before they appeared on the horizon. Shortly after daybreak we were running along on the quiet road when suddenly a kangaroo hopped out of the bush and across the road in front of us, then stopped on the white line on our side and started to eat the grass. Janette was running slightly ahead of Alan and was about 200 metres away from the kangaroo, who continued to stand on the white line munching away happily and quite oblivious of the approaching runners. Then the scene changed dramatically. There was a corner about 1/2 km beyond the spot where the kangaroo stood and around the corner came a big road train. Janette immediately went into action, running faster towards the Roo, waving her arms around and shouting at the top of her voice for it to get off the road. The Roo continued munching, totally oblivious to the impending danger. Alan meanwhile was running behind Janette and noticed that she had started to act somewhat erratically and wondered what was going on, not having noticed the Roo. As she got closer Janette saw that the road train was also closing on the Roo at an alarming rate and realised that the Roo could move onto the road instead of away from it, so she stopped running and stood on the side of the road, still waving her arms frantically and shouting at the top of her lungs. Finally, instinct kicked in and the Roo turned towards Janette. Immediately his ears twitched and he stood up taller to assess the situation, decided in an instant that he wanted no part of whatever was going on and in one hop covered half the distance from the road to the fence, the second hop took him over the fence and he didn't stop to look back. Meanwhile, the road train driver had seen Janette's antics and decided he didn't want any part of it either, so tooted his horn and swerved over to the other side of the road to pass the runners at a wide and safe distance. Alan caught up with Janette still not knowing what was going on, to find her laughing and pointing out into the distance as the Roo joined his mate and hopped out of sight. Five km later another road train came into view and immediately sounded his horn and moved well over into the other lane, waving as he passed. So we figured the first driver had put out an all alert on the UHF going something like this: *"Hey guys, you know those old geezers that are out running around Australia that we see every day on the road, well, I thought one of them had lost the plot this morning, better give them a wide berth when you see them!"* The long straight road for the first hour then a few corners giving way to real hills and trees. Temp 18-38 degrees then cooled to 33 degrees in the last 7 km. Marleen found some great spots to stop for breaks, John did a full clean out of all the vehicles and inventory of the produce so we could put in the order at Coles in Mt Isa. They will have fresh produce delivered from Townsville on Monday for us to pickup when we arrive in Mount Isa - fantastic service, thanks Richard in Townsville and Chris in Mount Isa. Ran an extra km to finish the run where John had set up camp. Distance 43.61 km Total Km 4646.26.

Marathon #109.

April 19, 2013. Landsdowne Hwy to Barkly Hwy roadside stop. Departed 5am in dark....

At daybreak the early morning mist creating strange shapes moving alongside us, the mist weaving it's way through the trees and rolling along the ground. The sound of hooves coming closer, breaking through the trees and out into the open, a herd of white horses, long manes flowing, galloping through the mist. Running free along the white sands of the Camargue, an ancient herd in an ancient land. I run with them, sensing their freedom, feeling their beauty....and then, one of them mooed...bringing me back, waaay back, to the red dust of the Outback. A herd of white cattle, crashing through the brittle bush, long tails swishing, an ancient herd in an ancient land. I run with them, sensing their fear, feeling their betrayal....majestic beasts from a foreign land, trapped in a void from which there is no escape....and the great white stallions were gone...

    Again the sun rose in a cloudless sky, again the flies joined us, swirling around our faces, buzzing in our ears, trying to get through the head nets. Again the cool misty morning became a dry, hot 38 degree day. Straight roads broken only by running through the town of Cloncurry. A quick stop and a shower in the service station while John and Marleen did the laundry and we were out on the road again. Climbing out of the town, Flinders Hwy became Barkly Hwy and the hills began. Good to be running hills again. Finished 42.3 km at a good spot away from the road where John had set up camp. Total Km 4689.87.

Marathon #110.

April 20, 2013. Gravel Pit in Middle Earth to Gravel Pit 40 km east of Mount Isa. Ran out the door at 4:55am under the starry sky, heading due south directly towards the Southern Cross for the first hour, then the first corner in the road had us heading due west. At daybreak we could see the road stretching out in front of us to the horizon, a long straight uphill road on undulating terrain, appearing like giant steps into the sky. As the sun rose and we ran down into each dip of the road, we turned around to watch the sunrise over the brow of the previous hill, giving us four sunrises in one morning! Then as the sun rose higher, the warm wind blew in the flies. We put our fly nets over our heads and continued running into yet another day of heat (22-35 degrees), warm following wind, rough and rocky tar melting road, and the flies. After a couple of hours, the terrain changed dramatically. As the road ascended ever upwards, the surrounding landscape filled the horizon with rolling hills and rocky outcrops. Tussock grass and sage brush gave way to larger shrubs and trees, the white trunks of the gums making a stark contrast to the red earth and rocks. The edge of the road dropped away sharply into sandy creek beds and rocky gullies, leaving nowhere for our vehicles to pull off the road for our breaks, so the first leg was 16 km and the second of 15 km got us to 31 km with only 12 km to go. We split the last leg into 2 of 6 km for more water stops as the temperature was rising rapidly. Stopped by the police to ask if we were OK, we said yes we had a support crew a few km away. He asked how far we were going and we replied, "Melbourne." "OK," he said, "then you'll need more water for sure!" He filled our bottles, we gave him a RunRAW2013 flyer and he said he would alert the other patrols to keep an eye out for us. With only 2 km to finish a young man pulled over and asked if we wanted water, he was from Mt Isa and had been competing today in the triathlon at the Dust & Dirt Festival in Julia Creek. We hope to see him and other Mount Isa triathletes as we go through on Monday. Finished today's run 8.4 km before where John had set up camp in a Gravel Pit by the side of the road. As the sun sets and the temperature drops to 30 degrees, we chase the flies out of the caravan and say goodnight... Distance 42,36km.

Marathon #111.

April 21, 2013. 8.4 km east of Gravel Pit, Barkly Hwy to 4.3 km east of Mount Isa. John drove us 8.4km back to where we finished yesterday. Started 5am in the dark, running by the stars. Stopped at caravan to pick up more water bottles as John and Marleen were preparing to leave. Alan was showing John the kms on the Garmin watch and hit the wrong button so the 8.4 km was reset as a separate lap. Restarted the Garmin again and continued on uphill through changing landscape, looking more like Arazona at every corner. More red rocky outcrops and hills dotted with ant mounds appeared over every brow of the hills as we ran ever upward. A sad day on the road as we had to remove quite a few kangaroos who had been hit. Also moved a razorback wild boar, very heavy, maybe 60 kg, but young as his tusk was only 1" long. We placed him in the shade under a tree and stroked his rough hair on his head and the soft hair behind his ears, his eyes glazed over no longer seeing, his beautiful camouflage no longer protecting him... We continued to climb hill after hill, it seemed like we would never get to Mount Isa, but eventually could see a cloud of smog above where Mount Isa lay, but could not see the town until we were only 4 km from it, huge chimneys from the copper mine dominated the skyline. Finished just 3.3km short of the campground where John and Marleen had set up camp. John drove out to meet us and drove us back, but can you believe it, Alan forgot to turn the Garmin watch off when we got in the car, so it registered the extra 3.3km.

Adjusted distance to 42.40 km. Temp 24-35 degrees. Total Km 4774.63.

Comments from Facebook/RunningRawAroundAustralia2013

- *I appreciate how you both see the beauty in all animals, and not just those 'few" designated as more worthy of our care and concern. Thank you for the compassion you show to all the wildlife you come across! Best wishes.* - **JJ**
- *Its so sad to see the animals, but overall you are about to run though my favourite country in Aus. I'm a city girl originally from Melb, but have a weird affinity for the red dirt and the rocks of central Aus, have had since a young child. Seen it, know I'll be running with you in spirit for the nest few days* - **Mandy**
- *I know this road; industrial as it is, it was a blessing to reach Mt Isa Greetings and encouragement from Old South Wales.* - **Doug and Dog**
- *Keep on running.* - **Peter**
- *47??km run your hearts away.* - **Dawn**

Marathon #112.

April 22, 2013. 4.3km east of Mount Isa to 39 km west of Mount Isa. Spent a restless night in Mount Isa campground, very noisy-people partying, kids crying, adults yelling, dogs barking, cars and bikes screeching through town, sirens wailing and machinery in the mine starting up and grinding, smoke belching from the chimneys. We could smell the mine and breath the dust in the air. John drove us back to where we finished yesterday, on the hill above the town. Started at 5am in the dark, running towards the glaring lights of the town and mine site. Set Garmin watch and ran down into Mount Isa, through the town and out towards Camooweal. Found it hard to breathe with grit in the air, made our noses bleed and our throats dry. By the time we got onto the road heading west, our arms and legs were coated with the fine dust, looked like we'd been painted with a pinky-white powder. Ran out past the airport where the fumes from the planes was overpowering, and on uphill past another mine where dust was heavy in the air. Stopped for the first break at 15 km then John and Marleen took the vehicles ahead, parked the ute and caravan, and drove back to Mount Isa to pick up the produce order from Coles and pickup the new blender from Froothie that was waiting at the Post Office. We ran on, all uphill and getting very hot (39 degrees) to where the caravan was parked. Had our midway break and left shortly before John and Marleen got back and drove past us for the third stop. Had a Skype interview for a German Sports Program then ran on into the sunset to finish 43.88 km at a great camp spot away from the road. Arrived in time to do another Skype with the folks in Kindness House in Melbourne for the start of 'We Love Life' Festival Week. John had stowed all the produce away and Marleen had made dinner with some of the fresh veg and a durian, what a treat! Total Km 4818.51.

Thanks for your comments everyone. Our post is an honest report of what it was like for us running through Mount Isa. We have been experiencing a great deal of dust in the air for several days before reaching Mt Isa and for the last couple of days since going through and leaving, we think it's from the loaded truck trains from the mines that come past us several times a day.

Marathon #113.

April 23, 2013. 39 km west of Mount Isa to Rest Area 81 km west of Mount Isa. Depart in the dark 4:50am. Got 2.5km into the run and realised hadn't started the Garmin watch, again! We're just so keen to start running! Hence adjusted distance from the Garmin data. Uphill, hot (39 degrees), radiant heat from road (48 degrees), hot wind, melting road and tar sticking sharp rocks to our shoes. Otherwise a great day on the road! Finished 42.99 km at another great camp spot off the road. John and Marleen had everything set up and dinner ready as they are departing today. After 3 weeks on the road with us, we are sad to see them go, they have been fantastic, looking after us with a smile. Thank you so much you two for everything, you got us through. Alan drove back to Mount Isa Airport with John and Marleen to see them off and meet our new crew, Rose and Narelle. Janette stayed at the camp to update FB as we have internet here! Everyone is now tucked up in various tents and bunks and we're off to sleep in 30 degrees. A big day awaits us all tomorrow... Total Km 4861.50.

Marathon #114.

April, 24, 2013. Truck Stop 95 km east of Camooweal to Split Rock Station 62 km east of

APRIL 2013

Camooweal. Slept well after a long day yesterday, Rose drove us back 16 km to where we finished yesterday. Started running at 5:30am in the dark (remembered to start the Garmin watch this time!) Beautiful daybreak and sunrise to reveal long straight road with scrubby bush on the sides and larger trees beyond. In the distance we could see something black on either side of the road and on approaching realised there were two steer standing right on the edge of the road. They did not move as we ran between them, one continued chewing the grass and the other, very large beastie, stared at us, appearing quite perplexed! They were absolutely beautiful with black shiny coats and bright curious eyes. So glad we didn't run into them(literally) in the dark. Not much further down the road we were passed by a guy on a motorbike going the same way as us. Then he turned around and came back to ask us if we were okay. We assured him that we were and thanked him for coming back to ask. He had the same perplexed look on his face as the young steer! We told him why we were Running Around Australia and he wished us good luck and went on his way. We ran on to the camping spot and spent a couple of hours with Rose and Narelle showing them the ropes, so to speak. Narelle drove the SuperRoo out onto the road, going on ahead to scout out the next break stop while Rose drove a few laps of the campsite with the ute towing the caravan, then she was off with us following behind (on foot of course). Got hot in the next few hours (39 degrees) and just as our water bottles were getting low, a car pulled over and the driver jumped out and said, "We have cold water for you, and fruit!" We must have had that perplexed look on our faces as he was speaking as if he knew us or about the Run. We thanked him as he gave us ice cold bottles of water, 2 bananas and a pear and he said, "You just enjoy your day!" Meanwhile two other vehicles had stopped behind his and were waiting with their lights flashing. He started to drive off and the others followed, as they went past they called out "You're doing a great job and now our Mayor has taken care of you, stay safe and enjoy!" ...and we did, thanks to the Mayor of Mount Isa! Finished the run at Split Rock Station, exactly 42.57 km and celebrated Rose and Narelle's first day on the road by eating 3 delicious durians! Rose and Narelle put up the tents while Janette made a quick dinner of zucchini noodles with tomato sauce. A memorable day on the road, now off to bed with a full moon...

Comments from Facebook/RunningRawAroundAustralia2013:
- *Enjoyed reading. Restful sleep.* - **Jamie**
- *Go hard! You guys are fantastic.* - **Roy**
- *Following your progress. Great job!!! Love to our friend Narelle who has now joined you.. From her art buddies* - **Laurel xx**
- *Still following from Old South Wales. It's my birthday Friday 26, and a full moon! I shall mark the spot where you are, and remember my (driving) trip across the Barkly Highway in 2010. Keep up the good work!* - **Doug & Dog**
- *Cool* - **Jessica**
- *Hi mum (narelle) pleased to hear to hear you have now joined up with Jeanette and Allan. Running in 39 deg heat... Wow... Wow, wow...! Good luck and keep going.-Monique xxoo*
- *Great to see sister Rose is on the job. Love to you all.* - **Judy**
- *So awesome effort amazing people & amazing athletes.* - **Sue**

Marathon #115.
April 25, 2013. Anzac Day. *Today's run is dedicated to all the Anzacs and especially to our parents... the real super heros. Thanks to our two Mums and two Dads for being great examples of devotion, commitment and love, every day we try to follow in your footsteps...*

Split Rock Station to Driveway 20 km east of Camooweal. Departed 4:50am in the dark, but able to see by the light of the silvery moon. Stopped at daybreak and reflected on how blessed we are and as the dawn coloured the sky with brilliant red and purple, the birds began the chorus. Beautiful orange moon set at 6:15am and sunrise at 6:40am above a flat landscape for 360 degrees. Small uphill for the first couple of hours then flattened out on the Barkly Tablelands with a slight downhill for the rest of the run. Easy running with a following wind and lower temp 26-35 degrees. Narelle spotted great break spots off the road throughout the day and Rose navigated the ute and caravan in and out of each spot with the skill of a pro. Met Walter who is cycling around Australia (bettenonbike.com.au) and his wife who was driving their support van. Pleasure to meet you both and best wishes on your trip. Ran past a huge wind wheel (to drive a water pump) on the side of the road and in the next field of long grass, dotted with tall red anthills, a beautiful scene with a family of 4 adult horses surrounding a tiny foal in the shade of a white trunked gum tree. Further in the distance, a single white stallion stood between two gums, tall and proud. For as far as the eye could see, the sculptured red anthills filled the landscape, standing tall amongst the yellow grass. With only 10 km to finish, the reverie was broken with sadness as we found a small cat lying on the road. I picked him up, a still warm furry bundle cradled in my arms, his soft paws tucked into his fur, his little head flopped to one side, his eyes closed. I took him well away from the road and laid him down, still curled up in the shade of a tree, wrapped his tail around his face and left him there, asleep forever....Life on the road can be beautiful and sad in one day...and we learn. Finished the run 42.38 km camped across a driveway. Rose and Narelle making fresh veg juice (carrot, beetroot and tops, fennel tops, apple and ginger) and a delicious grated salad for dinner (carrot, beet, broccoli, wombok, tomato, apple, avocado and sprouted mung beans with sesame orange dressing.

Marathon #116.
April 26, 2013. 20 km east of Camooweal to Gravel Pit 22km West of Camooweal. Departed at 5am in dark, running by the full moon. Daybreak revealed straight road ahead and behind with moon setting directly ahead and sunrising directly behind. A rare phenomenon to see as they set and rose simultaneously, the sun creating very long shadows of us stretching down the road ahead. Had a quick smoothie break at 13 km then ran 7 km into Camooweal. Went to P.O. to pick up our package of Vibram shoes sent from Barefoot Inc, but hadn't arrived yet. Graeme of the Camooweal P.O. & General Store was very helpful with suggesting ways to get the shoes to us on the road when they do come in. Came up with a plan of asking the local Police to bring them to us - just like the old days, only this will be Cop & Co, the mail must go through! Graeme also gave us a donation and assured us that he would get the shoes to us one way or another. All had showers and did the laundry at the campground, filled the vehicles with fuel and water, had some food and we were back on the road. Next stop was on the border going into the Northern Territories, into the Fifth State! Everything changed quite dramatically, the road was not as wide and no verge on the side, but also no rubbish anywhere.

The landscape became very sparse, very few trees, just yellow grass for as far as we could see, which we estimate was up to 7 km in any direction. Narelle found a great camping spot in a huge gravel pit, she and Rose had everything set up when we finished the run (42.82km) at sunset. The moon rose shortly afterwards, a big orange ball into an empty sky. Another great day! Temp 20-37 degrees. Total Km 4989.27.

Marathon #117.

April 27, 2013. Gravel Pit to Avon Downs Police Station. Depart at 4:50am by the light of the full moon. At 5:30am we saw a comet travel slowly, low across the North Eastern sky with a green and orange tail. Very little traffic so we ran down the middle of the road for most of the day through the flattest landscape we have ever seen. The road is rough and rocky with no shoulder in some parts, very hard and hot under foot. Finished 42.98 km just 3 km from Avon Downs, Narelle picked us up and drove back to a campsite across the road from the Police Station. Went over to meet the Police to organise the shoe delivery and eventually came up with the best way to get them to us by bus and local delivery. Phoned Graeme at the P.O. in Camooweal and he said he's got it covered - shoe saga to be continued! Temp 18-37 degrees. Total Km 5032.25 - finally passed the 5000 km mark!

Marathon # 118.

April 28, 2013. 3 km east of Avon Downs to Farm Driveway 39 km west of Police Station. Narelle drove us back to where we had finished yesterday, started 4:50am, ran past Police Station and everyone asleep in the campsite. Narelle and Rose passed us shortly after sunrise and we caught up with them for the first break at 17 km. We could see them down the long straight road for about 6 km. Hardly any traffic so ran down the middle of the road again for most of the day, accompanied by millions of flies of course. Rose and Narelle found a good camping spot in a farm driveway off the road only 1 km from finish so we ran up and back to finish at 42.57 km. We all took refuge in the caravan from the flies although a lot came in with us, most we've had so far. Sunset at 6pm flies disappeared at 6:30, as soon as it became dark. Where do they go? We know they're waiting out there somewhere to join us again at daybreak! Temp 21-37.5 degrees. Total Km 5074.81.

Marathon #119.
April 29, 2013. Farm Driveway to Radio Tower 100 km east of Barkley Homestead. Walked out to road and started running 5am, still good moonlight to run by felt cool (18 degrees). After daybreak could see houses in the distance and at 10 km came to Soudan Cattle Station where there was a public phone, so made a few calls to check in as we still don't have phone or internet coverage. Started to heat up with the sun and flies back swarming around our heads. Landscape had more bush and hills, second break at 26 km at the Soudan Bore where we filled up with water and gave some water to the small birds gathering around the bore. Temp 18-37 degrees. Finished run 42.98 km and camped at a radio tower half a kilometer off the road.Total Km 5117.79.

Marathon #120.
April 30, 2013. Radio Tower 100 km east of Barkly to next Radio Tower on Barkly Hwy. Walked down track 1/2km from tower to Hwy, started running 4.45am, with moon overhead, another lovely morning, no wind and 20 degrees. Running to the mournful sound of dingoes howling at the moon. Daybreak brought the flies again, more than yesterday, constant buzzing around out heads. Had to keep running as the flies go into a frenzy if we stop for any reason. Otherwise an easy run up and over 7 hill crests today, seems to be getting easier each day although the road surface is not. Very hard, pointy rocks for most of the way, we get very excited if the road surface changes to small stones! Finished 8.2km past another radio tower where Rose had set up camp. Temp 20-37 degrees. Running Distance 42.71km. Total Km 5160.50. Sun down at 6pm, flies disappeared at 6:30pm. Early to bed (7pm).

May 2013

MARATHON #121-151

May 18, 2013. Oh, the silence is deafening! Come back on line soon J&A! Whilst we know the reality is very unglamorous, long roads fighting flies and heat glare, here's a lovely shot from Townsville! Would love to hear your stories about how J&A are inspiring you this year, I mentioned going barefoot-because they like to, what things are you doing to live a more conscious lifestyle? Damn that internet!! Tell you what, let's do our darndest to bring the numbers up to 4000 before Janette gets back on line (probably tomorrow) That's just 97 more people!!Considering what they're doing on a daily basis, a few more arm chair marathoners won't be too hard! Eileen

Hellooo! We're back! Just having late dins and will post updates soon.

Comments from Facebook/RunningRawAroundAustralia2013:

- Looking relaxed! - **Mark**
- Enjoy dinner. Reading your posts are a highlight. Cheers. - **Jamie**
- Wow you guys look GREAT, SO looking forward to the updates - **Jenny**
- Going great guys! - **Roy**
- Still looking amazing and doing fantastic... - **Leeanne**
- Great photo! Hello again. - **Nalin**
- You guys are simply rawmazing xxxx love the love In this picture - **Sarah**
- Such love ... The eyes say it all - **Debbie xo**
- What a lovely picture-so much love! I like the word rawmazing, it suits perfectly....Sieghilde
- Pleased to hear you are getting on fine and feeling better pleased to see you enjoyed the hot pools. Its getting cooler here. - **Marleen**

Marathon #121.

May 1, 2013. Radio Tower to 20 km east of Barkly Homestead. Narelle drove us forward 8.2 km to where we finished yesterday, started 4:45am by the moon and stars. Another hot day on a rough road with our fly entourage. Spent the run looking at the amazing sculptures of the anthills alongside the road, ranging in size from 200 mm to 3 metres! Fascinating study and keeps us entertained. Finished run 20 km east of Barkly Homestead 42.57km. Narelle drove us in while Rose set up camp in the campground and phoned in our food order to Tennant Creek, which is 4 days away. Rose also tracked down our Vibram shoes which will hopefully arrive tomorrow morning by bus, fingers and toes crossed! All into the pool to cool off before showers, laundry and dinner. Temp 18-38 degrees. Total Km 5203.07.

Marathon #122.

May 2, 2013. Today marks one-third of the way, Wahoo! 10 km East Barkly Roadhouse to 23 km West Barkly Roadhouse. Drove back 20 km to where we finished yesterday and started 5am. Ran in dark with quarter moon and stars. Narelle drove out to 15 km to meet us with a green smoothie then we ran the last 5 km to the campground. The Vibram shoes had arrived, thanks Sally & Dylan of Barefoot Inc., and a big thank you to Graeme of Camooweal Post Office who tracked the shoes down in Mount Isa and put them on the bus to Barkly for us, donating his time and the bus fee. Your support is much appreciated! Spent a couple of hours on the internet, checking emails and updating the Facebook page, Alan and Narelle checked through the food store in the ute and Rose filled the water tanks. Food supplies getting low as there has been nowhere to buy extra food along the way since leaving Camooweal. We departed 11:15am, leaving Rose and Narelle to fuel up the vehicles before joining us on the road for water drop and going ahead to set up camp in a Farm Gateway off the road, 23 km west of Barkly. Janette running in new Vibram Bikila LS shoes, felt like slippers after running over 1000 km in the old shoes. Temp 20-38.6 degrees. Finish 43.23 km. Total Km 5246.3.

Marathon #123.

May 3, 2013. Today's run dedicated to brother Stephen, your love and support travels thousands of miles without a sound. Sorry can't call you, but thinking of you on your birthday and sending much love with every step. Looking forward to when you join us in Tassie, Meanwhile, on the Barkly Hwy, 23 km west of Barkly Roadhouse to 119 km East of Stuart Hwy Junction. Narelle drove us back 4.2km to where we finished yesterday. Started running at 4:45am in dark. Nice daybreak and sunrise as Narelle and Rose passed us to go to the first stop at 16 km. Second stop at a water bore to find three dogs who had been abandoned, I don't understand how anyone could do such a thing. The police man back at Avon Downs had told us that we would see abandoned dogs and cats on this stretch of road, left to fend for themselves. The three dogs were in good condition so hadn't been left for long, perhaps a few days, as they were patiently waiting, although clearly hungry and thirsty. Gave them a bowl of water each and felt so sad that we couldn't help them anymore. Good luck woofers. Back on the road we did see a cat walking across the road in front of us and it pounced when reaching the bush, then disappeared with it's catch into the scrub. Survival instinct taking over. We continued running at a good pace (must be the new shoes) with two legs of 16 km then a 5 and 6 km finishing at 43.15km. Total Km 5289.45. Temp 26-40 degrees (seemed cooler with a following SE wind). Narelle and Rose had set up camp in a Farm Gateway off the road, and made fresh juice with the last of the carrots, beets and silver-beet stalks. Now out of fresh bananas but using dehydrated bananas in the smoothies (we dehydrated several boxes of bananas ahead of starting the Run for this very occasion). We'll be at Three Ways in three days when we can drive to Tennant Creek to pick up our next bulk order of fresh food. Meanwhile, we're making some delicious meals with what we have left - oranges, grapefruit, apples, kiwifruit, tomatoes, raisins, dates, cabbage, fennel, cauliflower, sweet potato, nuts and seeds. Early night coming up out in the bush where the wild things are....

Marathon #124.

May 4, 2013. Farm Gateway 119 km east to Nextgen Plant 76 km East of Stuart Hwy Junction. Our early night was interrupted by the wild things just before midnight a dingo passed through our camp, his call waking us abruptly. Went out with a light but didn't see anything, although Rose and Narelle were sure they heard the dingo sniffing around their tent! We departed 4:50am in the dark and by the light of the crescent moon and stars. No sign of the dingo but we did hear the pack howling off in the distance. Onto the long straight undulating road, counting the 'crest' signs as we ran up and over the crest of each hill. Must have been seven or eight including the sign that was on the ground, or was that crestfallen? Much the same landscape as the last couple of days, same hot temperatures (35-38 degrees), same amount of traffic (a few cars with caravans or boats, camper-vans, delivery trucks, road (truck) trains, and motorbikes….and the same amount of flies. Running down the middle of the road for most of the day, could see for more than 10 km so able to gauge when to go to the edge of the road for vehicles to pass. Meanwhile Narelle and Rose found good break spots along the way, made an excellent smoothie with the dehydrated bananas for first break, we finished the delicious left-over salad at the second break and had fresh cut oranges at the third. We finished the run at 43.11 km with Rose filming and Narelle presenting us with a poster she had made, showing the Total Km and an Oz map for us to draw our progress on. They found a great place to camp for the night off the road in the bush, maybe we'll see the dingoes tonight. Total Km 5332.56.

Marathon #125.

May 5, 2013. Nextgen Plant 76 km east to Likkaparta Community 37 km east of Three Ways. Departed 4:50am in the dark, cloud cover over the moon and stars, so running along the white dotted line in the middle of the road. On the long straight, could see the lights of traffic from either direction at least 15 mins before the vehicle came within hearing and another 5 min before we needed to move off the road. Mellow daybreak and no visible sunrise because of the clouds, flies had a sleep in as there was no sun to wake them, so arrived in swarms about an hour later than usual. Temp started to rise as did the road in undulating hills, but still we could see about 20 km in either direction along the straight road. Rose did some filming and we just kept plodding on, step after step, until suddenly we could see a corner ahead! We were so excited when we reached the corner we had to stop there and look back along the 60 km of straight road we had finally run. ounded the corner and guess what was there? Yep, another long straight road reaching out to the horizon, where it became a hazy mirage, oh joy! Shortly afterwards, a couple stopped their car alongside us and asked where we were running to. When we answered "Melbourne" they wanted to know all about the Run. We stood in the middle of the road and chatted for about 5 minutes, they took photos and said they would stop by the caravan which was visible further down the road. They left, we ran on, Narelle walking back from the caravan to meet us with full water bottles and we all ended up chatting and eating oranges at our last break. Great to meet the Yeomans and hopefully will meet up again on the road. Finished the run 3 km past the road to Likkaparta Community where Rose was setting up camp for the night. Narelle drove up to pick us up at 42.53 km. Great dinner of pumpkin fettuccine and settled in for an early night. Temp 25-36 degrees. Total Km 5375.09.

Marathon #126.

May 6, 2013. (May Day in NT) Likkaparta to Three Ways. Last day on the Barkly Hwy. Narelle drove us 4.2km forward to where we finished yesterday. Started early at 4:30am, quite dark with a small crescent moon, but a sky full of stars. Heading west counted 50 shooting stars in the South, West and Northern sky, moon swinging in the Eastern sky behind us. Good running for 15 km, 13 km and 5 km off the Barkly and onto the Stuart Hwy, turned right towards Darwin and into Three Ways at the junction. Rose and Narelle had gone ahead and set up camp, thanks to Three Ways Roadhouse for the complimentary campsite. Janette, Rose & Narelle drove to Tennant Creek, 25 km down the Stuart Hwy to pick up the food order. Everything closed in the town for May Day except the food store. Did some extra shopping then loaded everything into the SuperRoo and headed back to Tennant Creek. Meanwhile, Alan cleaned out the ute in readiness to store the food, did the laundry and finished his run. On returning, Janette went out to finish her run, Rose & Narelle went for a dip in the pool, Alan returned from his run and started stacking the food in the ute, joined by Rose & Narelle after their swim. Janette returned from her run just after sunset, joined by a dingo for the last 1 km, came out of the bush and started running on the other side of the road while I was running in the middle. He kept pace all the way to the Roadhouse and then sat down under one of the picnic tables to catch his breath. The dingo must hang out at the Roadhouse as there was a dish of water under the table for him. What a treat to run with a dingo! Finished run at 43.72km and finished packing the stores at 7:30pm, quick dinner of chia and fruit pudding, cold showers then off to bed by 10pm.

Marathon #127.

May 7, 2013. On the Stuart Hwy 4 km north of Three Ways to Rest Stop 47 km north of Three Ways. Narelle drove us forward to where we finished yesterday. Started running 5:30am in the dark, moon getting very small but stars still lighting the way.

Felt quite strange to be heading North with the Southern Cross behind us. Daybreak revealed a changing landscape, red hills with rocky outcrops, different shrubs and trees and small leafy plants with a variety of flowers along the roadside. Many termite mounds on both sides of the road, all different shapes and sizes. More long straights so running down the middle of the road as the traffic was quiet on the road for the first 4 hours, then increased with campers, utes towing caravans, road (truck) trains, motorbikes and two army convoys. All the motorists very courteous and supportive with toots, waves and thumbs-up. Both feeling a bit weary from the long day yesterday (18 hours on our feet) and lack of sleep. Janette felt light headed at 30 km and said to Alan, "I'm depleted, I need a banana or some dates and I'm out of water, I'm going to have to stop and wait for Narelle to come and ask her to get some from the caravan." (we didn't have any phone coverage). Then, right in front of us on the road where we stopped, was an orange, an apple and a bottle of water. We didn't question it, just picked up the fruit and ate it. It was exactly what we needed and we were able to continue on for about 1/2 km when Narelle arrived with more water. We told her what had happened and she asked, "Do you still want a banana, because I have two in the car." So we ate the bananas as well and felt much better, enough to continue on to the next stop. So thank you to whomever left the fruit there, whether it was for us or not, the timing was perfect. Halfway to the next stop Narelle returned with more water, oranges and dates. Fully replenished, we got to the next stop where we ate 6 oranges each and had more water. With 6 km to go we had a good run to finish at Attack Creek Rest Stop. Temp 18-36 degrees. Distance 42.60 km. Total Km 5461.42.

Marathon #128.

May 8, 2013. Attack Creek Rest Stop to Gravel Pit 15 km north of Bank Banka. Departed at 4:45am in the dark with small moon rising. Quiet on the road for the first two hours, first break at 13.5km for a great smoothie with fresh bananas again. Feeling strong today, must be the bananas! Stopped at Banka Banka where the owners invited us to fill our water tanks and bottles with their spring water and have hot showers. Thank you for your hospitality and support, the water tastes wonderful! Continued on uphill to finish at 44.35km. Temp 22-35.6 Km. Total Km 5505.77.

Marathon #129.

May 9, 2013. 15 km north of Banka Banka to Renner Springs. Departed at 5am in the dark, no moon. A cloudy daybreak and sunrise. Hilly run all day. Saw a dingo run across the road ahead of us and as we approached where we had seen him, he ran back across the road the other way, must have forgotten something. Otherwise, no other wildlife seen apart from our crew at the breaks! Finished the run 42.96 km at Renner Springs where Rose and Narelle were waiting at the campground. Thanks for the donation. Set up near the pond with ducks, geese, turkeys and chickens wandering around. Nice setting with good facilities, laundry, showers and a pool. We all had a soak in the pool (very cold water) to cool off, (still 34 degrees at 7pm). Temp 19-38 degrees. Total Km 5548.73.

Marathon #130.

May 10, 2013. Renner Springs to 47km South of Elliott. Departed 5am, very dark with no moon. Very rough rocky road, Janette tripped on small rock embedded in the tarseal (we call them landmines) and fell landing on right hip, knee, elbow and shoulder. (Just as everything had healed from the last fall!) Walked for 30 min until the vehicles caught us up and took an early break to assess the damage. Nothing a good run wont take care of. Stayed to watch the solar eclipse, sharing the view through an Elton John CD, (works really well). Great eclipse too. Continued on, running slower with Janette's knee swelling, took longer breaks, icing and resting the leg and arm. Met Andre from France who is cycling from Melbourne to Darwin, ran the last 5km together, finished at 42.47 km and set up camp on the side of the road, had a delicious dinner together to the sound of Edith Piaff in honour of our guest. Temp 20-37 degrees. Total Km 5591.20.

Marathon #131.

May 11, 2013. 47 km south to 4 km south of Elliott. Departed 5:15am in the dark, no moon, used torch to see the road for 2 hours till daybreak. Cloudy sunrise, Janette running well despite swollen knee. Many caravans on the road all day, the gray nomads are on the move, all tooting and thumbs up as they passed us. Had a sad moment when we came across a wounded eagle, the updraft from the trucks had left him lying with broken wings, a questioning look in his deep blue eye as it glazed over and he closed his eyes for the last time... Finished the run at 43.22km, 4 km short of Elliott where Narelle was waiting and drove us to the campground in Elliott. Phone and Internet connection at last, phoning home, updating FB, showers, laundry, dinner outside under a fragrant frangipani tree...Temp 20-37.6 degrees. Total Km 5634.42.

Marathon #132.

May 12, 2013. 4 km south of Elliott to Grassy Farm driveway 40 km north of Elliott. Narelle drove us back to where we finished yesterday 4 km south of Elliott, Started at 5am in the dark but could see the lights of Elliott in the distance. No traffic so running in middle of the road to Elliott, everything quiet in town except for the dogs barking as we passed their gates. Stopped at the campground to set up the computer for Rose and Narelle to make their flight bookings while we continued on to the first break. Could hear dingoes howling just before daybreak as we headed out of town, onward and upward on the long straight road. Looking back we could see the water tower in Elliott for 10 km. Stopped at the Newcastle Waters Rest Area for our midway break, Rose and Narelle had driven to the Ghost Town of Newcastle Waters 3km away to see the museum. While we were having our break at least 20 caravans and campers arrived to set up camp for the night, the Gray Nomads had arrived! Met a few and chatted awhile before setting off again. Just left when a couple on motorbikes pulled over calling out to say hello. They are riding around Australia, had seen us on the Sunrise Show and had been looking out for us on the road ever since. Lovely to meet you Lisa and Rod, keep in touch and safe riding. Continued on to finish 42.75 km at a delightful spot well off the road on a grassy driveway to a farm about 3 km past Newcastle Creek Crossing, where Rose & Narelle had set up camp. We all sat on the chairs outside watching the sunset, drinking our freshly made juice (carrot, beet, apple, ginger), a Beet Treat hard to Beat! Late finish but a great day. Temp 20-37.5 degrees. Total Km 5677.17.

Marathon #133.

May 13, 2013. 40 km north of Elliott to Farm Gate 18 km south of Dunmarra. Departed 4:50am very dark so used the torch until daybreak. Could just make out that we were running through forest on either side of the road, and as the growing light brought the images clearer, we discovered a scene to behold.... *The blackened trees stood tall, their bare branches intermingling in an eerie image of the lush canopy there had once been. On the ground below, scorched bare of underbrush, standing in sombre silence, were the Guardians of the Forest. Their hooded robes flowing softly to the ground as they stood together paying homage to a once and beautiful forest. The scene caused us to stop, drawing us in to the sacred circle. We stood in silence amongst them, feeling the need to pay respect. The only sound a faint rustle of burnt leaves moving in the breeze across the ground where they had fallen. Slowly we left and we did not look back. We ran on in silence, there was nothing to say....The road went ever on, through the blackened forest until eventually green grass replaced the bare ground and the sunlight played on the trees, lighting up the lush canopy in shards of silver and green. The tree trunks white and red with life, standing tall amongst the vibrant undergrowth, shrubs bursting into flowers, yellow, pink, white and red...and below the trees, the Guardians appeared to be dancing, their robes swaying outward with flair, their hoods bouncing on their shoulders, their joyful laughter mingling with the music of the brightly coloured birds that flew amongst them. The scene caused us to stop, to reflect on nature's lessons and how crucial it is for us to protect the land and all that share it....*

A day of reflection and delight as we ran through the forests alive with the Guardian's sculptured homes, the most special termite mounds we have seen so far...

Finished at 42.27 km in a Cattle Ranch driveway were Rose & Narelle had set up camp.

We had just finished dinner and were ready to have an early night when a truck came down the driveway, red dust swirling around the tires as it approached the gate that we were parked in front of. We all rushed to move the vehicles but the kind rancher said, "No worries, I can drive past you," and promptly did so, a few inches from the caravan. He stopped and said that he had seen us on the road several times, so we told him about RunRaw2013 and he said he would go on the website and make a donation. Thank you for your support and for the safe campsite for the night. Temp 21-33.3 degrees. Total 5719.44.

Marathon #134.

May 14, 2013. 18 km south of Dunmarra to Truck Stop 25 km north of Dunmarra. Started at 4:55am in the dark, cloudy so no starlight, ran for an hour by the light of a flashlight. Narelle & Rose arrived at sunrise which we all watched together, a golden ball rising into red tinged clouds. Stopped at Dunmarra to fuel up the vehicles and take on water in the tanks and air in the tires. Met a beautiful Brahman cow who had obviously been raised from a calf as she was very friendly and curious about our water bottles. Janette gave her a drink of water from her bottle and she gave Janette a big kiss with her tongue! She was so gentle, her nose so soft, her eye so bright. A precious sentient being. Running on, I could still feel her soft touch on my hand and I felt blessed....Finished the run 43.59km at a truck stop called Dingo Hill, tucked away in a corner away from the road (truck) trains also stopped for the night, each with 3 trailers, 80 wheels, 55 metres long, 2 tiers high loaded with precious sentient beings, standing in the dark, waiting..... *Look into the eye of a sentient being and you look through the window to their soul...* Temp 17-31.5 degrees. Total Km 5763.03.

Marathon #135.

May 15, 2013. 25 km north of Dunmarra to Truck Stop 28 km north of Daly Waters. Janette awoke feeling nauseous and weary. Started running at 5am in the dark, but she was having trouble keeping going, just wanted to lie down on the road and go to sleep, lucky there was no traffic! When Narelle & Rose arrived at 7am we decided to take a long break, Janette had a carrot & beet juice and slept for an hour, then we set off again. Stopped at the Daly Waters

Hwy Inn where the staff gave a generous donation, thank you for your support. Took another long break at Daly Waters 7 km further on, Janette had another freshly made juice and a power nap while Alan and Rose met the locals at the Daly Waters Historic Pub, the owner giving a generous donation and a couple having lunch in the pub also gave a donation. Thank you all for your support. Narelle visited the local museum and gallery and they offered for us to use their phone and internet connection, but it was time to move on as we were already well behind time for the day. Continued on, Janette running slower than usual but feeling slightly better with each juice and sleep. Finished 42.68km very late at 8pm, running in the dark by the light of the crescent moon for the last hour, listening to the wild dingoes howl, the cattle lowing and the bats flapping around our heads. Narelle drove a few kilometres ahead of us so we had backup if needed while Rose went ahead to set up camp in a truck stop before it got too dark. More fresh juice for Janette and fresh tomatoes for dinner before turning in around 9pm. Temp 18-34 degrees. Total Km 5807.71.

Marathon #136.

May 16, 2013. 28 km north of Daly Waters to Farm Gate 18 km south of Larrimah. Narelle drove us back 1.4km to where we had finished last night. Started 5am by the light of the stars, the Southern Cross resting on the horizon now that we are 15 degrees south of the equator. Dingoes howling in the distance in all directions, odd because there is no moon, but a hauntingly beautiful sound. Another magical daybreak and sunrise. Janette back on form running well with only slight swelling to the knee. First break at 15km, had only run 100 metres into the second leg when Alan had severe stomach pains which brought him to his knees vomiting. He tried to go on but the pain had him doubled over. Back into the caravan and onto his bed, couldn't think of the cause as we all eat and live the same and the rest of us are fine, so Alan had half a glass of water with half teaspoon of bicarb soda in it, went to sleep for a couple of hours and woke up with no pain and no after effects. Back on the road 4 hours behind schedule, but taking it easy marveling at the amazing termite sculptures alongside the road. Narelle stayed with us again while Rose went ahead to find a good camping spot and we finished 42.43km in the dark at 7:30pm. Met a couple on the side of the road with their vehicle broken down, waiting for the tow truck. Narelle had told them to watch out for us and when we came by they gave us a donation and wished us well. Thank you Brian and Dagmar for your support, we look forward to catching up with you in Tassie. Temp 18-32.5 degrees. Total Km 5850.14.

Marathon #137.

May 17, 2013. Farm Gateway 18 km south of Larrimah to Wubalawun Station Gateway 55km Sth of Mataranka. Narelle drove us back 5 km to where we finished last night and we started 5am in the dark, no moon. Janette running slower, Alan back in full form. Running through changing terrain, more trees and still more termite mounds. Met Anne & Eric on the road when they stopped to fix their caravan window who gave us a donation. Stopped outside Larrimah Pink Panther Pub for midway break, visiting their animal sanctuary with many birds, snakes and a very large crocodile. All had been rescued or injured and now being cared for out the back of the Pub. Talked to many people who had also stopped there, including Pete and Donald who gave us donations. Thanks everyone for your support. Late leaving with 21 km to go, slow going as Janette feeling weary, finished 42.83 km at dusk just past the spot where Rose had set up camp. Narelle picked us up and drove us back. Another long day, and another marathon completed. Temp 22-35.5 degrees. Total Km 5892.97.

Marathon #138.

May 18, 2013. Wubalawun Station Gate to 10 km south of Mataranka. Rose drove us back to where we had finished last night, started 5am, very dark, moon had set and low clouds covered the stars. Running by torchlight until daybreak. Long straight road with tall trees and lots of termite mounds in many shapes and sizes, some resembling people and others looking like cathedrals with intricate spires. Both still running a bit slow but otherwise ok. Did long first and second legs to 29 km for midway break after which Rose drove off to Mataranka to shop for fresh fruit and veg, get set up at the campground and do the laundry. Narelle stayed with us for another break of oranges on the road then met us at the finish 43 km and drove to the campground. We all had half a watermelon that Rose had bought, then walked through the bush to the natural springs for a soak in the warm thermal water. What a treat! We all floated downstream with the current as the sunset on a great end to another day and another marathon.....Total Km 5935.97.

Eileen here...and they're off! The internet that is....till Tuesday... So it's just you and me again, but I have a shout out to DARWIN. We want to make a BIG DEAL of Janette and Alan's arrival there because I'm sure you'll agree these last few weeks have been super tough. The lovely Martin at Eat At Martins has agreed to open for DINNER from 6pm on Wednesday 29th for a special Meet, Greet and Eat with Alan and Janette. They'll do a bit of a talk on their travels to date and enjoy a meal with you. Martin is doing his regular a la carte for the non raw foodies but is happy to accommodate you if you are fully raw. He is generously donating 25% of the evening to RUN RAW and we encourage you to go along too and support this fantastic cause. PLEASE get behind this Darwin and share and invite friends, Martin has plenty of room! Please RSVP to him, see details on link. Janette and Alan will arrive into Darwin on May 28 and depart on the 30th. They'll be running in and around the area on Wednesday.

Marathon #139.

May 19, 2013. 10 km south of Mataranka to 2.2 km north Sturt Downs Station Gateway. Narelle drove us back 10 km to where we had finished yesterday. Started 5am, a nice run in the dark downhill to Mataranka, through the town while everyone slept, looking at the statues depicting characters from the book "We of the Never Never" which was written about this area. Out of town on the long straight undulating road, termite mounds abounding on either side of the road keeping us entertained as the temperature and humidity rose. Stopped for a 2 hour internet and phone break before heading out into the unconnected world again. Saw a fox run across the road in front of us, flocks of birds in the trees and flying overhead including the red tailed black cockatoos, several small wallabies hopping along and 2 wild boar who had not made it across the road. Last 8 km very hot and slow finishing 42.5 km as the sun went down. Narelle picked us up and drove 2.2 km forward to where Rose had set up camp outside the gates to Sturt Downs Station. Temp 26-36 degrees. Total Km 5978.47. Tomorrow we break 6000 km, stay tuned!

Marathon # 140.

May 20, 2013. 2.2km Nth of Sturt Downs Station to Cutta Cutta Caves 28 km south of Katherine. Rose drove us back to where we finished last night and we started at 4:45am, very dark with no moon. Heard the blue winged Northern Kookaburra but couldn't see them. First break had delicious smoothies made with dehydrated bananas as we're out of fresh until we reach Katherine tomorrow. Hot and humid again, Narelle checked on us every 4 km with water and dates to keep us going between breaks. Found a wild hibiscus with rosellas all over it, Narelle picked a bowl full for us to add to our salads, first bush tucker we've found that we recognise enough to eat. (Has a delicious bitter lemon flavour similar to sorrel). Finished the run 42.92 km in the heat a kilometre past the Cutta Cutta Caves Entrance where Rose had set up camp for the night. Narelle was waiting for us on the road and was talking with Chris from Katherine who had stopped to find out why we were running as she had seen us when she drove past earlier. Great to meet you Chris, we look forward to seeing you again when we come back through Katherine next week. Temp 22-36 degrees. Total Km 6021.39.

Marathon #141.

May 21, 2013. Cutta Cutta Caves to 10 km north of Katherine. Started 5am in the dark, good running and nice daybreak and sunrise. Had one break for green smoothies before running into Katherine where Rose & Narelle were shopping for fresh fruit & veg. Called in to the Police Station to refill our water bottles as it was getting very hot and humid with 2km to go. Had a good chat with the Police and they said they would look out for us on the road. We had our 2nd break in Katherine then met up with Tamara, the journalist for the Katherine Times for an interview in the park, took photos then ran on to finish 42.27 km. Made a special dessert for Rose & Narelle's last night with us. Temp 22-37.5 degrees. Total Km 6083.66.

Marathon #142.

May 22, 2013. 10 km to 52 km north of Katherine. Started in the dark at 4:45am, cloudy daybreak and sunrise. Very humid and getting hot. An emotional last day with us for Rose & Narelle, thanks to both of you for everything you have done for us during the past 4 weeks as support crew and for your friendship and love, so much appreciated. Our friends Myke & Melissa arrived mid morning to join us as support crew for the rest of the trip. We left to continue the run with Rose & Narelle showing Myke & Melissa the ropes then all leaving in convoy to join us for the next break, Rose & Narelle driving on to Darwin to fly home. Rest of the day went smoothly with Myke & Melissa finding good spots to stop and to camp for the night. Last 10 km became very hot and humid, finally breaking with a downpour of rain amid thunder and lightening. Very refreshing to run in the rain, haven't had rain for a month and a half. Finished 43.12 km. Temp 27-35 degrees. Total Km 6126.78.

Marathon #143.

May 23, 2013. 52 km Nth of Katherine to 7 km north of Pine Creek. Started 5am in the dark, rained throughout the night, cloudy daybreak and sunrise. Melissa caught us up at 8 km, Myke not far behind, cameras rolling as he passed us. Let the video footage begin! More traffic than usual on the road this morning, must be getting closer to Darwin. M & M found great spots to stop for breaks, made yummy green smoothies and a delicious salad for midway break. Ran into Pine Creek, met by Melissa on the side of the road outside the Pine Creek caravan park where she and Myke had set up camp in a complimentary site (thank you for your support). She had water, bananas and dates for us so we could continue running on to finish 7km past Pine Creek, while she and Myke got all the laundry done and made beet juice and zucchini noodle dinner. Finished at 42.57 km, Melissa picked us up and drove back to Pine Creek for showers, dinner and internet updates. Temp 26-36 degrees. Total Km 6169.35.

Marathon #144.

May 24, 2013. 7 km north of Pine Creek to 5 km south of Hayes Creek. Melissa drove us 7.9 km forward to where we finished yesterday, started 5am by the light of the moon. Cool morning, dry with much less humidity, much easier running, but still rough rocky road so hard underfoot. First break at 16 km, yummy green smoothies made with oranges, bananas, dates and silver-beet, then second leg to 30 km. Great tasting locally grown watermelon and a delicious salad of wombok, carrot, beetroot, tomatoes and cucumber. With only 12 km to go, the terrain changed quite dramatically to a more tropical look, hills covered with palm trees and bamboo growing amongst the gum trees and the termite mounds now huge, looking like tall cathedrals dotted through the landscape. Melissa ran out to meet us and we ran the last few km together to where Myke had set up camp in a secluded spot off the road. Finished 42.8 km and had fresh juice of carrot, beet, apple, ginger and silver-beet stalks. Delicious chia pudding with fresh fruit salad for dinner and bed at 8pm. Temp 25-32 degrees. Total Km 6212.23.

Marathon #145.
May 25, 2013. 5 km south of Hayes Creek to 17 km south of Adelaide River, NT. Started 5am running by moonlight, watching as the moon set in the West and the sun rose in the East. Cool morning, light dew on the ground and a dry wind. Rough and rocky road with very little edge for us to run on for most of the day, so had to move right off the road into the gravel or grass and wait while the traffic passed. Many huge termite mounds along the side of the road, some at least 6m tall and 3m in diameter. Finished the run 42.4 km where Myke had set up camp on the side of the road. We were just about to have dinner when a car stopped and 4 guys came over saying they were from Victoria and had seen us on TV back in January when we started and thought they might see us as they set out on their fishing trip together. They were staying on a cattle ranch nearby and were very interested to hear how we were running a marathon a day while eating raw vegan food. We showed them the bowl of fruit salad that Melissa had freshly made and told them that we were having it for dinner. They said, "But you can't run a marathon on that, can you?" We said, "Well, we just finished marathon #145," and they said, "that has got us thinking!" So, happy thoughts Greg, Grant, Geoff and Alan and thank you very much for your generous donation. Temp 18-31 degrees. Total Km 6254.61.

Marathon #146.
May 26, 2013. 17 km south of Adelaide River to Coomalie Rest Stop 25 km north of Adelaide River. Started 4:50am with a full moon lighting the way, no traffic for the first hour so ran down the middle of the road listening to the dingoes howling in the distance. Felt much cooler this morning, maybe winter has come at last! Stayed relatively cool all day although

sunny with a following wind, near perfect conditions. Delicious green smoothie at the 15 km first break then on 3 km to the small town of Adelaide River to fuel the SuperRoo and take on water from the Fire Station. There was a small craft market in the park so we stopped to chat with the people there, one dear lady who had a stall with handmade crocheted items, gave us a donation. Thank you for your kindness and support. Had telephone reception so phoned our son, daughter-in-law and grandkids to check in on how things are at home. All well as they eagerly await the birth of another precious little one, due to arrive within the next week or so. It's hard to be so far away at such a special time. Finished the last 5km at 43.87km, thinking of all our loved ones near and far, sending hugs with every step. Myke and Melissa had set up camp in a roadside rest area, a pretty spot with a stream running alongside. We sat on the edge and soaked our feet in the cold water until the sun set behind the trees. Met a gentle husky dog sitting by the campfire who happily gave us a kiss as we went by. Back to the van for another delicious dinner of pumpkin fettucine and salad, then off to bed to the soothing sound of the stream. Temp 18-32.8 degrees. Total Km 6298.48.

Marathon #147.

May 27, 2013. Coomalie Rest Stop to Strauss WW11 Airfield 44 km south of Darwin. Started 5am by the moon. Road very rough and rocky, virtually no shoulder with a jagged drop off onto gravel with large pointy stones, making it very difficult running. A lot of traffic both ways, mostly driving very fast and close to the edge on our side. Janette was moving off when she tripped on the edge and fell onto the gravel, banging up all the old wounds that had just healed- right ankle, knee, elbow and shoulder. Really not liking that split second moment of the road coming up to meet me and knowing this is going to hurt! Dusted off and ran on slowly until Melissa & Myke caught up with us, cleaned up and iced the knee. Continued on to first break, had green smoothies, iced knee again and applied fresh aloe vera to the wounds. Esther and Michael from ZDF TV Germany arrived to film us on the run. With Esther driving their car and Michael aiming the camera out the back, we ran behind them for a few km, then caught up at the second break for more filming and interviews. Finished the run at 42.44km at WW11 Airfield site, Melissa had delicious fresh juice ready for us and Myke set up camp amongst the trees off the road. Early dinner of beetroot salad and marinated mushrooms, then an early night as we'll be running into Darwin tomorrow with more filming and interviews on the way. Temp 18-33 degrees. Total Km 6340.92.

Marathon #148.

May 28, 2013. Strauss WW11 Airfield to Darwin. Michael and Esther from ZDF TV arrived at our camp 4:45am to film us getting ready to go and for a few kilometres along the Hwy. Started 5am in dark, moonlight enough to see by and lights on the hwy as we got closer to Darwin. Finished 42.69km, 5 km from the info centre downtown Darwin. Myke drove us in to where Melissa waited in the caravan parked near the Esplanade. ZDF TV crew there to say goodbye and good luck. Footage will be aired next week in Germany and internationally. Drove out to Nightcliff to stay at friend Terry's place near the beach. Met up with Tony from Ireland who is running around the world and his crew Michael, also staying with Terry. Chatting into the evening, swapping road tales, we discovered that the orange and apple we had found on the roadside a few weeks ago had been left by Michael for Tony the night before. So how great was that! Into the pool for a cool down before going to bed, watching the bats flying around the palms and feeling relaxed now that we've made it to the Top. A great feeling to know that when we leave Darwin, we'll be heading for home. Temp 23-36 degrees. Total Km 6383.65.

Marathon #149.

May 29, 2013. Darwin, NT. Started at 6am running with Terry and friend Beth along the trails around Nightcliff. Back to van for a green smoothie 8am then drove into the city to pick up Janette's books at the Post Office. How exciting to see it in print! Continued run along the esplanade until 2pm when we met up with Lorella from ABC Radio for a live interview on air. Picked up the local newspapers Darwin Sun and NT News with articles in about our arriving in Darwin. Drove back out to Nightcliff, continued the run along the beach trails until it was time to go to our dinner speaking event at 'Eat at Martins' Restaurant. Great turnout of around 70 people, enjoyed a delicious raw meal prepared by Martin and his kitchen crew then spoke for an hour. Wonderful to meet everyone and best wishes to you all on your own journeys through life. Many thanks to Martin for your support, generosity, hospitality and donation. Totally recommend everyone in Darwin to get on down to Eat at Martins to experience Martin's great menu and delightful hospitality. Combined the dinner evening with Janette's book launch and the first 11 books went into Darwin homes. Finished the run 42.69 km after the evening at Martin's Restaurant, drove back to Nightcliff and ran along the beach trails under the lamplight. A great day, thanks Darwin for your support.

Marathon #150.

May 30, 2013. Darwin, NT. Started at 6am running under the street lights to the beach and along the trails following the cliff edge and down along the beach. No-one around so we made the first footprints on the sand, apart from the birds and crabs of course. Very picturesque coves with brilliant blue water lapping on the white sand. First time we've seen the Timor Sea. Ran back to the van for a green smoothie then drove to city and ran the Esplanade in between doing some shopping, posting mail and doing interviews. Many people recognised us from the newspaper article yesterday as we ran through the city streets and called out or stopped us to chat. Left the city and drove out to Mindel Beach, stopped for an hour to take in the market on the beach. Great market with entertainment, so Janette drove out to pick up Myke and Melissa and bring them back to enjoy the fun, just in time for sunset at the beach. Finally got back at around 9pm and ran down to the beach trail to finish the run at 42.41 km. Another world record milestone - 150 consecutive marathons completed. Temp 20-32 degrees. Total Km 6468.85.

Marathon #151.

May 31, 2013. Darwin, N.T. Started at 6am down to the beach trails out to Lee Point, the Northernmost point that we will go on the Run Around Australia. 12.20 degrees latitude. Last 4 km going out went through tropical rainforest with old bunkers from World War 2 standing stark amongst the green vines. Ran back to van for first break at 20 km, had green smoothie and then drove to the beach with our banner to take photos for Marathon #150. Back to the van and the computer to upload the daily blogs and pics. Continued the run around the neighbourhood and on the beach trails. Back to the van again to be there while the brakes and tires were checked and serviced, all good and ready to roll. Onto the road again for the last 8 km along the beach trail at sunset amidst families having picnics and watching the sun sink into the sea. Finished 42.26km, another beautiful day in Paradise…Temp 20-28 degrees. Total Km 6511.11.

June 2013

MARATHON #152-181

Marathon #152. June 1, 2013. Darwin, N.T. Terry invited us to run with him this morning so we drove to Parap Village where there will be a Market and started our run from there at 6am. Terry took us along the trails to East Point, down past the Botanical Gardens and back to the Market, where we stopped for some papaya and jackfruit and some fresh juice. Bought some papaya, passionfruit, avocado, spinach and basil, which Terry took back in the car while we continued on the run. Stopped at Martin's Restaurant for a fresh juice and a last chat with Martin as we will be leaving Darwin tomorrow. It's been great to meet so many Darwin folks, especially Martin and his Team at his restaurant, 'Eat at Martin's'. If you haven't already experienced the hospitality and friendly atmosphere there, as well as Martin's passion for creating delicious vegan food, you are in for a treat when you go. Thank you Martin for your support and friendship, we will keep in touch. Continued on with the run back to the van where Melissa had made a yummy Thai salad. Eating outside on the patio beside the pool with a gentle breeze keeping us cool, it was hard to get up and finish the run, but we did. Down to the beach and along the coast trail, the sea breeze blowing in our faces as the sunset coloured the sky a brilliant red. Finished the run at 44.63 km back at Terry's house. Myke and Melissa had been to the local 'Fresh Produce Market' and bought a variety of fruits and veg for the next part of our trip to Western Australia. Melissa was making zucchini spaghetti with basil and spinach sauce and Alan started preparing a tropical fruit salad of banana, passionfruit, pineapple, red dragonfruit, papaya, orange, ginger, poppy and sesame seeds. Now it's time to cool off in the pool before sharing dinner with our host and friend Terry, who has made us feel at home in his Darwin home, thank you Terry, it's been a wonderful few days here in Darwin before we hit the road again tomorrow. Temp 19-29 degrees. Total Km 6555.74.

Marathon #153.

June 2, 2013. Darwin, N.T. Started from Terry's place 5am and ran up and down the Nightcliff coast trails until 7:30am then up to Rapid Creek Market for a fresh juice, great produce market to stock up on fruit and greens. Continued running the coast trails and going back to the van for water and fruit until finished the run at 45.38 km, did a few extra kms to meet up and chat with Darwin folks along the way. Lovely to meet you all, thanks for your support (and the yummy watermelon juice and persimmons!) Back to the van where Melissa had fresh juice made and everything ready for us to leave. Had a last dip in the pool, said goodbye to Terry and drove out, leaving Darwin and heading back along the Stuart Hwy towards Katherine where we will resume our Run towards Western Australia. Stopped in Adelaide River for the night, camped at the showgrounds, ready for tomorrow's run to Robin Falls. A long day and into a long night getting there and settled in, Wrote the details down in our log from the Garmin Watch, then accidentally wiped off all the Data for the day before saving it for uploading! Written Data 45.38km, Running time 6hr 45min, Average Pace 9.00. Temp 22-32 degrees. Total Km 6601.32.

Marathon #154.

June 3, 2013. Adelaide River to Robin Falls on Dorat Rd and back to Stuart Hwy. Started at 6am at daybreak running down Dorat Rd towards Robin Falls. So good to be on a small country road with hills instead of running back on the rocky Stuart Hwy. No traffic except a few tourists when we got to the trail for Robin Falls. Ran in to meet up with Myke and Melissa who had driven ahead with green smoothies and fresh pawpaw. We all hiked in on the trail to see the falls, very pretty although not much water. We ran out and back uphill on Dorat Rd to the van while M & M drove back and got everything ready to leave. Stopped for our second break at 28 km, Melissa had made a delicious Thai salad with fresh greens from yesterdays market. We continued the run back on the Stuart Hwy, heading south for the first time, with a strong head wind but a good pace of 7.51. Felt well rested from the Darwin break, even though we have run 44, 45 and 44 km on the last 3 days. Only had 16 km to finish so ran in two 8 km legs, Melissa staying with us for water the first water break and to pick us up at the finish. Myke drove on with the van to set up camp in Katherine. Finished the run 42.92 km at a spot where we had seen the tallest termite mound when we were running up to Darwin. Saw a young dingo running amongst the termite mounds while we were there, then we piled into the SuperRoo and drove to Katherine. Interesting driving the road that took us 7 days to run, seems an awful long way! Good to be back at our point of resuming the run from Katherine towards Western Australia, one day here and we'll be on the road heading south west. Thanks to the Riverside Campground for your support and a great place to stop for two nights. Temp 22-32 degrees. Total Kms 6646.24.

Comments from Facebook/RunningRawAroundAustralia2013:

- *J&A!! You both are going well! Keep it up. Your green smoothies have been a real hit in our family!* - **Monique**
- *I love following your updates well done, keep juicing and carry on!* - **Ashlee**
- *Great run! Well done both.* - **Sandy**
- *Keep up the brilliant job you two at doing.* - **Dianne Marathon #155.**

Marathon #155.

June 4, 2013. Katherine, N.T. Started 5am in the dark running under the street lights from the campground to the town centre. A cool morning (17 degrees, but reaching 37 degrees mid afternoon). Ran around the town then out on the road towards Katherine Gorge to the historic Knotts Crossing on the Katherine River. Back into town along the bike trail and out to the camp-ground for our first break at 17 km. Melissa had made green smoothies which were delicious with the fresh market greens. Back out on the bike trails around Katherine and the small roads through the town, eventually finishing the run along the river trail to the hot springs near the campground at 42.43 km. Myke and Melissa drove out to see the Katherine Gorge while we ran around in circles all day! They picked up 4 boxes of bananas from the local plantation and stocked up at the store with enough fresh fruit and veg for 12 days until we get to the border of Western Australia, as we're not allowed to take any fresh produce through. We all walked down the river trail to the hot springs behind the campgrounds and spent an hour soaking in the mineral rich waters before coming back for another of Melissa's delicious salads. Tomorrow we're off on the next adventure, heading west on the Victoria Hwy towards Broome, and so, the next chapter begins....Total Km 6688.67.

Marathon #156.

June 5, 2013. Katherine to 45 km west of Katherine on the Victoria Hwy. Started at 5:20am heading west on the Victoria Hwy by the street lights for an hour until daybreak. Very little traffic on the road, good smooth surface but very pronounced steep camber which made our feet ache after running on the flat trails around Darwin. Ran on the other side of the road whenever it was safe to compensate for the camber. Melissa caught up with us at 7 km to give us water then we continued to the first break at 17 km for green smoothies. The landscape seems different, more trees and long grass with fewer termite mounds, more hills, but still the long straights. Had about 20 cyclists pass us early on, they were in the group cycling around Australia and thought it was a bit extreme for us to be running around Australia! Midway stop at a rest area where Myke filled the water tanks from the rainwater tank there. Met two couples traveling in their campers, thank you for your support and the donation Brian. Finished the last 15 km in 2 legs of 8 km and 7 km, hard going and painstakingly slow in the heat. Myke and Melissa had found a good spot off the road at exactly 42.24 km. Melissa had made a fresh juice of carrot, beet, apple and ginger which revived us immediately. Soaked our feet in ice cold water with epsom salts, had a delicious pawpaw, banana, lime and ginger smoothie for dinner and heading off to bed for an early night as the sun sets at 6:30pm. Temp 17-37 degrees. Total Km 6730.91.

Marathon #157.

June 6, 2013. Remembering our dear Grandma on the anniversary of her birthday and sending love to our son and daughter-in-law for the imminent birth of their third child and our 5th grandchild, thinking of you every step. 45 km west of Katherine on the Victoria Hwy to Farm Gate between Scott's Creek and Willeroo. Started at 5am in the dark, the crescent moon rising in the East behind us. No traffic for the first two hours, silently running by starlight down the middle of the road. Met Jan from Melbourne cycling around Australia and later her husband support crew. See you both December 31 when we come in to Melbourne! First break at 15 km for green smoothies, second break at 30 km for delicious green salad, 3rd break at 35km for oranges, then finished the run at 42.96 km at a farm gate off the road. Melissa had made fresh juice and zucchini noodles with tomato chili sauce for dinner, yum! We're heading for an early night again, hopefully in bed by 7pm, after we've moved the swarm of bees that are all around the caravan searching for water, Myke is on the job giving them water further away so they wont come in when we open the door. Meanwhile off to sleep to the lulling sound of buzzing...buzz, buzz, buzz, I wonder why he does.....Temp 27-34 degrees. Total Km 6773.87.

Marathon #158.

June 7, 2013. Farm Gate between Scott's Creek and Willeroo to 52 km NE of Victoria River on the Victoria Hwy. Started at 4:50am in the dark, smaller crescent moon rising behind us. No traffic again for the first 2 hours, no sound, no-one knows we're out here, running into another day on the road. Daybreak brings the morning chorus of birdsong, and the distant hum of an approaching road train. By the time we got to 11 km at the first break in a roadside rest stop, we had only had three trucks and four cars pass us. However, there were 20 campers and caravans at the rest stop, everyone just starting to get up, have breakfast and pack up ready to leave. We had our green smoothies while Melissa and Myke filled up with water from the raintank, then back on the road for a 17km leg with all the campers and caravaners tooting and waving as they passed us. After they had gone it was back to a quiet road, a few cattle grazing by the side of the road running off into the bush when they saw us. At the last break we met Dennis and Lynette, the Indigenous Schools Supervisor for the District, who invited us to visit two of the schools that are on our way, so looking forward to that in a few days. Temp went from 25 to 36 degrees from the start to the finish of the run, last 12 km being slow in the heat. Finished the run at 42.32km where Myke and Melissa had set up camp by the side of the road. Had a fresh juice of beetroot, apple, kiwifruit, green stalks, lemon and ginger and half an avocado each (we're on rations to the border, making sure we have eaten all the fresh fruit, veg, nuts & seeds by the time we get there as we cannot take them into Western

Australia). For dinner we're having chia pudding with apple, kiwifruit, bananas (fresh and dehydrated), sultanas, nutmeg, cinnamon, almond pulp and fresh almond cream, yum! Then off to bed at sunset for another early night, sending sweet dreams to our little family as we eagerly await news of another grandchild's arrival due yesterday, but we have no phone or internet for 2 more days, so every step we take will bring us closer to news of the little one.... Total Km 6816.19.

Marathon # 159.

June 8, 2013. 52 km NE of Victoria River to 17 km east of Victoria River on the Victoria Hwy. Started 5am after drinking a smoothie of 22 bananas, 2 grapefruit and 6 dates. All our bananas (4 boxes) have ripened at once so it's banana bonanza time! First stop at 15 km had a green smoothie with bananas, oranges and a variety of greens. Ran on up hills to 30 km second break had half rock-melon each and another of Melissa's delicious green salads with curry dressing. Landscape changed to high cliffs with flat tops and red rocky outcrops on either side of the road coming into Victoria River Crossing. Very warm and humid for the last 12 km, finished at 43.35 km and Melissa drove us into Victoria River Crossing Campground where Myke had set up on a complimentary site, thanks Roy & Theresa at the Victoria River Roadhouse for your support and hospitality. No phone or internet coverage but a public phone so phoned home to see if there was any news of our grandbaby's arrival, but no answers, so hope they're either asleep or otherwise occupied!

Met most of the campers there including a couple cycling from Perth to Darwin, thanks for the donation Peter. Laundry done, long hot showers all round, dinner and bed. Temp 25-36 degrees. Total Km 6859.64.

Marathon # 160.

June 9, 2013. 17 km east of Victoria River to 60 km east of Timber Creek on the Victoria Hwy. Made a 22 banana, 2 grapefruit & 6 date smoothie to drink while Melissa drove us out to where we finished yesterday at 1km. She dropped off water bottles and a bag of dates and bananas at the 12 km mark. Started 5am in the dark, no traffic running down the middle of the road by starlight. Southern Cross already set, still not far enough south yet! Approaching the 12 km mark just after daybreak, we could see something moving by the dropbag and bottles under the sign, then as we got closer we realised it was a dingo. It must have sensed us because it ran across the road, stopped then ran back again and disappeared into the long grass beside the sign. We got there to find that he had chewed through the bag and eaten part of a banana, no doubt would have eaten the lot if we had not come along right then. We left his banana on a rock for him to come and get once we were gone as we're sure he was watching from the grass. Continued on as the sun rose changing colours on the rock escarpments around us. Stopped on the Victoria River bridge and saw a crocodile in the river, our first croc in the wild, took lots of photos of course! Called in to the Roadhouse to phone home again, but no baby yet. Had a chat with Tom, Lydia and baby Adelaide from Kununara (thanks for the baby cuddles Adelaide!) and Aunty Lou all on holiday in the area, hope to see you again when we get to Kununara. Continued the run through dramatic landscape of red rocky escarpments on either side of the road and the river winding it's way through the gorge. Stopped with Melissa to take photos of our first boab tree, very unusual shape. The rest of the day was hot and humid again, temp 27-36 degrees, making for a slow finish at 43.29 km. Camped alongside the road. Total Km 6902.93.

Marathon #161.

June 10, 2013. 60 km east of Timber Creek to Roadside stop 23 km east of Timber Creek on Victoria Hwy. Had our usual banana & grapefruit smoothie before starting at 5am in the dark. No moon, no traffic, no sound, a quiet 2 hour run before daybreak. No colour in the sunrise and no clouds in the sky, promise of another hot day.

Yummy green smoothies at the first break at 14.5km and delicious salad with the last of our fresh salad greens at 29 km for the second break. Landscape changed again with the escarpments further off in the distance and small rocky hills by the road. Met Lynette & Dennis on the road again and confirmed arrangements for going to the schools at Timber Creek tomorrow and Bulla Camp in a couple of days. Turned hot and humid again (temp 27-36 degrees), finished at 42.41 km at roadside camping spot where Myke and Melissa had set up, made fresh juice of beets, oranges, apples, greens & ginger and a fruit salad for dinner with bananas, kiwifruit, oranges, pineapple, grapefruit, ginger, chia and poppy seeds, cinnamon and dates. Brilliant red sunset with a crescent moon and Venus aligned. Total Km 6955.34.

Marathon #162.

June 11, 2013. 23 km east of Timber Creek to 21 km west of Timber Creek. Started at 5am in the dark to the sound of dingoes howling in the distance and others close by returning their call, a haunting yet plaintive sound. Are they letting each other know where we are? We call to them, but do not see them and their cries abate, leaving the only sound we hear as that of our own footsteps on the road. No traffic as we run silently along, following the stars and listening for the first call of the crows to signal the break of day. A gentle breeze wafts across the road, first one way then the other, first cool then warm, bringing with it the musty smell of hickory smoke and then it was gone. The darkness softens around us and a faint glow in the eastern sky fades the brightness of the stars, the constellation of Scorpio slowly sinking in the west and the crows call, heralding another day on the road...Stopped for our first break of smoothies 5 km before Timber Creek, then continued in to the small town, immediately phoning home for news of our little grandchild's birth, but no baby yet. Spent a couple of hours on the internet catching up with emails and updating the Website and Facebook page. Then we all drove down to the Timber Creek School to visit with the kids, great fun to talk with them and answer their questions. Also met the folks from Indigenous Hip Hop Projects who were also at the school on project. Departed at 3:45pm with 21 km to go, easy run into the sunset with the moon and Venus setting, a beautiful evening running alongside the Victoria River in the twilight and the darkness bringing a full starry night sky. Finished the run at 42.89 km (46.89 km with 4 extra km when we did not turn the Garmin off while driving to the school). Fresh juice, carrot, beet, apple, lemon, ginger) and an avocado when we arrived, then banana chia pudding with fresh almond creme for dinner. A long day from morning till night, but a good one, especially the visit to Timber Creek School and all the while thinking of our little one due to arrive anytime... Temp 18-36 degrees. Total Km 6998.23.

Marathon # 163.

June 12, 2013. 21 km west of Timber Creek to Baine Picnic Area 57 km west of Timber Creek. Started at 6:30am at daybreak after checking the food supply and deciding that we needed to buy more to get us to the WA border. Melissa drove back to Timber Creek to buy out the small 'supermarket' of their oranges, bananas, avos and greens. She arrived back in time for the first water stop and drove on to meet Myke and make smoothies for our first break. Another hot day on the road 18-38 degrees, really glad we came here in the winter! Several travelers stopped to ask if we were OK or needed water, most wondering what we were doing running in the heat, but some had heard about us and wanted to take photos and ask questions. One couple stopped to take photos and we chatted for a while, Thanks Val and Darryl for your kind donation and for the veg before you go through the border! Continued running through interesting landscape of red rocky escarpments, yellow grass Savannah and bizarre shaped boab trees. Stopped at Bulla Community too late to see the kids at school, but chatted for a while with some folks who gave us their spring water when they heard that we were running around Australia. We gave them a RunRAW2013 flyer and they commented " that must be an old photo, you are much more healthy and fit now!" That was nice to hear! Stopped for third break after running through the 7000 km mark, wrote up the banner and took some photos, then continued on into the sunset for the last 6 km to finish at 7:15pm, 42.84 km. Melissa came to pick us up and drive back to the picnic area where Myke had set up camp for the night. Another long day, but finally made it past 7000 km! Total Km 7041.07 wahoo! Still no phone or internet so no baby news, but we're sure the little one has arrived...

Oh Janette and Alan life is so dull without you! Is there a new Grandbaby yet? Hopefully, Kaje managed to get a call through to you in the middle of 'somewhere'! Well, I am turning my back on winter and hopping a flight to Istanbul in the morning, I'll check in from time to time and I am armed with Run Raw flyers to leave surreptitiously around Europe - if you find one, drop us a note on Facebook! MEANWHILE, please keep up the momentum for me, if you have any media contacts, give them a wee nudge, if you have groups you can share the story with, share away, between now and Perth (early September) it would be good to get some hype happening to celebrate the HALF WAY milestone! See you in a few weeks! Eileen

 Hello from Western Australia! We came across the border yesterday (Sat 15), still out of internet and phone range until arriving in Kununurra today. First news we heard was that our fifth little grandchild arrived last Tues 11 and she's very cute, of course! We made it to the sixth State - VIC, NSW, ACT, QLD, NT and now WA...and we're almost half way round, past 7000 km and just finished Marathon #167. Now it's late and we'll post updates and pics and catch up on emails tomorrow.

Comments from Facebook/RunningRawAroundAustralia2013:

- *Congratulations! Both my thumbs up for you!* - **Petra**
- *Legends ....Well done wow, what an inspiration you have on us in Oz. Sweet dreams and a well earned rest.* - **Bell xxx**
- *Amazing stuff guys!* - **Bradley**
- *Congratulations and welcome to WA!* - **Melanie**
- *Welcome to WA* - **Naomi**
- *Greetings & congratulations from Lithgow, NSW. I read about your story in That's Life mag a few weeks ago. You are such an amazing inspiration.* - **Adele**
- *Amazing!* - **Afra**
- *Yeah I cant wait till you get to Perth, you are epic.* - **Amy**
- *Enjoy seeing the best part of Oz!* - **Bromwyn**
- *Now hurry up and run about 3000 km directly south to the SA border where the best state begins.* - **Shane**
- *Welcome to WA! Congrats on your amazing achievements.* - **Kylie Xx**
- *Congratulations! Always good to have a safe arrival* - **Wendy**
- *Congrats!* - **Anni**
- *Congrats - Border today - new Grandchld last Tuesday. What will be the third important thing you do..... Keep up the good work, run tall and straight, not much further to the half way mark!* - **Barbara**
- *So amazed at what you are achieving !!!!! Go Raw!!!!!* - **Jenny**
- *Welcome to the Wild West. Us sandgropers welcome you and your amazing achievement*

with open arms. - **Anthony**
- *Congratulations on the arrival of your little granddaughter. I am in awe of you both, what an achievement! I love this pic, it looks like very interesting countryside. I am envious of you both in shorts and t-shirts, it is freezing here in Geelong, Victoria and I have my heater on full blast.* - **Lisa**
- *Congrats all around........your new arrival of your little granddaughter ......and arriving at the border is Western Australia.........you keep amazing me how you do it......* - **Anne**.
- *Amazing achievement, guys!!* - **Lennie**
- *Welcome to WA.* - **Caroline**
- *Hi to you both. Congrats on your new grandchild!* - **Lynette**
- *Hey congrats for grand child no 5 you guys are still going hard stay safe and God bless your efforts.* - **Mark**
- *Congrats for your new granddaughter and congrats on your journey!* - **Brenda**
- *We have seen you guys on the road.. We are the crazy cyclists cycling around Oz ... Stay safe!!*- **Jacquei**
- *Great to hear you are still powering along.We are happy our friend Narelle is back with us and enjoying her great stories of your journey..congrats on your magazine article and on your new grandchild.* - **Laurel**

Marathon #164.

June 13, 2013. Baine Picnic Area to Saddle Picnic Area 110 km from Kununurra. Melissa drove us forward to where we finished last night, started 5:30am after half hour sleep in after two late nights as we were both feeling a bit weary. First leg of 15 km had smoothies, second break at 30 km, long straights all flat, but rolling hills for the last 4 km finishing at 43.93 km. Melissa drove us on 7 km to a beautiful picnic area beneath red escarpments. Filled up the water tanks and washed the vehicles from the rainwater tank so we'd be clean for going through the border (no soil, no fruit & veg, no cane toads allowed) Also, no phone or internet! Temp 20-36 degrees. Total Km 7085.00.

Marathon #165.

June 14, 2013. Happy Birthday to our oldest grandson all the way over in Canada, we're thinking of you every step we run today, this one is for you buddy, welcome to the teens! Saddle Picnic Area to roadside spot 75 km east of Kununurra. Melissa drove us back 7.3km to where we finished last night, started 5:30am in dark till we got back to camp, quick water stop, then continued on through high escarpments with huge rocks balanced on top of the bluffs and large boab trees growing randomly amongst the rock, very dramatic landscape. Road surface changed to rough rocks and no edge past the white line so had to stop and wait in the rough gravel when traffic went past. Our feet were still tingling at 8pm from the day-long reflexology session! Finished 42.31 km at roadside spot, had pumpkin spaghetti with botanical cuisine Victorian olive dressing for dinner. Still no phone or internet, no news of bubs... Temp 20-37 degrees. Total Kms 7127.31.

Marathon #166.

June 15, 2013. 75 km east of Kununarra to 33 km east of Kununurra. Cool start at 5:30am in the dark (Temp 18-32.5 degrees) running towards the border of WA, so with a time difference of 2 hours, will it suddenly become light as we cross? Also, wondering about the little old fruit fly, do they stop mid flight at the border and turn around? Obviously the cane toads have it figured out, we came across one sitting in the middle of the road between the double white lines, just waiting for a vehicle to come along so he can jump up and hang on underneath as it goes through the border - honest! Thought he was a rock in the dark until he turned and looked at us. We suggested he high-tail it back where he came from, but he didn't seem too sure where that is...Had a smoothie at the first break and Melissa left to drive into Kununurra to buy fresh produce for the next couple of days until we get there. We ate up all the remaining fruit and veg at the second break, then ran the 5 km to the border. Had a good chat with the Border folks about RunRAW2013 and filled up the water tank as Myke came through with the van, put the clocks back one and a half hours and into WA we came. Melissa was there waiting on the other side with fruit and veg, we ate a few ripe bananas while we checked the messages on our phone that she had taken with her to

Kununurra to get reception for the phone. Sure enough, there was the message we've been waiting for, a brand new baby girl, our fifth grandchild born last Tuesday, June 11. Oh, how we wish we were there...but on we ran, amid the tears of joy, how blessed are we... Finished the run 42.35km. Total 7169.66.

Marathon # 167.

June 16, 2013. Happy Birthday to sister Rose, who since being on board RunRAW2013 as support crew has been eating mostly raw vegan and "feeling great" and no doubt getting younger every birthday! 33 km east of Kununurra to 7 km west of Kununurra. Started at 5:30am at daybreak, after a long sleep due to the extra time change coming through the border. So now we wont be running in the dark in the mornings, unless we start earlier of course...So excited about everything that we forgot to start the Garmin and didn't notice until after we had done 5 km (by the odometer in the SuperRoo) when Melissa caught up with us. Ran easy all day, felt relaxed now that we've made it to WA and only 2 weeks to go before we'll be officially half way around Australia. First leg of 14 km went well had a green smoothie with fresh greens from the Kununurra market that Melissa had got yesterday, yum. Myke and Melissa drove on into Kununurra 17 km to set up camp, found the distance a bit slow as the temp was rising quickly from the coolest morning we've had (Temp 15-32.5 degrees). Stopped 2 km from town when the phone reception came in and called home, happy to hear our son and grandson's voices with all the baby news. They were happy to hear that we are "still alive and running!" It was a long time without connection, we'll be staying an extra night in Kununurra to catch up on internet and stock up on food for the next trip to Broom. Thanks to Town Campgrounds for the complimentary site, we appreciate your hospitality and support. Went into Coles Supermarket to arrange for a food pickup tomorrow, but decided to do it tonight while the produce is fresh, so thanks to Josh for organising the order while we finished the last 7m of the run (42.42km with 5 km not recorded on Garmin). M & M picked us up and we all drove back to Coles to get the order. Thanks again to Josh and Coles Kununurra for your support and wonderful fresh fruit and veg that will fuel us to Broome. Total Km 7212.08.

Marathon #168.

June 17, 2013. Kununurra. Started at daybreak 5am, running around the streets of town and back to the campground for smoothies. Interspersed running with shopping and internet catchup throughout the day. Cooler day (Temp 15-30 degrees) with a cool breeze. Towards the end of the run we followed a dirt trail out to the lake, with the only footprints belonging to birds, dingoes and wallaroos, all of whom we came across along the way. The birds were mostly waterbirds and they ran rather awkwardly through the soft sandy dirt, flapping their wings and squawking noisily. The wallaroos boinged out of the way thumping their tails behind them and the dingoes retreated a few feet into the long grass, their watchful eyes following us as we passed. The trail ended at the lake where a white pelican floated gracefully on the water amongst the purple waterlilies. As the sun set over the lake turning the distant hills a water-colour pink, the bats in the trees above unfolded their wings, let go of the branch they had been hanging from and swooped down, squealing as they flew through the trees and up into the darkening sky. Another magic moment on another marathon day. Total Km 7212.08. Distance 42.37km.

Marathon #169.

June 18, 2013. 7 km west of Kununurra to 4.9 km south of the Victoria Hwy and Great Northern Hwy turnoff. Departed campground with all vehicles, drove to service station to fuel up with Autogas then out to where we had finished when we arrived in Kununurra on June 15. Started running 6:15am at sunrise. Cool morning (Temp 15-34 degrees), changing landscape with more hills and red rocky escarpments, boab trees in a variety of shapes and sizes and the road goes ever on. Much more traffic on the road than before Kununurra. Getting waves and toots from the motorists, mostly those who had seen us on the road in the past few days. Had a few people stop to give us donations, thanks for your support folks, we really appreciate you stopping. Decided to camp overnight at the Cockburn Rest Stop at the junction of Victoria and Great Northern Hwys even though we still had almost 5 km to go, so turned left and started running down the Great Northern Hwy, heading towards Halls Creek and heading south at last! We'll have to go west again to get to Broome, but for now, it's great to be running in a Southerly direction, heading for home! Finished the run at 42.59 km with the bluffs ahead of us glowing red in the sunset. Melissa came to pick us up and drive back to the Rest Stop for the night. The ole SuperRoo was running a bit hot and we found that it was leaking water from the radiator. Alan cleaned the motor, refilled the radiator and put some 'supergoo' in the water, hopefully it will hold until we get to where we can replace it, possibly not till Broome. Total Km 7254.67.

Marathon #170.

June 19, 2013. 4.9 km south of Cockburn Rest Stop on the Great Northern Hwy. Melissa drove us forward to where we had finished yesterday, SuperRoo's radiator not leaking, fingers crossed...Started at 5am just before daybreak. Surrounding bluffs of the O'Donnell and Car Boyd Ranges on either side of the road turning pink as the sun rose in the East. Beautiful scenery all day and good run on the winding hilly road through the Ranges. Came across a dingo that had been hit on the road, it was not long dead so we removed the still warm body off to the side, then noticed a second dingo running across the road just up ahead. The poor thing appeared confused, running back and forth several times, most likely not understanding why his mate did not get up and follow him. So sad...Running along an open stretch when a 4WD stopped ahead of us and two runners came out to meet us asking "Are you the vegans?" Well, they were the Gibb River Rd runners we had heard about from campers in Kununurra who had seen them on the road and thought it was us. So had a great chat on the side of the road, swapping a few stories and commiserating about the road conditions and high temperatures for winter! Great to meet you, keep in touch and stay safe on the road. Ran through a canyon between high bluffs and saw a small black dog (perhaps a pup) sitting in the middle of the road ahead. He ran off into the long grass when he saw us so couldn't tell if he was a dog or dingo, are there black dingoes? Run wild little fella and stay off the road! Ran an extra 2 km to finish 44.88 km at a parking spot off the road, with a view of the Bungle Bungle Ranges in the distance. Total Km 7299.55.

Marathon #171.

June 20, 2013. Cockburn Rest Stop to a 3G Transmitter 220 North of Halls Creek. Awoke at 3am to the smell of smoke and a red glow of a bush fire in the distance. Started at 5am just before daybreak and shortly afterwards saw the little black dog on the road up ahead again. As we approached, we realised it was not as small as we had first thought and it was not a black dog, it was indeed a dingo. With the fading light yesterday and the early dawn this morning, the dingo looked darker than it really was. Again it ran off the road into the grass, but stopped only a few metres away, a questioning look on it's face. Perhaps it was the same dingo we had seen yesterday, still waiting for it's mate to catch up...We ran on 9 km to Doon Doon Roadhouse, Myke and Melissa arrived at same time with the vehicles. Alan checked the SuperRoo radiator, still leaking water. Melissa noticed a small hole on top where the water was leaking from, so Alan stopped it up with a 2 part epoxy he bought from the Roadhouse. Meanwhile Janette phoned the Subaru dealer in Broome and the Garage in Halls Creek to let them know when we'll be there to check it over. Then hopefully it will get to Broome with the temporary job and we can replace the radiator there. Only 220 km to go SuperRoo, you can make it! Thanks to Marijke at Doon Doon Roadhouse for her friendly hospitality and for the use of her phone. Melissa and Myke stayed for another 40 minutes to let the epoxy harden off while we ran on 10 km. Big uphill climb but wide shoulders on the road, great scenery with huge rocky outcrops on the surrounding Ranges. Stopped by the Main Roads guys just before a steep incline and told we can't run up the hill on the road, but offered to drive us up there. So we had to explain that wasn't an option for us, so he said we had to walk on the other side of the barrier as it was too dangerous with the road trains. Has it happened no trucks came while we ran up, so all was well. Saw them on the road further up and stopped to tell them more details of RunRAW2013 and they gave us a donation, thanks guys for your concern and support. A nice change in the weather to cool, cloudy and showery for the rest of the run, haven't had rain for months! Just a few km to go and we saw a dingo on the road ahead again, is he keeping pace with us? Finished run at 43.62 km where Myke and Melissa had set up camp off the road next to a 3G transmitter. Off to bed at 6:45pm for an early night, listening to the rain on the roof...Temp

27-29 degrees. Total Km 7342.17.

Marathon # 172.

June 21, 2013. 220 km Nth of Halls Creek to Truck Stop 175 km north of Halls Creek on the Great Northern Hwy. Rained most of the night, started 5am in the dark, heard a dingo call just after leaving, daybreak at 5:30am. Cool today (Temp 18-27 degrees), fresh smells of damp earth and wet foliage permeate the air. Spectacular scenery of huge rocks balanced precariously on top of cliffs on one side of the road, rows of high pointed hills looking like giant sleeping dragons on the other side. Stopped for bananas and dates at 11 km and Melissa told us that she and Myke had seen the dingo at our camp before they left. We ran on and then saw him one last time running off into the hills...Stopped at 15 km for green smoothies, Alan checked the SuperRoo, no leaks in the radiator so all good there. Stopped at 29 km break and found we had phone coverage so phoned home, good to hear that all is well with our little family. Also phoned the store at Halls Creek to order some fresh produce for when we arrive in 4 days time. Meanwhile the fruit and veg we have on board is holding out well with Myke and Melissa managing the storage and preparing delicious smoothies, juice and meals. We all got really excited to see a herd of wild horses near where we stopped, so beautiful to see them running wild and free. Finished the run at 43.44 km, set up camp at a truck stop on the side of the road. Total Km 7385.61.

Marathon # 173.

June 22, 2013. Truck Stop 175 km north of Halls Creek to Hilltop 132 km Nth of Halls Creek. Started at daybreak 5:15am, moon had just set. Easy downhill run to first break at 10 km and as we approached the roadhouse at Warmun, the road leveled out. Plan was to take on LPG Autogas fuel, but although they had the gas tanks full, the pump was not working. We were not concerned as we had enough to get us to Halls Creek, but found out that the pumps there are also not working. So the nearest place for us to fuel up is at Fitzroy Crossing and we're not sure that we'll make it there before we run out. Phoned the RACV & RACWA who advised us to keep going and if we don't get to FC they will come out at tow the ute there to fuel up.

Apparently this has happened to several motorists recently as the pumps have been down for a while. So we're taking precautions with the driving, moved the weight forward and keeping the speed down to use the least amount possible and we'll see how we go. Meanwhile checked the SuperRoo and the radiator is holding in there, so fingers and toes crossed! Back on the road climbing uphill again, but because it took a couple hours doing the phoning, we finished the run (46.08 km) in the dark with a steep hill climb at the end. Dinner and bed by 8:30pm. Total Km 7431.69.

Marathon #174.

June 23, 2013. Hilltop 132 km north of Halls Creek to Roadside Stop 88 km north of Halls Creek. Started at 5am daybreak. Hilly and beautiful landscape but sad day with several dead animals on the road. Removed two kangaroos, one of them still warm, must have only just been hit. Then we came across a cow lying on the road, the blow to her head had killed her, otherwise there was no other visible injury. Of course we could not move her off the road, but luckily a road train came along as we got there and pulled over with some precision driving to stop alongside the animal. The driver told us that one of the earlier truck drivers had seen it happen and had radioed to let him know so he could move her when he came through. We stroked the cow while he tied a chain to her, then thanked the driver and left as he dragged her off the road. Such a beautiful animal, her face so sweet, even in death....It was a day for cattle on the road, but thankfully the rest we saw were all alive, wandering along the roadside feeding on the grass. They were oblivious to the danger of the traffic on the road, taking no notice as vehicles passed by them, but would run away when we approached. The scary part was not knowing whether they would run across the road in front of traffic, but luckily that did not happen. Roam free beautiful beasts, but please stay away from the road....There were a lot of road trains this morning, mostly traveling to and from the mines, all the drivers waved and tooted as they passed. Had phone reception as we passed the entrance to a huge nickel mine, so phoned home to talk to the family who were out for a Sunday walk with the three little ones, lovely to hear their voices. Another uphill finish today 43.66km. Delicious tomato soup for dinner as the moon was rising and in bed by 6:30pm! Temp 17-32 degrees. Total Km 7475.35.

Marathon #175.

June 24, 2013. 88 km north of Halls Creek to Roadside Stop 44km Nth of Halls Creek. Started at daybreak 5am, cold morning 10 degrees (went up to 31 degrees), had to wear our gloves! Beautiful sun rise as the moon was setting when we reached the top of the range at 6am. Had the last of the bananas at the first water stop, went through three boxes in six days! Green smoothies at the first break made with bananas that we had dehydrated six months ago, tasted like caramel. At the second break we had melon salad made with 3 different types of melon that were grown in Kununurra, very sweet tasting. Ran on through road works for a few km, talked with the guys who were working the machinery, thanks for the donation Kevin. Running easy uphill most of the day, 4 oranges for the last break and finished the run at 44.03km. Delicious green soup and carrot salad for dinner, bed 6:30pm. Total Km 7519.38.

Marathon #176.

June 25, 2013. 44 km north of Halls Creek to Halls Creek Campground. Started at daybreak 5:15am, another cold morning 10 degrees (went up to 32 degrees). Moon still high in the sky at sunrise. Ran at a good pace to get to Halls Creek by 2:30pm. Easy run into town, did last 14 km with no break as Myke & Melissa had driven in ahead to set up in the Halls Creek Campground complimentary site, (thanks for your hospitality and support). Finished the run 42.38 km, got hot and muggy and looks like it will rain soon, we heard there is heavy rain in Broome. We have not seen heavy rain in 3 months, have crossed many creeks and 10 major rivers, all dry and sandy, so hope the rain comes and fills the tanks for us to fill up on our way. Drove SuperRoo to the garage for a radiator checkup (should hold together till we get to Broome) and fueled up with petrol (luckily SuperRoo is dual fuel so we can do an emergency run for phone reception between Halls Creek and Fitzroy Crossing if the ute runs out of gas before we get there). Went to the IGA to pick up the fresh food order (thanks for the discount) and back to the campground to catch up on the internet as we wont have it again till we get to Fitzroy Crossing in a week, and by then we'll be halfway Running Raw Around Australia! Today's Total Km 7561.76.

Marathon #177.

June 26, 2013. Halls Creek Campground to Roadside Stop 145 km east of Fitzroy Crossing. Very late night catching up on the internet, but still started at daybreak 5:10am. Slow day on the road, very flat with only a few trees, still up in elevation (around 400 metres) so we're running on top of the tablelands. Phoned the Subaru dealer in Broome at the first break to order a new radiator and book it in for installation the day after we arrive (July 11), so we'll be staying there two nights. Also phoned home, all kids and grandkids are fine, our two little families talking to each other on Skype, the Canadians seeing our littlest one for the first time. It will be our turn on Sunday, if we have internet! Finished the last few km of the run (43.65km) in the twilight, hot and humid (29 degrees in the caravan at 6:30pm) Temp 17-34 degrees. Total Km 7605.41.

Marathon #178.

June 27, 2013. 145 km east of Fitzroy Crossing to Summit Lookout 200 km east of Fitzroy Crossing. Very dark and stormy and warm all night (minimum 26 degrees) but no rain. Started at 5am daybreak and a clear sky. Janette had a thorn in her forefoot which made for slow progress until removing it at the first break. It can be a prickly business around here walking into the bush! Landscape changing all day, long distance views over the tablelands and sweeping curves in the road. Ran through another area of road works where they insisted on escorting us through, (following close behind us as we ran, since we refused a ride), thanks guys. Finished the run 43.76 km at a summit lookout where you can see 360 degrees for 50+ km, grassy tablelands surrounded by distant hills, and there's internet! Checked the vehicles, all okay with SuperRoo, looks like we'll run out of gas in the ute on Saturday, so we'll be getting a tow to Fitzroy Crossing to fill up, stay tuned! Temp 27-32 degrees. Total Km 7649.17.

Marathon #179.

June 28, 2013. Summit Lookout 200 km east of Fitzroy Crossing to Roadside Stop 155km East of Fitzroy Crossing. Started at 5:15am, slight drizzle of rain that cleared within 10 minutes, still warm and humid (temp 21-30.4 degrees). Phoned RACV/WA at first break to book a tow to Fitzroy Crossing for the ute this afternoon to get autogas fuel as it's getting too low to safely go on. Decided to run the marathon without anymore breaks so we can finish earlier and Alan can go with the tow truck. Myke and Melissa drove the vehicles on to the final destination for the night at a roadside stop about 30 km ahead. We continued running with Melissa coming back to bring water and bananas. Janette had the phone and took the phone calls from RAC while Alan ran ahead. So there we were, running outback in the middle of nowhere along the Great Northern Hwy and a runner appears coming the other way carrying a torch! We had heard that the Sri Chinmoy Peace Run was on and the Aussie Team were in the area, so were expecting to see them sometime today. Stopped for a quick chat, held the Peach Torch, made a wish for World Peace during our lifetime and took a photo before continuing on in opposite directions, but running for the same reasons. Finished the run 43.45 km, drained all the water out of the ute tank into the caravan tank so Alan can restock on water when he gets to FC, unhitched the ute and waited for the tow truck to arrive. They departed around 4:30pm so we'll see Alan back with full tanks, gas and water, in a few hours. Meanwhile, we have internet out here in the outback and we're only 4 days away from running through the halfway point when we reach Fitzroy Crossing! Total Km 7692.62

Marathon #180.

June 29, 2013. 155 km east of Fitzroy Crossing to 111km east of Fitzroy Crossing on Gt Northern Hwy. Started 5am, dark clouds and light rain. Cool following wind pushing us along, felt a little sore and weary from our fast run yesterday and late night with fueling the ute. No traffic to speak of so mostly ran down the middle of the road to stay off the rough rocks on the edge. Long straight road and flat scrubby landscape with lots of termite mounds as far as the eye could see, some really huge surrounded by many smaller mounds with thousands of termites and small ants racing around building as fast as they could go. What will happen when the small mounds get bigger? The landscape will be one big mound! Finished the run 44.56 km at a farm gateway, all in bed by 7:30pm. Temp 25-29 degrees. Total Km 7737.18.

Marathon #181.

June 30, 2013. Farm gateway 111 km East of Fitzroy Crossing to Roadside Parking 68 km east of Fitzroy Crossing. Started 5am, no stars, dark and stormy but no rain. Strong cold following wind, wearing 3 layers of clothes for the wind chill factor. Beautiful red sunrise lighting up the black clouds and creating a pink rainbow. Landscape changed to a huge outcrop of red cliffs and lime green grass growing amongst the red termite mounds. Ran through a gorge with red cliffs on one side and black rocks on the other. Sides of the road getting very wet and soft, almost got stuck twice so not safe to park the vehicles any more as we were told by the tow truck driver that the ground is wet all the way to Broome from the storms over the last few days. One of the road maintenance guys who had seen us on the road every day during the last 2 weeks stopped to talk. Thanks for stopping, great to meet you and we look forward to seeing you in Perth. Had a good strong run to the finish at 43.93km at a roadside parking place. Temp 17-30 degrees. Total Km 7781.11.

July, 2013

MARATHONS #182-212

Marathon #182. July 1, 2013. Six months on the road today, so officially halfway by months! 68 km east of Fitzroy Crossing to Joy Springs Community 25 km east of Fitzroy. Started 5am, stars in a clear sky, but very windy and cold. Seemed strange to be heading north! Wind got stronger and more head on as we turned a few corners to the right, heading NNE. Wind so strong at our first break we had to take the pop-top of the caravan down. Another day of long straights in the road and tiring with the head winds, but we recovered quickly after each break. Finished the run 43.30 km at the gateway to Joy Springs Community 25 km from Fitzroy Crossing. Temp 19-28 degrees. Total Km 7824.41.

Comments from Facebook/RunningRawAroundAustralia2013:

- *You guys are AMAZING well done.* - **Kat xx**
- *Just to Awsomeeeeedde for words.* - **Bell**
- *Good luck and continuing good health to the two of you... I am so envious!! I read of your feats in amazement....*- **Bill**
- *Keep going guys....*- **Brendon**
- *Go ahead, guys ... you are of great inspiration!* - **Matteo**
- *Well done guys!!* - **Brendan**
- *Very inspiring guys, well done.* - **Sylvia**
- *Rawesome! Enjoying following your progress. Well done!* - **Jenna**
- *RAWsome.* - **Rose**
- *Rawesome indeed!* - **Matt**
- *Incredible! Would love to know how you are feeling physically. Is your recovery still good? How are your feet? Questions....questions...* - **Tisha**

- *All good Tisha, getting better every day...*
- *Wonderful news J&A - looking forward to joining you on the run back into Melbourne with a few other Kids Under Cover staff.* - **Martin**
- *You guys are rawmazing very inspirational.* - **Magda xx**

Marathon #183.

July 2, 2013. Passed through the official halfway point for Marathons (182.5- half of 365) at 21km into today's run from Joy Springs to 20 km west of Fitzroy Crossing. Started 4:45am in dark, clear and starry, cool 18 degrees. Ran 24 km into Fitzroy Crossing with a quick smoothie break. Very busy 6 hours in FC fueling the vehicles, filling the water tanks, picking up and stowing away the food order, doing laundry and uploading the daily updates on Facebook Page. Departed caravan park in Fitzroy Crossing to finish the run, ran 10 km and picked up some dates and water so Myke & Melissa could drive on to find a camp spot for the night before it got dark. Finished the last 6 km into the sunset and watched as the stars filled the night sky. Finished at 42.33km on side of road. Temp 18-28 degrees. Total Km 7866.74.

Marathon #184.

July 3, 2013. 20 km West Fitzroy Crossing to Farm Gateway 62km West of Fitzroy Crossing. Started 5am, cold, clear sky and long hilly straights on the rough rocky road. Little to no shoulder on the edge and thick red sand. Tried running on the sand but we were sinking into it too much, leaving interesting footprints alongside the dingo's. Beautiful bird calls at daybreak and throughout the morning, couldn't see them but sounded like warblers. As the temperature rose, so did the flies, yes, the flies are back! We each had about 50 flies hovering around us, hitching a ride on our backs, shoulders and heads, buzzing up and down in front of our faces, landing and crawling in our eyes and noses, into our ears and mouths. I must have crossed myself a hundred times trying to shoo them away, the Pope would be proud of me, except I'm not Catholic. When they all decided to take flight at once from my cap and swarm around my face, the shooing became a frantic wave, the motorists waving frantically back and probably wondering what that was all about, since they are comfortably traveling along in their air conditioned vehicles with the windows up oblivious to the flies. Might be time to start wearing the nets again....and the road goes ever on, landscape changing from wide expanses of long grassy savannah to thick bushy hills. The last 6 km of the run was magical. First we spied a single boab tree, not having seen them for a few weeks, we were elated. Then, we saw another, and another, and around the corner we came across the biggest plantation of boab trees we've ever seen. Running through an enchanted forest, hundreds of beautiful boab, all sizes and shapes standing tall amongst the anthills, and then like magic they were gone, replaced by a bright yellow haze of wattle trees in bloom, the heady scent laying heavily in the air. Finished at sunset 42.81 km. Temp 15-28 degrees. Total Km 7909.61.

Marathon #185.

July 4, 2013. 62 km west of Fitzroy Crossing to Truck Stop 105 km west of Fitzroy Crossing. Started 5am, cool, starry and small crescent moon. Both felt good after good night's sleep (9 hours), ran well on long straights again, rocky road but good edges and not much traffic. A motorist following our vehicles stopped when he passed us on the road to say how great he thought what we're doing is. Turned out he is working with placing aboriginal people in work on cattle stations, working with the horses. When he read our flyer and noticed that we are vegans, he said that we all want what is good and positive so we should all be working together towards a sustainable future for the planet. He was amazed that we're running a marathon every day around Australia and said it was good that we're raising awareness for the charities and a more sustainable future for the animals and the kids, and he would spread the word and make a donation on line. So that was encouraging to know that the positive message we are running for is getting through, thanks for stopping and for the donation, made our day. Finished at a Truck Stop for the night 43.36 km. Temp 15-33 degrees. Total Km 7952.91.

Marathon #186.

July 5, 2013. Truck Stop 105 km west of Fitzroy Crossing to Grader Stop 75 km east of Willare Roadhouse on the Gt Northern Hwy. Started 4:55am in the dark, starry sky and crescent moon. We'd been running in the dark for about an hour, daybreak just starting to glow red in the eastern sky when suddenly we noticed animals on the road up ahead. Presuming they were cattle we continued running, but as we got closer we discerned that they were wild horses. We slowed to a walk as we approached and whistled to let them know we were there. Immediately the largest of the herd stood across the middle of the road, while the others (all 9 of them) crowded behind him, luckily there was no traffic in sight. Janette spoke quietly to the horses as she continued to approach and they slowly moved to the side of the road, the largest still protecting the others as he stood his ground while they moved further back towards the bush. Janette continued to approach slowly, her hand outstretched and talking to the horses in a quiet voice. Alan walked quickly past them all and stopped, turned back to witness an amazing scene. Janette still talking quietly to the animals, was surrounded by all the horses, all of them standing several hands taller than her, pushing their noses forward to nuzzle her hand and face. The scene was surreal in the early light of daybreak, a herd of wild horses surrounding a small woman, strangers in the dark and no trace of fear, only trust. The softness of their velvet noses lingered on my hand, the gentle nudge on my face will stay with me forever....the rest of the day's run paled in comparison to the feeling of love and trust expressed by these gentle giants, we can learn so much from animals...may the light in their eyes shine on...forever free. Distance run 44.35 km, Temp 15-32 degrees. Total Km 7996.92.

Marathon #187.

July 6, 2013. Passed through the 8000 km mark today. Grader stop 75 km east of Willare Roadhouse to Roadside Floodway 33 km East of Willare. Started 5am, another dark, starry morning, coldest yet at 7 degrees, the strong scent of wattle heavy in the air. We knew we were on a long straight when it took 8 mins for an oncoming car's lights to get close enough to hear the car before it passed by 2 mins later. Another day of long straight rocky road climbing hill after hill, lined with golden flowering wattle, huge boab trees, monster anthills and red dirt. Myke and Melissa found roadside stops all the way where the grader had leveled, between us we consumed 4 smoothies, 10 bananas, 10 dates, half watermelon, 4 bowls of tomato soup, 2 avocados, 4 bowls of veg curry & rice (made from cauliflower). All to bed just after sunset 6:30pm. Distance run 43.48 km. Temp 7-33 degrees. Total Km 8040.40.

Marathon #188.

July 7, 2013. Roadside Floodway 33 km east of Willare to 9 km West of Willare. Started 5am, back on the rocky road with no edges, rough running all day. Temperature range 15-33 degrees. Finished 9 km past Willare Roadhouse where Melissa picked us up and drove us back to the campground at Willare where Myke had set up in a complimentary site and room for the night, also free laundry and hot showers. The girls at the roadhouse set up a donation jar for RunRAW2013 at the bar. Thanks for your hospitality and support, and for the donations. Today's run 42.46 km. Total Km 8082.86. *Speaking of donations, we found some coins on the roadside as we were running the last 9 km which amounted to $8.20, the onroad donations for the day. When we passed the halfway point a few days ago, we counted up the donations that we have received 'onroad' during the past 6 months. These donations have come from passing motorists who stop to talk to us on the road, fellow campers in campgrounds and roadside stops, people we meet in the street when we're running through towns and coins we've picked up alongside the road. Interestingly, there were more roadside coins in Victoria mostly 5c pieces, in NSW the denominations went up to 10c, 20c and 50c pieces and in Queensland we got really excited when we found $1 and $2 coins. Overall the coin pickup daily average amounted to $2.40. We have found none throughout NT and none in WA so far, until today. Altogether, the 'onroad' donations have amounted to $1000.00 for the 6 months. Online donations made through the website have also amounted to $1000.00, but at that rate the four charities will only receive $1000 each at the end of the Run. We've run over halfway round Australia, 188 consecutive marathons, more than 8000 km and the donations amount is equivalent to 25c per km! Now we know that what we're doing and the positive message of RunRAW2013 is inspiring thousands of people and making a difference in their lives and that is wonderful, but we'd really like to also make a difference for the four very worthy charities that we're raising awareness for. So we're asking for your help with this, because we're starting to feel like we're Running Out of Time! So please, if you haven't already done so, take the time to make a donation through our website. It will take less time to do than it takes us to run 1 km! Please share our website and facebook page links with all your friends, family and colleagues, ask them to Like, Share and Donate. Please help us to keep RunRAW2013 on the road and keep the donations rolling in! Thanks everyone, we really appreciate your support.*

Marathon #189.

July 8, 2013. 9 km west of Willare to side road 53 km west of Willare. Melissa drove us 9 km where we had finished yesterday and we started in the dark at 5:15am. Quite a few cattle on the sides of the road and crossing the road all day. There are no fences here so the cattle roam back and forth on the road looking for food. One had been hit and appeared to have an injured leg, she had moved off the road and was sitting under a tree, but could not get up when we approached. The look she gave us was as if asking for help, but there was nothing we could do. We hope she will recover, but unfortunately we see too many who have not. Finished the run 44.09 km. Temp 15-33 degrees. Total Km 8126.95.

Marathon #190.

Just another number, just another marathon. Only 10 days and we'll have run 200 consecutive marathons, setting another world record, stay tuned...July 9, 2013. 53 km west of Willare to Gravel Pit 70 km East of Broome. Started 5am in dark, warm and brilliant sunrise. More long straights on a rocky road. Highlights of the day was the food breaks, thanks to Melissa and Myke. The bananas have ripened so we had many bananas and some dates at first stop, green smoothie at first break, paw paw and fresh tomato soup midway, oranges at last stop before finishing the run 43.56 km at roadside gravel pit. Cabbage wraps for dinner and bed after sunset. A quiet night away from the traffic, but millions of mosquitoes outside, some managed to get through the netting and joined us inside the caravan so not a great sleep. Temp 16-33 degrees. Total Km 8170.51.

Marathon #191.

July 10, 2013. 70 km east of Broome to Farm Gate 26 km east of Broome. Started at 5am, very dark, no moon, no traffic, no sound, just the constant slap, slap of our feet on the road. Much the same as yesterday, long straights and no shoulder. Got very hot by midday, 36 degrees and muggy. The workers laying the culverts stopped to give us some ice cold water, thanks guys. Came to the Broome junction with 34 km of road works to Broome. The smell of fresh tar on the road made us feel ill and the soft red dust on the side of the road covered our shoes as we ran through it. When the cars came past, the dust filled our eyes and noses, not a pleasant run. The road workers escorted us through the areas where the heavy machinery was working, driving behind us as we ran holding up all the waiting traffic, but the motorists were very patient and gave us the thumbs-up as we passed. Had to run past the roadworks to finish the run 44.10km at a Farm Gateway. Temp 16-36 degrees. Total Km 8214.61. Average Marathon 43 km.

Marathon #192.

July 11, 2013. 26 km east of Broome to Broome and around the city streets. Started 5am in dark through roadworks, very hard to run off the edge of the road in sloping soft dirt and stony sand, very dusty. When the roadworks patrol trucks arrived at daybreak they wanted to take us through in their vehicle, but when we declined, they escorted us on the road by driving behind us as we ran, thanks guys. Our Broome hosts Brett and friend Nicole drove out to meet us on the road, Nicole offering accommodation and parking at her house, thanks so much for a safe and comfortable place to sleep and catch up on everything, not to mention the wonderful hot shower and being able to do the laundry. Myke and Melissa got settled in to the guest house while we parked the van in the driveway, hooked up to the power and then continued the run through the streets of Broome. Went straight to the Post Office to pick up our new Vibram shoes, thanks to our sponsors Barefoot Inc. Called in to the Subaru dealer and all is good to have the new radiator installed tomorrow, good old SuperRoo made it. Ran to Coles and put in the fruit & veg order for pick-up tomorrow, ran through Chinatown and out to the ABC Radio Studio so we'd know where it is for the live interview tomorrow. Airing at 1045am, tune in! Finished the run 42.24 km as the sun set, a long day but a lot done. Melissa had dinner ready, delicious tomato and mushroom soups and everyone off to bed except Janette who is catching up on the internet! Hopefully we'll have better reception for internet and phone from now on and we'll be able to keep everyone updated on a more regular basis as we head south to Perth. We'll be putting the updated schedule on the website tomorrow and sending off the Half Way Running Raw Around Australia Press Release to all the media, so watch for media coverage soon. Meanwhile, please keep Sharing our FB posts and the website link for donations and thanks for the Shares, Likes and Donations to date. We and the Charities really appreciate your support. Total Km 8256.85. Temp 17-36 degrees.

Marathon #193.

July 12, 2013. Broome, WA. Drove the SuperRoo to the garage to have a new radiator installed this morning then started at 4:30am running around the neighbourhood under street lights to get some distance in as we have so much else to do today. Quick smoothie back at the caravan then back out on the road, running around the town until 10:30am when Janette went to the ABC Kimberley Studio for a live broadcast, which went well. Alan meanwhile checked in at the garage to find SuperRoo ready to leave with the new radiator in, although not recommended to drive until the head gasket is checked, which is a big job, big $$ and big wait-2 weeks. So that's not happening, SuperRoo came quietly and we'll be doing daily checks to make sure everything is OK, taking a risk but then we're doing that every day anyway! Back on the Run out to Cable Beach, over the sand dunes, down to the Indian Ocean and into the warm water. We ran along the beach for a couple of kilometres and decided we'd have to come back to spend more time in Broome. Started running back into town and met a few camels heading down to the beach, hope we get to see them in the wild as we run down the coast. Ran back to the caravan in time to go out for a raw potluck with the local raw vegan foodies. Great evening, delicious food and wonderful to meet new friends - thanks for your hospitality and support everyone, we'll be back! Had to finish the last 3.76km afterwards at 11pm. Garmin Data recorded the day's run (43.01km) in two laps, 39.25 and 3.76 posted separately. Temp 19-35 degrees. Total Km 8299.86.

Marathon #194.

July 13, 2013. Port Hedland turnoff at Roebuck Roadhouse to Truck Parking at 44.26 km south on Gt Northern Hwy. Drove from Broome to where we had left the Gt Northern Hwy on Thursday to run into Broome and started at the Roebuck turnoff to Port Hedland at 7:30am. SuperRoo performing well so far. Terrain on both sides of the road changed to open dessert except there is still floodwater after the recent rain storms which occurred the week before we arrived. Myke and Melissa pulled off the road for the first break and got both vehicles stuck in the soggy soil. Thanks to the passing motorists who helped push SuperRoo out and to Ray and Lesley for stopping to help disconnect the caravan so we could drive the ute out and reconnect to pull the van out. Way too much excitement! Warm and muggy day on the road, both tired after the long day yesterday. Road is rocky so we were running on the sandy verge when Alan tripped on a stump that was hidden under the sand, bit the dust literally, red dust rising in a cloud as he hit the ground. but was soon up and running again after brushing off. He's now sporting road rash on his forehead, right shoulder, elbow and knee and feeling bruised ribs. Finished the run 44.26 km at a truck stop as it was getting dark. We were invaded by thousands of mosquitoes that buzzed and stung all night, oh it's great to be back on the road! Temp 19-35 degrees. Total Km 8344.12.

Marathon #195.

July 14, 2013. Truck Parking to Roadside Runoff 200km North of Sandfire Roadhouse on the Gt Northern Highway. Started 5am in the dark after a restless night with the mosquitoes. Both still feeling tired, especially Alan after his fall yesterday and the road is very rough again so running a bit slower today. Hot and muggy, temp 18-37 degrees. Checked SuperRoo after the first break and found a loose hose clamp so lost some coolant from the radiator. Topped it up and checked again later, all okay. Finished the run 43.62 km as the sun set behind the cars and caravan where Myke and Melissa had set up camp for the night on a roadside runoff. Fresh juice was ready for us and Melissa had made a delicious curried veg dinner. A couple of hours catching up on the internet before going to bed at 10pm, another late night, but not so many mozzies here so here's hoping for a good sleep. Total Km 8387.74. Daily average 43.01 km.

Marathon #196.

July 15, 2013. 200 km north of Sandfire to 154 km east of Sandfire. Started 5:10am in dark heading SW until dawn. Still on the rocky road, both running slow with lack of sleep and Alan's painful rib. Stopped at a roadside stall selling melons, first one since the Queensland coast. Met 4 Kiwis on motorbikes who also stopped there, great to meet you, thanks for the walnuts! Hot and muggy again, temp 19-36 degrees, finished the run 42.85 km parked on the side of the road for the night. Bed by 6:30pm. Total Km 8430.59.

Marathon #197.

July 16, 2013. 154 km east of Sandfire to 110 km east of Sandfire. On the road again 5:10am after a good sleep last night with not so many mozzies. Alan's rib still very painful, strapped it with a bandage at the first break which made a big difference for the rest of the day. Met a few very large bulls on the side of the road and saw a dingo in the distance crossing the road. We were pleased to see dingo footprints in the sand again, it's good to know they are still around as we haven't seen them for a while. Hot and humid again (temp 19-36 degrees), a bit of a discouraging day with slow progress and wondering what difference we're making by being out here, running a marathon a day on the edge of the Great Sandy Desert. Why are we out here talking (to) a lot of bull about being kind and compassionate to others (including the animals) as the cattle trains thunder past, their precious cargo heading for slaughter? Why are we out here pounding on the rocks with everything hurting and our feet screaming for us to stop, when we could be at home with our precious grandchildren? How is it that one celebrity can raise $25,000 for one cause in one day by riding a one-wheeled bicycle around one track in one town, while we've each been running a marathon every day for 197 days, through 7 major towns, 4 states and 2 territories, and have raised less than $5000? We're thinking, "Seriously, does anyone really care?" I listen to my feet and come to a stop, rip my shoes off and grab my toes shouting at them over the roar of the road trains, "Will you stop screaming at me, I know the rocks are rough but it will get better, so give it up!" I hear myself shouting at my own toes and the words resound in my ears, "so give it up"...and I start to cry. Alan stops, walks back to me, wincing as he holds his rib in place and asks, "What is it?" I answer him with a loud sob, "What's the point? Why are we doing this? Do you really think we're making a difference?" The sound of a road train gearing down caught our attention and as we looked up into the cab of the huge truck, the driver waved and gave us the thumbs-up signal, he was asking if we were okay. We waved back, gave him the thumbs-up and he pulled down on his air horn as he geared back up to speed. His compassionate concern and kind actions answered my questions. I put my shoes back on, we straightened up and started running…As the sun set the sky filled with a red tinge and we finished the run at 43.54 km, a total of 8474.13 Km, an average of 43.02 km per marathon. DONATIONS to date $3706.60

Comments from Facebook/RunningRawAroundAustralia2013:

- *Just so you two know you've made a difference in my life. Keep it up, you have admirers from all over the world. Regards from Canada!* - **Alan**
- *Don't give up! What you are doing is amazing. The world needs more compassion towards our fellow man and towards animals and you are slamming that truth home with every, albeit painful, step. All the best from a Pom in NZ.* - **Kirsty x**
- *You guys are so inspiring ~ and you ARE making a difference! In many people's lives!* - **Andrea**
- *I have SERIOUS respect for you both. You both are the true definition of ROCKSTARS!*- **Michelle**
- *You are both strong. and you did pretty awesomely GREAT so far. This will do a change. As it does for me. Keep it up! I'm positively thinking for you guys.* - **AnneSophie.Canada (Québec)**
- *I've donated!* - **Kristina**
- *you are amazing people,you are doing it because you care and so compassionate,a BIG hug from a Dutchy in Australia* - **Willeke**
- *YOU make a difference to me. Everytime I read another of your updates, you inspire me to keep my voice loud. I too feel that deep sadness for the all too many humans who are asleep and the millions of animals that are forgotten, ignored, enslaved, abused. I too feel pained at those who say they love animals but in reality continue to sit in their denial and hypocracy as they still seem quite content to treat them only as food. Your posts and your runs make a difference to me. YOU, Your Runs make me want to keep talking, keep demonstrating, keep trying to wake up a world that operates in ignorance and contradiction. You, your runs continue to make me want to be a better, stronger healthier person. YOU, your runs, make a difference to me and the hundreds who I continue to inspire on my journey. Love to you both.*

Look forward to meeting you when you reach South Australia. - **Lynda xx**
- *I can't believe that Australians who are so much about sports and fitness would not care more about 2 wonderful people who do not put it into their own pockets instead enduring all the pain in the hope to build up awareness about what's really going on with our relationship with animals! Please Australians wake up and honour these 2 Light-Beings with the donations and attention they deserve! There will not be anyone who CAN do the same any time soon! This is a record already!!!!!! -* **Sieghilde**
- *Every now and then when my world feels like it is falling apart for whatever reason...I take myself back to Federation Square on New Year's Day... And remember how I felt as you guys left and think of how much you have achieved. I look at the map consider where you are now and pick myself up dust myself off and get over myself. Big love. -* **Lada**
- *Keep up your amazing work, I love reading your post. You are both so inspiring. -* **Indee**
- *Go on! -* **Anja**
- *Keep shouting at your toes!! -* **Jackie**
- *Deep bow my friends,from the holy land. -* **Nico**
- *I feel You both & have posted this on A Current Affair, Sunrise, Weekend Sunrise & The Today Show, i tried to post on "Today Tonight" but they do'nt allow posts. I am willing You onwards & Praying that these Shows will pick up Your Story & "Run With It," No pun intended. Keep Up The Good Work, i don't have much money on a disability pension but Ive done what I can do and I love You both. -* **Lee**
- *You are legends. You make a big difference to me. You are the pioneers. Love to you both .... and your sore feet! -* **Wendy**
- *When it comes down to it the only people you can count on is yourselves..who better than to be your best fans. -* **Milt**
- *Keep going guys your an inspiration!!! -* **Brendan**
- *Every day, new people hear about you - I heard on Monday and told my friend Rachel Hogan who is training to run her first marathon to raise money for orphaned gorillas and chimps in Cameroon. She is finding running in the Cameroon city of Yaounde difficult and the distance is daunting, but you guys are now inspiring her to keep going when her feet are screaming for*

her to stop! So don't give up, you are making a difference across the world in lots of ways..... Cameroon and the UK are with you! - **Caroline**
- That was an amazing update that actually brought a tear to my eye... Whether you 'give up' (which wont really be giving up as you've already achieved so much) or not, what you've done is incredible - and something I'm certain your precious grandchildren will be immensely proud of... How do we donate? With love from the UK. - **Nadia x**
- I think what you are doing is inspiring and I think you are both amazing. When I read your posts I am amazed that you are running this marathon everyday, so don't give up what you are doing is making a difference. Even if it inspires someone to just get out there and doing something out of their comfort zone your doing that everyday so keep going!!! - **Alli**
- The difference in raising some quick cash and making a statement that will last many decades is what you are doing. Your legendary status as runners will be very powerful to those who sit and watch. Your raw food diet will serve as a beacon to those searching for a better life. Potentially every footstep can be thought of as changing for better another person. Gandhi and Mandela got jailed for changing the lives of as many people!! - **Stuart**
- I felt so sad that you were hurting I nearly burst into tears myself. You are both so awesome (terrible word but cant think of a better one!) I know that you will find that inner strength to keep you going to reach your goal. Even when you think what you are doing is no more than a butterflys wing beat, remember it can be the start of a tornado. Your message will prevail - you will succeed - people will learn more about compassion and love and how raw foods can sustain them and help the planet - all because of YOU TWO! - **Madeleine**
- What you're doing is far more inspirational than any celebrity raising quick cash. I am a young woman from Poland and you've had a great impact on me - you give me motivation to change myself and the world around me. Your message travels far further than the actual distance you've run! - **Milla**
- What you are doing isn't about money. - **Lee**
- All I can say is "The best is yet to come". You'll see. - **Doug and Dog**
- I care :) - **Karen**
- Please keep going if you can. You are truly inspirational. I have never been a runner, In fact

hated it and didn't think I could do it. I now can run 10 km. It is nothing at all compared to what you do but you have been an inspiration to me and I am sure to so many others.-Lucinda
- Lots of great support here - kind and thoughtful words Keep on plodding on - set your sights on the next termite mound or tree or rock and your feet will keep on chewing up the miles. - **Kaje**
- You guys are changing the world with every step. You are influencing people who are influencing people like sparks setting off little spot fires.I talk about you guys a lot and people are fascinated. Like yourselves I am disheartened by the small amount but I truly believe that the impact you have had so far is currently not represented monetarily, but, it ain't over yet I have a feeling! - **David**
- This post has been your most inspirational yet!! You totally touch me with your honesty, determination and compassion. I am shocked to hear you have only raised that small amount of money!!! And to be honest I had planned to wait until you came to Perth to give you my donation in person-but now I am totally inspired to help you raise the money! My aim is to double the amount you have raised-I'm not sure how I will-but my thinking cap is on. You both just put all your energy into running and moving forward and the community will get the donations coming in. - **Jazz**
- If it means anything you have certainly increased my awareness and practice of both raw food -especially in my own battle to return to health - and compassionate living. You rock, and am so grateful of your existence is this world. Wishing you the best. - **Katy Xoxo**
- Much love to you both. IT matters. Those who are last will be first someday. You're wonderful. Keep going. - **Dave**
- You are even more of an inspiration to me now that I know you have doubts!!!!! (Of course I should assume that you do, but then again, what you are doing is so unbelievably superhuman that I couldn't help wondering if maybe you are completely beyond normal fears & doubts) What you are doing is mind blowing and wonderful. I will do my best to spread the word of your amazing story! - **Dougal**
- You 2 are S U P E R inspiring!! - **George**
- You've been a huge inspiration for my raw vegan diet, and for my running. I can't go nearly

as far as you guys go, but I know it's possible and I keep striving because I always have you in mind. Your impact is so much greater than the donations you raise. Keep up the amazing work! - **Jennifer**
- Go on, even if you can't see the results. If you make it sincerely with love - and it's clear that you two do it - there will be good results. Go on! - **Lara**
- Thanks for your kind comments and concern, don't worry, we're not stopping yet, almost at Marathon # 200...

Marathon #198.

July 17, 2013. 110 km east of Sandfire to Roadside park on the desert sand 67 km east of Sandfire. Started 5:15am in the dark, stars but no moon. Both running better after a good sleep, Alan's rib feeling a bit better. Watched the sun rise through the shrubs, Alan has renamed the Great Sandy Desert, the Great Scrubby Desert, on the Great Northern Hwy everything is great! There is red sand beneath thick scrub and stunted wattle, no sign of any camels yet, would be great to see them in the wild! Our bananas are getting very ripe so had 5 each in our pre-run smoothie with 2 grapefruit, 4 each at 8 km and 3 each at 20 km. Then 2 melons for midway and 3 oranges for third break. All the motorists must have read yesterday's blog as they all tooted, waved and gave the thumbs up as they passed. We noticed several taking photos and videos as they drove past and one couple stopped to take a photo of us with them, they had seen us several times on the road but were not able to stop before. It was nice to stop and chat and be told "it's a great thing you are doing." Thanks for stopping, it made our day. We've been checking SuperRoo at every break, reinforced top radiator hose with rubber and plastic ties after finding a leak in the hose which had not been replaced in Broome when the new radiator was installed. Ordered a new hose from Port Hedland and will have it sent to the next roadhouse at Pardoo. Finished the run 42.82 km, had a fresh juice of carrot & beet and a green salad with avocado for dinner. Camped at a sandy roadside park off the road, an ideal spot except for the mosquitoes which we can hear and see surrounding the caravan. So off with the light and dive under the sheets and hope for a good sleep. Temp 18-34 degrees. Total Km 8516.95. Average 43.01 km per marathon.

Marathon #199.

July 18, 2013. Desert Park 67 km east of Sandfire to 24 km east of Sandfire on the Great Northern Hwy. Started 4:55am in the dark, very cold wind, should have put on jacket and gloves as we were cold by the first water break, but warmed up once the sun was up. More long straights and rough road with low scrub on the sides. Saw a bird on the edge of the road that had been injured on the leg, didn't look broken but it couldn't stand up to fly away. It was trying to move off into the scrub by flapping it's wings, dragging it's long legs underneath it and crying out. We heard another bird calling from the scrub so picked the injured bird up and carried it into the scrub, stroking and talking softly to it. The bird did not move off when we put it down, so hopefully it was waiting for the other bird to call, perhaps it was it's mother as the injured bird looked young. We left it there, hoping that the mother would feed it until the leg was mended enough for it to fly away. Looked up our book on birds when we got back to the van and found it was an Australian Bustard, which is a big bird when fully grown, good luck big bird, hope you make it... Alan's chest was still painful at the beginning of the run but eased off later, at least it's not stopping him from running. Finished the run at 43.89 km, camped right beside the road as there was nowhere else to pull off further. Sounds like the road trains are coming right through the van...happy sleeping! Temp 17-27 degrees (wind chill factor minus10 degrees). Total Km 8560.84. Average 43.02 km per Marathon.

Marathon #200.

July 19, 2013. Another milestone (or is that kilometer stone)? 24 km east of Sandfire to 20 km west of Sandfire. Started at 5:15am, very dark and starry, cold (Temp 16-24 degrees) but we're wearing jackets and gloves so kept warm enough. Road rough and rocky again and Janette tripped on a 'landmine' at 6 km and took the fall on her right elbow and knee again. Very frustrating as everything had just healed up after the last fall, but she got up and limped along for a bit before starting to run again. So now we have two running wounded, makes for a lot of toots and thumbs-up from the motorists anyway! Arrived at Sandfire Roadhouse midway through the run, thanks for the complimentary 4hr stop to do laundry, shower and take on water and fuel. SuperRoo still limping along (that makes 3 running wounded), but we're checking every break and should get to Pardoo to replace the radiator pipe. Back on the road for the last 20 km, finished up running in the dark by the light of the moon for the last 10 km, finishing the run at 42.77 km. Myke and Melissa had set up camp by a farm gateway off the road, fresh juice and dinner was ready for us and we were able to get off to bed by 9pm. A long day and another World Record for Female and Couple 200 Consecutive Marathons, one of those limping across the line marathons! Total Km 8603.61. Average 43.02km per marathon.

Marathon #201.

July 20, 2013. 20 km west of Sandfire to 75 km east of Pardoo Roadhouse. Started at 5:05am in dark. Daybreak was very long before the sun rose into a clear sky, migratory birds flying from the desert sands towards the ocean, the sound of their honking very different to the morning chorus we've been used to. Both of us running okay despite our injuries. Had 5 bananas each at 8km, green smoothies at 15 km, ran another 10km to the turnoff to Eighty Mile Beach. Remembered to turn off the Garmin and drove to the beach for a quick foot bath in the Indian Ocean. Beautiful white sand and shell beach, very isolated except for a few campers picking up shells. Spent about an hour at the beach then had some melon and a raw pumpkin and carrot soup that Melissa had made and put in the sun to warm it up. A delicious interlude. Drove back to the Hwy, started running and forgot to turn the Garmin on for about 1 km! Heading SW with 18 km to go, good run to finish at 42.62 km after a brilliant sunset around 7pm. Myke and Melissa had camp set up, juice and pumpkin noodles for dinner all ready for us again. Got to bed at 9pm, another long day but worth the stop at the beach. Temp 13-25 degrees. Total Km 8646.23. Marathon Average 43.02km.

Marathon #202.

July 21, 2013. 75 km east of Pardoo to 33 km east of Pardoo. Started 5am in the dark, walking out to road and headed East instead of west for about 150 meters before we realised we were going the wrong way! Thought it strange that the light of daybreak was ahead of us! Road and terrain much the same as before, wind much stronger blowing us along from behind. When the road trains passed us the wind force doubled and picked our pace up to twice the speed causing shin splints by the end of the day. We were thinking that someone could start up a great adventure tour where you bring the adventurers out to the Great Northern Hwy alongside the Great Sandy Desert, line them up on the side of the road in the red sand, wait for a great big road train to come along from behind, start them running and the wind will pick them up, double their speed and they'd be running on air, Great Fun! Continued to run on air for the rest of the day, finished at 42.42 km to camp off the side of the road in the sand. Fresh juice and salad before going to bed at 7pm, yay 9 hrs sleep tonight! Temp 13-28 degrees. Total Km 8688.65.

Marathon #203.

July 22, 2013. 33 km east of Pardoo to 10 km west of Pardoo Roadhouse. Started 5am in dark with moon setting ahead of us. Today was a rescue day, herds of cows and furry caterpillars all over the road. The cow herd were on both sides of the road ahead of us when a road train was approaching them, honking to stop them from crossing the road. They all stayed where they were, the road train came through and we heaved a sigh of relief, only to realise that another road train was coming from behind us and some of the herd had started to cross the road. We were much closer by then and we shouted and waved frantically to make them move faster and to alert the truck driver. It worked for the driver who geared down and honked the horn, but the truck was going too fast to stop. So then the cows stopped right in the middle of the road and our hearts stopped right in the middle of our mouths! We yelled and screamed at them as the road train came closer, they didn't even look up, but did decide to amble across the road, reaching the other side just as the truck rolled through missing them by only a meter. By then we were also upon them, chastising them severely as the rest of the herd started to wander across the road to join them, completely oblivious to our presence! We stopped shortly afterwards for our break and gathering our nerves, went back out on the road, only to find herds of furry caterpillars crossing the road! There were hundreds of them, all crossing the road as fast as their little legs could take them, apparently fully aware of the danger but determined to cross nonetheless. We started picking them up and carrying them across, putting them in the bushes well off the side of the road, but there were too many. Luckily they were concentrated in a small area of about 1 km stretch, so hopefully most of them made it to wherever they were going. Way too much excitement for us in one day! We arrived at Pardoo Roadhouse with 10 km to go, Myke and Melissa set up in a complimentary campsite (thanks for your hospitality Ian and Sarah) while we ran on to finish at 43.70 km. Melissa came out to pick us up and we drove back for an early dinner of delicious zucchini pasta with beetroot and watermelon juice. The radiator hose for SuperRoo had arrived so Alan put that on, all looking good under the bonnet for now. Laundry, showers and bed. Temp 15-24 degrees. Total Km 8732.35.

Marathon #204.
July 23, 2013. 10 km west of Pardoo Roadhouse to 54 km west of Pardoo on Floodway. We all departed Pardoo Campground with both vehicles and van at 5:10am, drove 10 km to where we had finished yesterday. Started running 5:20am heading west towards the setting moon. Much warmer this morning (Temp 17-34 degrees) and the wind not so strong or cold. Melissa and Myke caught us up right on sunrise for a quick water break then drove on to the 15 km stop to make green smoothies. Rough rocky road all day so hard on the feet, but otherwise both running well with less pain from our various injuries. Good thing we don't get injured from running, it's the stopping abruptly that does the damage! However, everything is healing quickly and not affecting our running. Had watermelon for midway break and finished the run at 44.29 km, set up camp off the road in the middle of a floodway that is hard packed so safe as long as it does not rain. Nice early finish with juice and salad ready, Myke and Melissa off to the tent to watch a video while we eat and get an early night, 6pm the sun has set and we're off to bed. Total Km 8776.64.

Marathon #205.
July 24, 2013. 54 km west of Pardoo to Gravel Pit 42 km east of Port Hedland. Started 4:50am in dark, running by the light of the moon. Both running well all day including a 7 km hill

climb. Rough road with no shoulder again so having to get off and wait for the traffic to pass before continuing on the road. A lot more traffic as we get closer to Port Hedland, mostly mining trucks and road trains carrying iron ore to the Port. Nice weather, 36 degrees but feels lower with a cool following breeze and no humidity. Our food is right down to the last banana, only one day's food left, but we'll be at Coles tomorrow to stock up. Melissa doing a great job of making delicious meals out of few ingredients. Stopped at a rest area by a river with water in it, good to see after so many dry riverbeds. Met Louie from NZ who had seen us on the road a few times since Broome, quote of the day, "There's just us grey nomads and a few trucks out here," thanks for the donation Louie & Colleen. Only a few km to go and a truck pulled over, the guys offered us some cold water and said, "If no-one has already told you, I'm telling you, you're mad!" Nice one guys, thanks for the water! Finished the run 45.23 km opposite the entrance to a quarry with loads of trucks coming and going, not suitable to stay the night so we drove another 1 km and there was a track going off to a dream camping spot under a rocky outcrop about 1 km from the road. Still no phone or internet connection so off to bed at sunset and with the dark came the mozzies... Total Km 8821.87.

Internet....where are you? Eileen here. I can report that J&A are safe and well, almost in Port Headland and endured an 8 km hill yesterday through the iron ore mines. Crazy temperature fluctuations with cold mornings and humid 36degC in the afternoons, that's the desert for you! I am starting my summer running campaign and did 7 km yesterday (I only managed about 10 runs in 5 weeks overseas!) - how about you? J&A's goal is to help people live more consciously and that includes (for me) getting off the couch!

Marathon #206.

July 25, 2013. 42 km east of Port Hedland to South Hedland Cemetery. Melissa drove us out to where we had finished yesterday and we started at 5am, running towards the moon and the lights of Port Hedland in the distance. A cold wind had got up in the early hours and blown the mozzies away, but we had to wear our jackets until the sun rose and warmed us up. Very busy on the road with road trains and mining trucks again, no edge to a very rough road, felt like we were tip-toeing through the stones. Toots and waves from the drivers and most slowing down as they passed. One stopped where Myke and Melissa were parked waiting for us and gave a donation, thanks Laine & Jenny. As if the road wasn't rough enough, we came into road works for most of the run into South Hedland. The first group of road workers stopped what they were doing and cheered us on as we ran through, then we recognised the guys who gave us water yesterday amongst them, so they must have told their workmates. Thanks for the encouragement guys! Between the two major road works we were crossing a small bridge and were surrounded by hundreds of swallows flying out from under the bridge and into the air above us. We looked below the bridge and sure enough, there were the mud nests attached underneath in the culverts. So beautiful to see the little birds in flight, but sadly one was caught in the updraft from a passing truck and was thrown to the ground in front of us, mercifully he died instantly. Janette picked him up and laid him to rest under a tree, his little flight pattern is done. But our run was not over, so we headed back out and just past the turn-off to Port Hedland we came into major road works again, very little space for us to go and very rough, back to tiptoeing through the stones and rubble. Running in single file with Alan in front, the unexpected happened. About 2 metres ahead of him on the edge of the road was a large socket spanner. As he drew nearer, suddenly the spanner flew upwards into the air, a truck wheel having just touched it and sent it spinning. It seemed like the next few seconds went into slow motion, as the spanner spun over and over, higher and higher, then stopped midair and hurtled towards the ground landing only inches away from Alan's feet. Shaken but not stirred, he picked it up and threw it further off the road, muttered "that was close, could have taken off my leg and that would have put me out of the running." Just when we thought it couldn't get much worse, we came into some serious road works and the roughest piece of road on the whole trip so far. We were reduced to a fast walk along the edge of newly sealed road, with extremely sharp little stones scattered on the dirt. The stones were being thrown up by passing trucks onto the edge where we were walking, Janette was hit in the knee and back of the neck and said, "A little bird told me that this was a dangerous road..." We battled our way across the road to a cycle path and finished today's run at 43.75 km outside the local cemetery, both very close to dead (pun intended). Had a quick juice to revive our spirits and drove into South Hedland township to do food shopping at Coles and

Alan took SuperRoo to see the local mechanic who pronounced the car good to go, "Probably just needs a good long run." Classic! Myke & Melissa drove SuperRoo back to where we had finished the run, we drove YouBeautUte and Van to fuel up and take on water then back to set up camp in the Dead Centre of Town. Should be a quiet night tonight, not much action by the local residents...bed at 11:30pm. Temp 16-34 degrees. Total Km 8865.62.

Marathon #207.

July 26. 2013 Sth Hedland Cemetery to Truck Stop 59 km east of Whim Creek. Started at 6am after sleeping in to 5:30am, not much movement or noise from the cemetery but the road noise went all night so must have eventually fallen asleep when we should have been getting up! Walked out of the cemetery onto the road amongst the heavy traffic, huge 4-trailer road trains carrying iron ore, 4-trailer super tankers, oversized truck trains 60 metres long with 86 wheels carrying giant mining equipment and of course, the Grey Nomads in their campers, fifth wheelers and 4WDs towing caravans, all larger than our vehicles but appearing squished and undersized in between the monster trucks. Still amongst road works and very rough road, air filled with dust from the trucks filling our eyes and nose, and we could feel the grit between our teeth. Worst morning run yet until we got to the turnoff to Newman where all the trucks were going to and coming from the mines there. Stopped just past the turnoff for our break and were relieved to see the road was smooth, wider verge and the air clean. We had been on the Great Northern Hwy for 1683 km came off it at the Newman turnoff, we were shattered from the constant traffic noise, wind from the trucks, the dust and the iron ore in the air, but now on the Nth West Coastal Hwy with very little traffic, the contrast was overwhelming. Finished the run at 42.97 km at a Truck Stop off the road, got to bed by 8pm. Temp 10-33 degrees. Total Km 8908.59.

Marathon #208.

July 27, 2013. 59 km to 14 km east of Whim Creek on the NW Coastal Hwy. Started 5am, running by the light of the moon. Sunrise at 6:40am, getting later as we go further west. Road smoother, but still no shoulder. Had one close encounter with a car coming from behind passing another vehicle right were we were running (single file on the other side of the white line) missed us by inches and must have been doing 130 km per hour, there was a clear straight road ahead of us which you could see for about 10 km. We both had to stop to catch our breath after that one. Later we had an oncoming vehicle slow down and out of the passenger window is a hand waving a donation! Thanks Alex and Janet for your support and for stopping to say hi, made the rest of the run very peaceful. Landscape changing with the desert more sandy and a few hills, also huge pyramid shaped heaps of rocks which we think may be the result of prospecting on a large scale. Stopped for our last break on the desert floodway, wildflowers are springing up everywhere, tiny white bouquets, masses of bright yellow and bunches of purple, brilliant against the red sand. Finished the run at 43.23 km where Melissa was waiting to pick us up and drive forward to the camping spot in a disused driveway to an old quarry opposite a 3G repeater station, so catching up on the internet and off to bed by 8pm. Temp 16-30 degrees. Total Km 8951.83.

Marathon # 209.

July 28, 2013. 14 km east to 30 km west of Whim Creek on NW Coastal Hwy. Melissa drove us back to where we finished yesterday, started 5am under the moon. Myke drove ahead to Whim Creek Roadhouse to do laundry, take on water, have shower etc, only to find a ghost town, everything closed up, no-one around except confused travelers! We had run 118 km to find this, too bad we were looking forward to showers, oh well, next roadhouse 85 km away in Roebourne. Phone and internet connection very strong at the abandoned roadhouse so stayed for a couple of hours to catch up. Had our smoothies and were heading back to the road when our Kiwi friends Louie and Colleen rolled in, you caught us up again, see you further on down the road! Phoned in our food order to Coles in Karata, it will be one of the longest stretches we'll be doing without any towns, roadhouses or stores from Karata to Carnarvon, so it will be a big food shop too. Continued on through changing landscape, more rocky outcrops on the wide expanse of sandy desert, looking like a Zen Garden with all the grass and wildflowers in bloom. Finished the run at 42.96 km, set up camp on the desert sand alongside the road. Delicious dinner and off to bed 7:30. Temp 14-33 degrees. Total Km 8994.79.

Marathon #210.

July 29, 2013. 30 km west of Whim Creek to 8 km East of Roebourne. Started at 5am, running west in the dark, half moon giving a little light. Stopped to watch the sun come up, standing still in the desert Zen garden and listening to chimes on the wind in the distance, felt like we were somewhere in Tibet. Think we might go there after we finish the Run, or maybe to an Ashram in India, and just Be for a while. Meanwhile, back on the NW Coastal Hwy in the Pilbara, Western Australia, we're running another marathon through a red sandy desert bursting into colour with thousands of wildflowers, pink, purple, yellow, red and white amongst the lime green grass.

Far in the distance the scene is surrounded by flat topped hills, deep red and purple in the sunrise, a dramatic effect on the landscape. A small herd of deep chestnut horses, 3 adults and 2 tiny foals, cantering across the field of green, wild and free. Two dingoes amongst the scrub watching the horses and howling as the sun rises into an azure sky. We linger awhile taking in the scene and count our blessings to be here on this day, a special time and place. Today's run finished at 43.02 km, camped on the desert sand across the road from the Mingullatharndo Community. As we drank our fresh juice we received a visit from the Community Pastor who came to make sure we were okay and give his blessing on our day. Our special day, 210 consecutive marathons and a total of 9037.81 Km.

Marathon # 211.

July 30, 2013. 8 km East of Roebourne to Gravel Pit 1 km west of Karatha Turnoff. Started 5am, another starry morning running in to Roebourne Caravan Park. Arrived too early for the manager to be around, but met Graeme who lives i the Park while working on the drilling rigs in the area, "They wont tell us what we're drilling for, but we think it's gold!" He had seen us on the road for the past few days and wondered what we were running for, "I figured you've got to be doing it to raise awareness for something, no-one would be doing it for fun!" We explained that we were wanting to have showers and do the laundry and he said, "Help yourself, I'm sure that will be fine and if not, I'll pay for it." Thanks Graeme, but we did see the manager before we left and she was more than happy to help out, even gave us coins for the laundry, thanks Shaun, Kylie & Tru for your hospitality and support. Sure felt good to have a hot shower and wash off all the red dust and road dirt. Back out on the road again, run through the historic township of Roebourne and on towards Karatha. Very heavy traffic all the way, almost got hit several times by vehicles passing road trains from behind us. There was no verge on the side of the road so we had to get right off onto the sloping rough area alongside, lots of stones and stumps so it was a nerve-wracking run to finish 1 km past the Karatha turnoff at 42.22km. Myke and Melissa had set up camp in a disused gravel pit area off the road for a quiet night away from the traffic. Bed 8:3pm. Temp 16-31 degrees. Total Km 9080.03.

Marathon #212.
July 31, 2013. 1 km west to 41 km west of Karatha Turnoff. Started 5am running SW on the NW Coastal Hwy for 7.5km where Melissa drove to pick us up. Drove back to Karatha, Myke following in the Ute & Van as we passed the camp spot and into Coles at Karatha to do the food shopping for two weeks as there are no shops between Karatha and Carnarvon. The food order consisted of fresh raw fruits and veges; 5 boxes bananas, 4 boxes oranges, 6 whole watermelon, 1 box grapefruit, 1 box kiwifruit, pears, lemons, pawpaw, avocadoes, tomatoes, zucchini, cucumber, corn, carrots, beetroot, cauliflower, broccoli, silverbeet and other greens, should keep us going for a couple of weeks!. Four hours later we had the food stored in the vehicles and rolled out with the vehicles low to the ground! Drove back to where we had finished this morning, Melissa dropped us off and they drove on another 7 km while we got back on the road to continue the run. Met a traveler parked at a rest stop, we chatted for a while and he gave us a donation, thanks Peter for your support. Myke and Melissa drove on to set up camp before it got dark, Melissa drove back to meet us as the sun was setting, bringing food and water which we ate watching the sun go down. Then she left us to finish the last 2

hours of the run in the dark, it was a thrill to see the caravan light at 42.46km just off the road at a farm gateway, finished at 8:30pm, a 17 hour day. Temp 16-34 degrees. Total Km 9122.57.

August 2013

MARATHONS #213-243

It's tough going up there! Eileen here. J&A are without the basic necessities of life: phone coverage and internet (imagine), but managed to get a message through to me via morse code. They did a 17 hour day yesterday while they passed through Karatha so they could load their enormous food order. They're on their way to Canarvon now and it's 15 days without a single shop! They advise it's a lovely day in the dessert today with a bit of a tail wind- ya gotta take what you can get!!!

Marathon #213.

August 1, 2013. *A very special day, we dedicate today's run to our granddaughter who turns 7 today, Happy Birthday Sweetheart.* Farm Gateway 41 km west of Karatha to 17 km east of Fortesque Roadhouse. Started 5am in the dark, both felt tired this morning after the long day yesterday and not enough sleep. Very quiet on the road, running in the middle as the edge still very rough. Very dark but lots of lights in the distance of gas plants with flame towers glowing, making an eerie scene. Ran past a huge gas plant at daybreak, looked like a small town with hundreds of lights and the smell of gas heavy in the air. Into early morning rush hour with hundreds of small trucks going to the mines and gas plants, all traveling very fast and passing the road trains all at once. We're wearing our high-visibility vests throughout the day as we had a few close encounters from behind yesterday. Traffic thinned out after a couple of hours and we were into rolling hills with purple wildflowers everywhere. Stopped to chat with Bill, a truck owner/driver pulled over with his road train for his compulsory 20 min break. He asked, "Where did you come from?" and we replied "Melbourne." "You must be mad" he said, "where are you going?" "Melbourne" we said again. "You are mad!" he declared. We told him why we were running and about the Charities that we're raising awareness for. He immediately said, "I better get you some money for that," and climbed into his cab to get a donation, thanks Bill for your support. See you on the road! Finished the run at 42.93km, camped for the night just off the road in a Zen Garden of grass clumps and purple wildflowers. Temp 17-35 degrees. Total Km 9165.50.

Marathon #214.

August 2, 2013. *Another very special day, we dedicate today's run to our grandson who turns 4 today, Happy Birthday Little Man.* 17 km east to 26 km west of Fortescue River Roadhouse. Started 5am in dark, starry sky but no moon. Stopped at Fortescue River Roadhouse to take on water, do laundry and have showers, thanks for your hospitality and support. We were able to connect to the internet to read emails but not to upload data. Received devastating news of a dear friend's sudden death, found it very hard to stay focussed to finish the run at 42.64 km. Myke and Melissa had set up camp on a roadside spot amongst the rocks and flowering shrubs, another of Mother Nature's Zen Gardens. So we built a cairn to honour and remember our friend, out in nature's garden somewhere in the desert in Western Australia. Temp 16-34 degrees. Total Km 9208.14.

Marathon #215.

August 3, 2013. 26 km west of Fortescue to 89 km east of Nanutarra Roadhouse. Started at 5am, after stopping briefly at the cairn and sending love to our other dear friend who will be grieving the loss of a dearly loved, kind and compassionate man. The early part of the run was slow with our hearts heavy with sadness and thoughts filled with memories of times spent together with our dear friends. The temp rose from 16 to 36 degrees as we plodded along the rocky road, feeling very down and finding it hard to pick up momentum. Just before the midway break we were met by Alice, a raw foodie from Perth currently working here in the mines, who had heard of us through the Perth Raw Group. She was so excited to see us as she passed on her way to work, she stopped and wrote an encouraging message on the pink tape she uses to mark possible mining sites. We arrived just as she was finishing, so we had a great chat, her enthusiasm for what we are doing was so uplifting, thanks Alice. We finished the run at 43.59 km, a Total of 9251.78 Km and an average of 43.03 km per marathon. We now have only 150 marathons to finish 365 in 365 days.

Marathon #216.

August 4, 2013. 89 km to 43 km east of Nanutarra Roadhouse. Started at 5am in the dark again, very starry sky with no moon. Today we stopped to talk with several people, it was good to have the diversion from our sad thoughts and feeling of loss. We met Chris who is following us on FB after hearing about RunRAW2013 from the other drivers on the road every day in this area. Chris pulled over after seeing us several times on the road the last few days, great to meet you and thanks for the donation. Also met Fiona, another Pilot driver whom Chris had told to look out for us on road., great job you two are doing, keeping us all safe on the road, thanks. Alice caught up with us again, she and her colleague Paul stopped to sign our book and take photos. Hope we catch up with you in Perth! Peter who is biking around Australia stopped to talk, he comes from a place not far from where we lived in Canada, "it's a small world amongst the crazies." With no backup crew and only a small bag attached to the bike bar and a smaller bag with his hammock tent tied on the back, he is the lightest traveler we've met yet. Stay safe on the road Peter. We finished the run 43.35 km at the rest stop by the Onslow turnoff and met 2 couples in camper and bus (1 couple live about 5 km from us, when we're home that is!) who had seen us on Sunrise TV and were wondering "whatever happened to that old couple who were going to run around Australia?" We had a laugh and chat about the Run so far and they gave us donations and best wishes, thanks for your support. Must be time to get back on Sunrise again! Temp 15-35 degrees. Total Km 9296.13. Ave 43.04km. 150 marathons to the world record for 366 consecutive marathons, stay with us!

Marathon #217.

August 5, 2013. 43 km east to Campground Nanutarra Roadhouse. Started 5am in the dark, following the stars and thinking of our dear departed friend and another dear friend and running buddy, and friends so far away, love travels countless kilometers to be with you today, this one is for you...

Tragedy...when you're feeling strong but you can't go on...

Tragedy...the words of the song keep hurtling through my head...
Stopping by the roadside to read who else is gone...and Jamie the Rock Star is dead,
His guitar attached to a single white cross, marking the spot where he died.
A note on the back "I tried to save you but I couldn't"...and I cried.
Strumming the song in my head, the sound of his guitar echoing on and on...
Tragedy...a Friend is gone but his Love lives on...
We shared so much and now we share the pain and sorrow, the grief, the loss.
Tragedy...when the feelings gone and you can't go on...
We're thinking of you while pounding the pavement...and going nowhere...
Tragedy...a Friend is gone, but we must go on.
Tragedy...the words of the song keep pounding through my head
With every step I take, reminding me of you...we will Run On my Friend.
A dear Friend and running buddy, lost but not forgotten, your light will shine on.
Tragedy....

Today's Run 43.39 km. Total Km 9339.52.

Marathon #218.

August 6, 2013. Nanutarra to 43 km west of Nanutarra. Started 5am in dark and had a lovely surprise at daybreak to find we were surrounded by wildflowers, mostly blooming on shrubs and small plants alongside the road. Got the camera at the first break and took photos all day, so many different varieties and colour that we didn't notice the rough and hilly road so much. Met a very large bull on the side of the road whom we coaxed away and back into the bush, a beautiful beast roaming free, please stay away from the road. Came over a hill to see a long straight ahead with signs and white markings on the road, a designated airstrip for the Royal Flying Doctor Service. We stopped at Cave Creek for our last break, visited the cave above the dry creek bed looking out along the road we had traveled. Finished the run at 43.03 km camped in a roadside Zen Garden. Temp 15-34 degrees. Total Km 9382.55. Ave 43.04km.

Marathon #219.

AUGUST 2013

August 7, 2013. 43 km west of Nanutarra to 137 km east of Minilya Roadhouse. Started 5:10am, no moon but many stars and constellations to watch as we ran in the middle of the road until daybreak. Decided to have a 4 Froothie day as the bananas are ripening fast; first smoothie bananas, grapefruit, dates and ginger, second smoothie bananas, grapefruit and greens, third smoothie bananas and pawpaw, fourth smoothie bananas, pawpaw and avocado. Also had 5 bananas at the water breaks so consumed 25 bananas each today. Met up with Kim and his crew cycling round Australia for MND (motor neurone disease) < nomnd.com.au > We all stopped for midway break out in the desert together, great to share some stories, stay safe on the road and stay in touch. Also met the Riksmans at a rest stop, thanks for your donation and support. Finished the run at 44.31 km in another roadside garden. Temp 16-34 degrees. Total Km 9426.96.

August 8, 2013.
Back on the road midway through Marathon # 220, more updates later......Running on...

Comments from Facebook/RunningRawAroundAustralia2013:

- *Awesome!* - **Dan**
- *Yes, great fun to see!* - **Jeff**
- *You are amazing!* - **Solar**
- *Wow! I cant believe you two.* - **Jason**
- *Gosh. you guys are amazing.* - **Anika**
- *Think of you guys every day driving to Onslow .. miss seeing you on the road.* - **Chris**
- *Can't believe you guys - Walter (cycling around Australia for Dementia Research & I met you 2 months ago!! Well done!! Our journey ends in 3 days and you have so many more!!-* **Deanne**
- *God bless u 2!* - **Nico**
- *Wonderful live.* - **Tatiana**
- *Fantastic effort. Keep up the energy!!* - **Laurel**
- *Inspiring, and what an experience! Love that countryside.* - **Lisa**

Marathon #220.

August 8, 2013. 137 km to 94 km east of Minilya Roadhouse. Started 5am in the dark, starry sky till daybreak, a brilliant red line in the Eastern sky. Watched the sun come up as the birds sang the morning chorus. Terrain undulating hills, fascinating landscape of green pin cushions (spinafex) on red sand in the gullies and bright pink tea tree shrubs lining the cuttings through the hilltops. Smooth road with plenty of shoulder until the Exmouth turnoff, then back to rough stones, no line on edge and rocky drop-off. We have to get off road and stop while the vehicles go by from either direction, it's too dangerous to keep running on that terrain. It's also safer for us to see the vehicles coming from behind in case they are passing and in the lane that we're running on facing the traffic. So we're losing quite a bit of time and momentum with all the stops, but at least we're getting lots of toots and waves, especially from all the truckies who are very considerate and try to give us a wide berth when they can. The wind they create can knock us back 2 or 3 meters sometimes so we have to brace ourselves when they come along, especially the very long road trains. So a special thanks to all the truckies on the road who really make our day when they pull on their air horns! We keep ourselves amused by reading the names on the trucks, here's a few from today: 'Duz Tha Job', 'End of the Line', 'Bushroo', and 'Still Hungry'. That one needs to eat more bananas! Myke and Melissa parked the vehicles for the last break amongst a field of white flowers that looked like snow on the ground, the first of the everlasting daisies. We had a strong head wind for the last couple of hours run, finished at 42.76km camped on the side of the road. Temp 14-32 degrees. Total Km 9469.72. Marathon Average 43.04 km.

Marathon #221.

August 9, 2013. 94 km to 50 km east of Minilya. Started at 5am in the dark, cool and damp mist with very wet dew, 15-32 degrees today. Long straights on road disappearing into a mirage about 15km ahead, very few corners but a few hills and gullies that define the strange landscape. Less and less bushes and more red sand visible. Mostly yellow wildflowers en masse art ground level and a few purple bushes. Met up with the PedalitForward Team, 2 cyclists and 1 driver biking around Australia to raise awareness and funds for World Bicycle

Relief, a charity dedicated to providing bicycles to developing communities in Africa. Great to meet you three Joel, Jordan and (Paralympian) Luke, showing the world that you are never too young to be kind and compassionate and that actions speak louder than words. Stay safe on the road, you're almost there, we'll see you in Perth. Finished at 42.88km, Myke & Melissa had found a nice spot off the road to camp for the night, off to bed by 8pm. Total Km 9512.60. Marathon Average 43.04km.

Marathon #222.

August 10, 2013. 50 km to 6.5km east of Minilya Roadhouse. Started at 5:10am, dark, no moon but clear starry sky. Daybreak revealed a vast landscape of scrubby bush and red sand with mauve wildflowers on the side of the road. We're back amongst the wild animals, kangaroos and emus evident, but haven't seen any alive yet. So sad to see so many piles of bleached bones lying in the sand. Another Froothie smoothie day, 25 bananas and 15 kiwifruit each - 4000 calories. Finished 43.11km and Melissa drove us on to Minilya Bridge Roadhouse where Myke had set up camp in a complimentary site, thanks for your hospitality and support, Mark & Danielle, Nicole and Wayne and for the donation. Great to get the laundry done and have hot showers. Janette was up till 11pm catching up on the internet. Temp 16-32 degrees. Total Km 9555.71. Marathon Average 43.04 km.

Marathon #223.

August 11, 2013. 6.5 km east of Minilya Roadhouse to 100 km North of Carnarvon. Melissa drove us back 6.5 km to where we had finished yesterday and we started 5am in dark, cool (15-31.5 degrees). Strong head winds all day making our running slow and Janette tired from only 5 hours sleep last night. Received a phone call to tell us that Kim from No MND had been interviewed on Macca's morning show on ABC Radio and mentioned RunRAW2013. For the rest of the morning we received toots and thumbs-up from the motorists passing us, seems like everyone listens to Macca on Sunday mornings. Hope we will get to be interviewed on the show soon. Meanwhile, we kept plodding on into the wind on a rough road, finishing at 43.80 km at roadside spot for the night. Soaked our feet in Epsom salts and off to bed by 8pm.

Total Km 9599.57. Marathon Average 43.05km.

Marathon #224.

August 12, 2013. 100 km south of Minilya to 56 km north of Carnarvon. Started at 5am, cold (16-31 degrees), but wind not as strong as yesterday. Daybreak revealed red sand on either side of the road, some scrubby bush but more like desert than before. Had to remove a large kangaroo from the road that had been hit only minutes before we got to it, mercifully it must have died instantly. Later we witnessed a very sad and heartbreaking scene where a bull had been hit, must have gone to the side of the road where he collapsed. When we got there, a cow and calf were walking around him, the cow stopping and gently pushing him with her nose, trying to help him get up, the calf standing beside the bull, with his head on one side staring into the bull's eyes with a questioning look - "come on Dad, get up, please get up"...but his father could not move, his front legs had given way beneath his huge body, the weight of the enormous beast had pushed him forward, his head pushing into the sand, his eyes no longer seeing his little calf's pleading look. The cow pushed him again with her nose, gently coaxing him to get up, but there was no longer any movement from her mate. We watched as she tried one last time, then nudged her calf and turned away, walking slowly into the bush, her calf following her, his head turning back just once to look at his dying father and then they were gone. The great beast lying alone by the side of the road gave a shudder and breathed his last breath. Never in all our years and even with Alan's years on a farm, have we witnessed such a touching show of affection and deep sadness from a loving family faced with their sudden loss. We were so moved by what we had seen that it was difficult for us to leave the scene, but there was nothing we could do and so, we ran on. Meeting a local cattle farmer further along the road, we talked for a while about the cattle 'industry' and how the live export ban was affecting their lives. She said that all the farmers were very concerned as they were still caring for their animals but had no income. Her husband had gone to work in the mines so they could afford to stay on the farm but were not sure how long they could keep going. We suggested that they turn their farm into a sanctuary and plant fruit trees instead and she said they were open to options as they did not want to walk away from their farm and leave the animals to fend for themselves. She also said that she was interested in finding out more and would go on the RunRAW2013 website so that was encouraging. We are hopeful that some conscious thinking will bring about change that will make a difference to the lives of all living beings in a kind and compassionate way, because clearly from the scene we had witnessed earlier, we are all sentient beings who care deeply about each other... We finished today's run at 43.98 km. Temp 16-31 degrees. Total 9643.49km.

Marathon #225.

August 13, 2013. 56 km to 3 km north of Carnarvon. Started at 5am in the dark, a cold and windy morning, the strong head wind hard to make headway into and pushing us backwards when the trucks go past, making for a slow, long day on the road. We're down to the last of our food, had an orange before starting the run, dehydrated bananas at the first break, dates at the second and overripe watermelon juiced for the midway stop. Meanwhile, Melissa had driven ahead to Carnarvon to buy some fresh locally grown produce from the plantations and arrived back with sweet organic bananas, oranges, grapefruit, tomatoes and black sapote, that was exciting and delicious! First time in 5 months we've been able to get fresh local fruit and veg from the growers. She and Myke drove on again to set up in a complimentary site at the Wintersun Tourist Park in Carnarvon, thanks for your hospitality and support Tracey. Melissa went back to some of the plantations for more fruit and veg then picked us up where we finished the run at 44.91 km, just 3.5km from the campground. We all had a delicious meal of fresh tomato and zucchini pasta and salad, then hot showers, laundry, internet and bed. Temp 16-30 degrees. Total Km 9688.30. Marathon average 43.06 km.

Marathon #226.

August 14, 2013. 3 km north of Carnarvon to 78km Nth of Wooramel. Melissa drove us back 3 km to where we had finished yesterday and we started running at 5:15am back towards Carnarvon, but turning to stay on Hwy 1 and bypass the town, a mass of lights in the darkness. Ran past the big Satelite Dish above the town that was used during the Apollo Space Missions and out for 10 km where Melissa met us and drove us back to the town to meet up with Myke and do the rest of the food shopping. Four hours later we left Carnarvon loaded up with fresh fruit and veg for the next 11 days run to Geraldton, Melissa dropped us off where she had picked us up earlier and we started out running again while she and Myke drove on for the next break stop. The road was rough with no shoulder again and we were running into strong head winds for the rest of the run. Melissa and Myke drove ahead to set up camp and she came back to give us water and melon at sunset, it was a very long and arduous day finishing at 42.88 km in the dark for the last 10 km. Bed at 10pm.Temp 18-27 degrees. Total Km 9731.18. Marathon Average 43.06 km.

Marathon #227.

August 15, 2013. 78 km to 34 km north of Wooramel. Started 5:30am in the dark, both a bit tired from yesterday's run and not enough sleep. Slow going again with strong head winds and rough road., kept ourselves awake by emu spotting, saw one running a lot faster than us, also saw a dingo cross the road in the distance. Had midway break outside a farm gate where there were very tall sheep, must be so they can walk through the desert landscape which has changed to mostly red sand and low scrub. We later saw a few herd of wild goats grazing on the grass by the roadside, they were very wary and ran back into the bush when they saw us coming. Thanks to Brian and Lorraine who stopped on the road to give us oranges from off their tree, they were delicious and thanks to the couple at the rest stop for their donation. Finished the run at 44.80km parked off the road on the desert sand. Temp 16-25 degrees. Total Km 9775.98. Marathon Average 43.06km.

Marathon #228.

August 16, 2013. 34 km north to 13km south of Wooramel. Started at 5:10am in the dark and cold (14-25 degrees) morning with strong head wind again, but running well today after a good sleep. No traffic for the first hour so ran in the middle of the road with the wind howling, couldn't hear the traffic but could see their lights for about 20 km on the straight road. Daybreak gave us a 360 degree view of the desert horizon, a cloudy sky with a beautiful sunrise turning the clouds pink and purple. Lots of goats and some sheep along the roadside today, the little kids running and kicking their hooves in the air and the lambs wagging their tails behind them, have I heard that somewhere before? Their cuteness at being wild and free, lightened our day's slog into the wind. Stopped for our midway break at Wooramel Roadhouse, thanks for the water and offer of a campsite and showers. Thanks to Bernie and Martin for your donation while we were at the roadhouse. We ran on another 13 km where Myke and Melissa set up camp off the road amongst a field of bright yellow wildflowers, a herd of wild goats grazing nearby. Decided not to go back to the Roadhouse but thanks for the offer. A great dinner of black sapote and mixed green salad with fresh tomatoes, in that order! Finished the run at 44.80 km. Total Km 9818.18.

Marathon #229.
August 17, 2013. 13 km south of Wooramel to 19 km north of Overlander Roadhouse. Started 5am, tired after very noisy night parked by the road and trucks going through all night. Very cold with strong head winds again. Scenery changing as we are nearer the coast, big sand hills and dried up estuaries, we ran up one of the hills to a lookout and could see where the tide comes in about 5 km to the foothills leaving sandy mudflats to the sea. Janette developed pain in the groin (we call it groin groan due to the steep camber of the road and running into strong head winds) which continued to slow progress through the rest of the run. Very busy on the road with traffic today, had to get off and stop as they passed as there is no shoulder and the edge of the road is very rough underfoot. Saw herds of wild goats in the foothills and amongst the scrubby bush beside the road. The sand is changing colour from deep red to a more mellow light apricot, the light in the sky reflecting the sandy shades at sunset. Finished the run 42.69 km in a good spot well off the road, at least 100 metres in on the sand, so a good night's sleep tonight! Bed 8:30pm. Temp 15-28 degrees. Total Km 9860.87. Marathon Average 43.06 km.

Marathon #230.
August 18, 2013. 19km Nth to 23 km Sth of Overlander Roadhouse. A Day on the Road - 4am Get up and dressed, Janette wearing tension bandage to ease the groin groan.

4:30am Make and drink smoothie: 15 bananas 5 dates, 2 grapefruit

5am Out the door running in the dark

6am Daybreak

7am Sunrise. First break: 10 bananas

8:30am At Roadhouse with free showers, laundry and internet. Green smoothie: orange, dates, bananas, silver-beet. Visit from Roadhouse cat who tried to stow away with us.

12:30pm Back on the road running

3pm Midway break: green pawpaw salad

4pm Back on road running

5:30pm Finish run 42.61km

6pm Fresh juice carrot, beetroot, green stalks and watermelon

6:30pm Avocado salad

7pm Download Garmin Data and daily blog

8pm Bed

Comment: At the 20 km mark we could see back to the start of the day's run and forward to the finish, one long straight road, accompanied by flies all the way.

Temp 14-28 degrees. Total Km 9903.48. Marathon Average 43.06. 136 marathons to go.

Marathon #231.

August 19, 2013. 23 km south of Overlander to 166 km north of Northampton. This one is for our son who is celebrating his birthday today, every step we take reminds us of you… Started 5am, very cold and strong head winds again. Janette's groin groan easing but Alan is experiencing it today. Got to 8.5 km at 7am sunrise, on to 17 km for green smoothies and to Billabong Roadhouse at 28 km, thanks for the water Jacque. Met a couple of the Linfox truck drivers who we see on the road every day, thanks for the donation Eric and for your consideration when you pass us. No phone or internet connection at the roadhouse so went to the Billabong Hotel next door where the owners kindly let us use their phone to make a Happy Birthday call and to use the internet for a couple of hours, many thanks for your support and hospitality. Left Billabong at 4pm to finish the last 16 km. Finished running by the full moon at 6:45pm, 44.71 km. Fresh juice and salad then bed by 9pm. Temp 13-28 degrees. Total Km 9948.19. Marathon Average 43.06 km.

Marathon #232.

August 20, 2013.166 km north to 122 km north of Northampton. Started at 5am with the moon setting and sun rising simultaneously. Landscape changing to more hilly, more trees and the sand colour a pale yellow. Yellow was the colour of the day, tiny yellow wildflowers on the ground and bright yellow 'gyrocopter' bugs that hover noisily above our heads then dive bomb Alan's orange high-vis vest, clutching onto him as he runs along. These beautiful bugs are quite large (2"), their yellow wings are edged with electric blue and the body is soft and fluffy like a bee, they cling on very tightly with barbed legs, Alan wasn't sure about them landing on him and clinging on for the ride, but they flew off into the trees after a while. They seemed to be coming from the gum trees that we're now seeing along the side of the road, beautiful olive coloured trunks and branches, bright red tips to the branches shiny olive leaves and pale yellow flowers. Haven't seen this variety before and it's lovely to see the old gum trees again. It was a day of surprises, later coming across what looked like a prehistoric dragon (complete with little horns sticking up on his body) standing on the road imitating a dead branch. On looking closer we could see his eye moving so tried to coax him off the road, but he was intent on staying right where he was. So Janette carefully picked him up, her fingers encircling his soft body, his little legs stuck out stiff as if he were made of stone, no part of him moving not even his eyes. She put him down on a rock well back from the road and he stayed still for a second then suddenly dashed a few inches forward onto a patch of dead leaves. Then an amazing thing happened, slowly he started to change colour and the pattern on his back completely changed to match the background on which he was standing so that we could hardly tell that he was there at all! Just like a chameleon...such an amazing display of nature at it's best. Hope he doesn't try to cross the road again, even if he did get that camouflage down it wouldn't help much. Had a nice surprise donation from a motorist who stopped and said she had seen us on the road the last few days then heard us on ABC Radio, thanks for your support! Finished the run at 43.70 km. Temp 13-25 degrees. Total Km 9991.81.

Marathon #233.

August 21, 2013. Going through the 10,000 km mark at sunrise this morning. 122 km to 79 km north of Northampton. Started at 5am, coldest morning yet (temp 11-26 degrees) but wind not so strong. Very hilly (uphill), road still rough but the groins have stopped groaning, so we're happy. Had 2 radio interviews while on the Run, 3AW Melboune and Perth Radio, both aired today with great response.Met up with Jimmy, Debbie & Ryan who are on Jimmy's Walk around Australia, going the opposite way so we were able to swap stories. Great to see the young folk putting their passion into action, way to go Jimmy! Keep your feet close to the road and stay headstrong into the wind across the Top, see you in April when you come through Melbourne. Also met Judy & Richard from NZ on the road, thanks for your donation and offer of help with support crew, stay in touch we'd love to have you along with us as we start across the Nullabor. Finished the last 11km uphill at 42.82 km in Kalbarri National Park. Marathon Average 43.07km. Total Km 10,034.63.

Marathon #234.

August 22, 2013. 79 km to 36 km north of Northampton. Started at 6am, another cold morning but wind not strong. Today we left the desert behind, climbing the rolling hills away from the sand and scrub and into fields of wheat and canola plantations, countryside looking very like scenes from France with the bright yellow canola flowers and wheat moving in the wind. We were looking out over the landscape and saw 4 emus running through a field of wheat, their feathers sweeping around them in the wind making them look like Jesuit priests with hoods on. Stopped at the Binnu Store to take on water and met Vickie who is involved in a raw retreat at Geraldton this weekend, these Raw Foodies are turning up everywhere! Thanks for the donation Vickie. Finished the Run after sunset 43.67 km, another long day and late night, good thing we're well fed during the day thanks to our support crew Melissa and Myke, thanks guys. Food consumed today, Carnarvon bananas, green smoothie, green salad, custard apple, kiwifruit, watermelon, veg juice carrots and beetroot, watermelon juice, avocado, tomatoes, fruit salad pears and bananas, all fresh from the Carnarvon growers, yum! Temp 10-20 degrees. Marathon Average 43.08 km. Total Km 10,078.30.

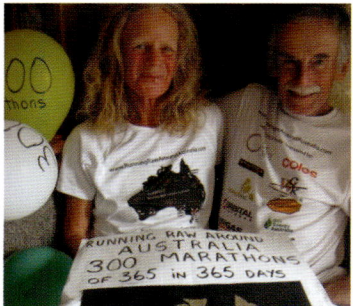

300 marathons.
(Photo courtesy Narelle Chesworth)

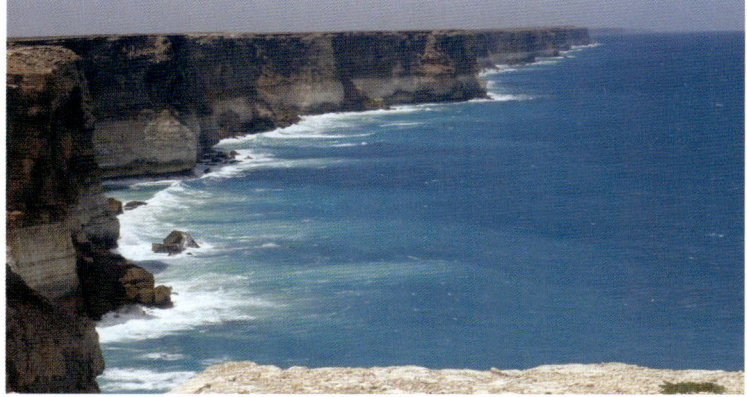

Southern Ocean meets the land, SA (Photo courtesy Narelle Chesworth)

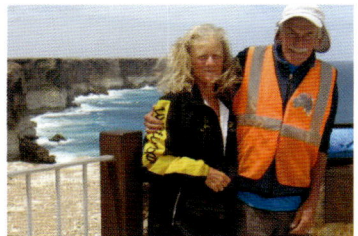

A windy day
(Photo courtesy Narelle Chesworth)

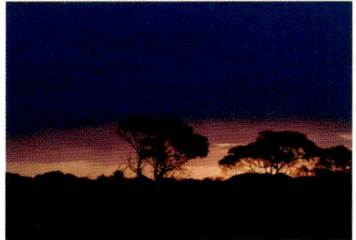

Nullarbor Sunset
(Photo courtesy Narelle Chesworth)

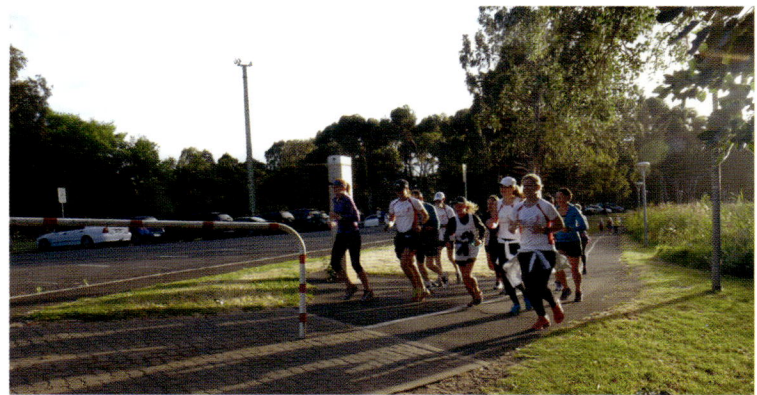

Running in Adelaide, SA (Photo courtesy Michael Gillan)

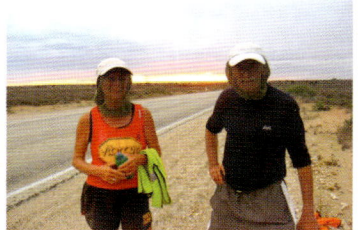

Sunset through flynets, SA
(Photo courtesy Narelle Chesworth)

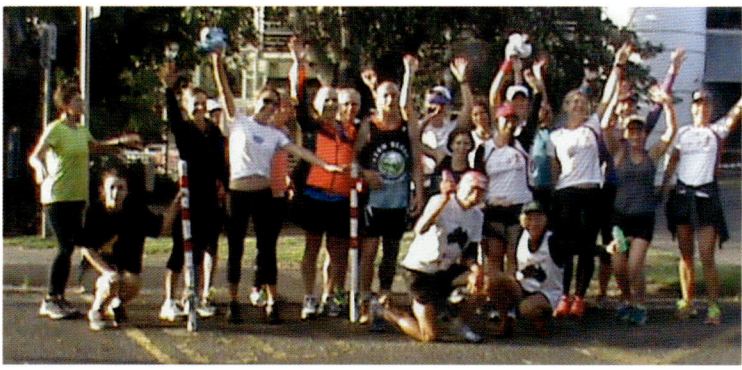

Adelaide runners. (Photo courtesy Michael Gillan)

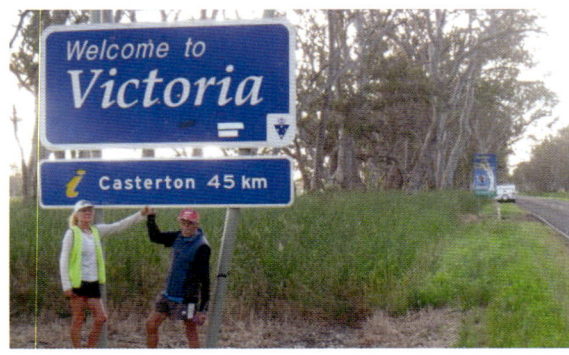
A momentous moment (Photo courtesy Michael Gillan)

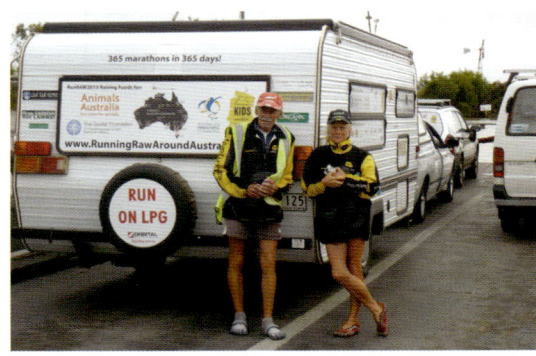
Crossing the Murray River, VIC (Photo courtesy Sylvia Pringle)

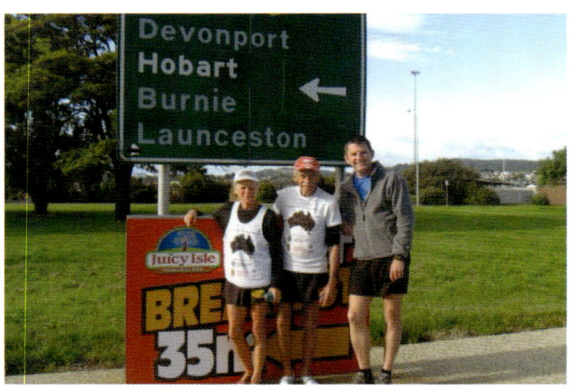
To Hobart, TAS. (Photo courtesy Sylvia Pringle)

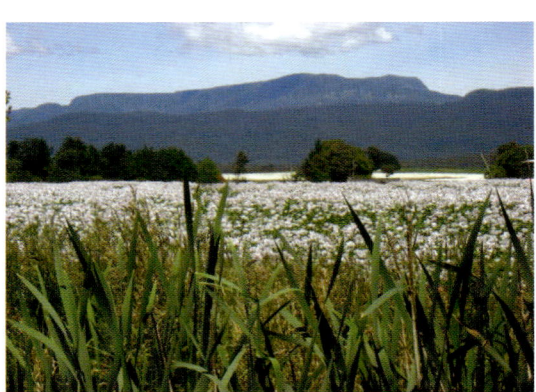
Tasmania Poppies

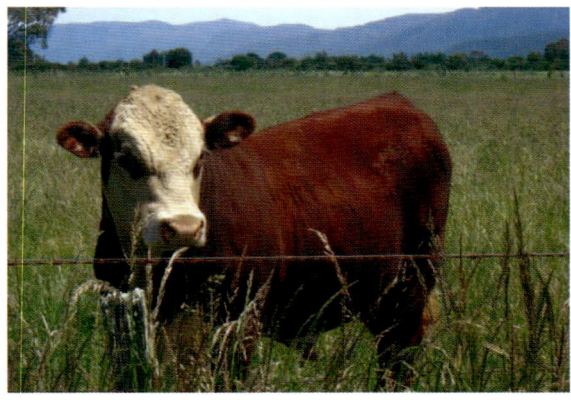
Tassie Moolaroo.

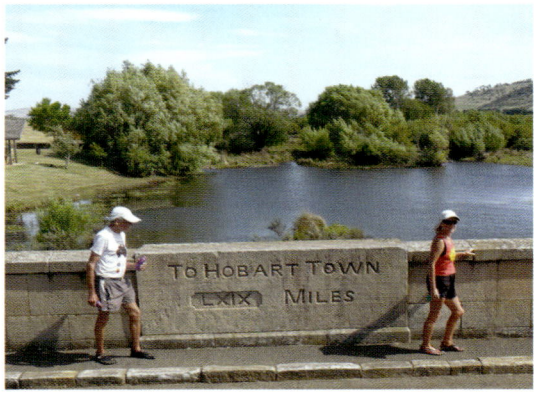
Bridge to Hobart. TAS (Photo courtesy Sylvia Pringle)

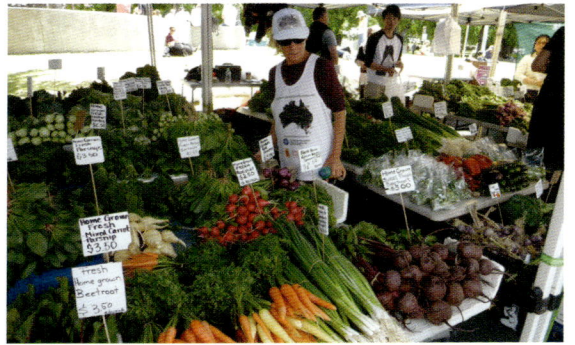
Hobart market, TAS (Photo courtesy Sylvia Pringle)

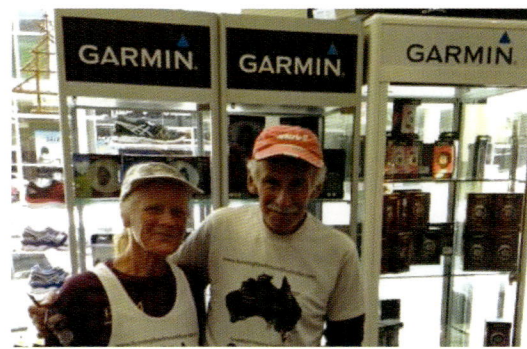
Thanks Garmin

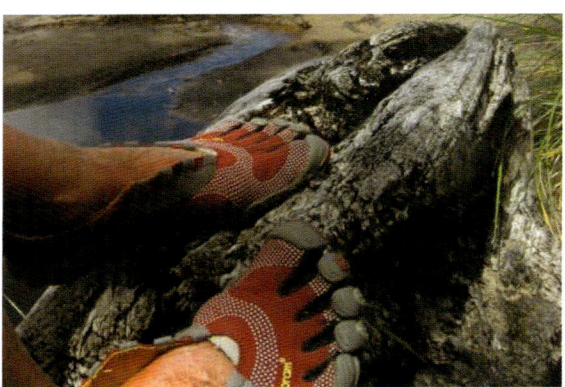
Thanks Vibram

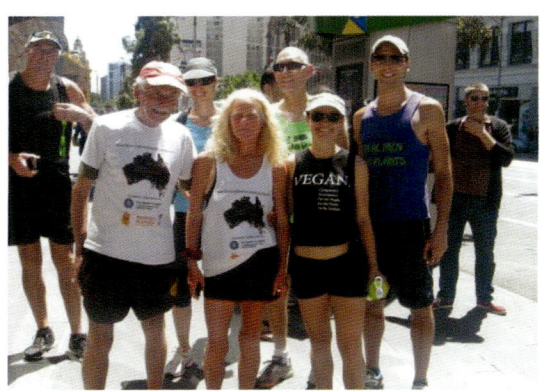
Finish 365 Marathons, Melbourne, VIC. Dec 31, 2013

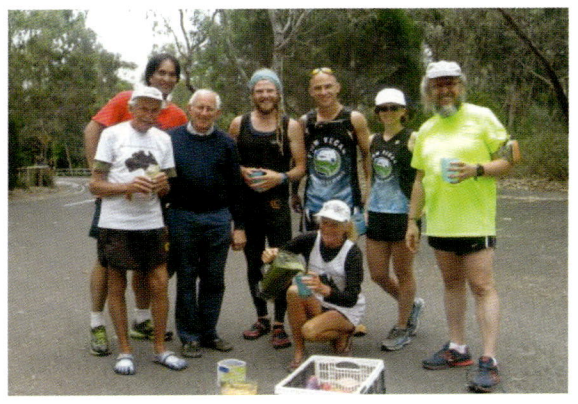
Smoothie break on #366 (Photo courtesy Melissa Kilkelly)

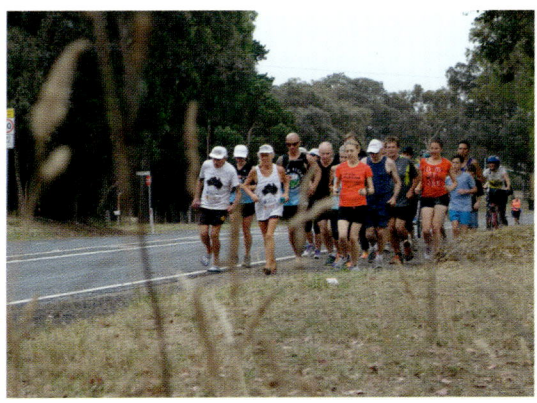
Running home (Photo courtesy Rob Berry)

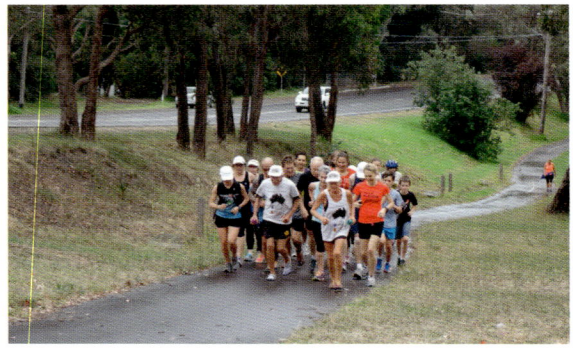
Back to the hills of home (Photo courtesy Rob Berry)

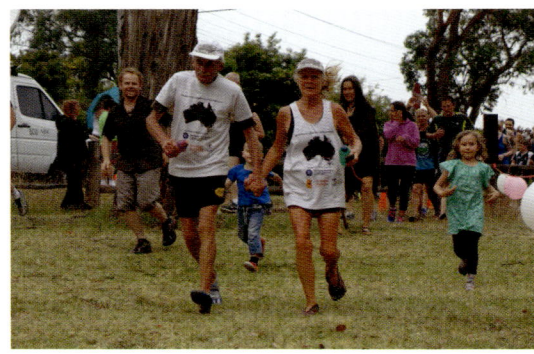
Heading for the finish line (Photo courtesy Rob Berry)

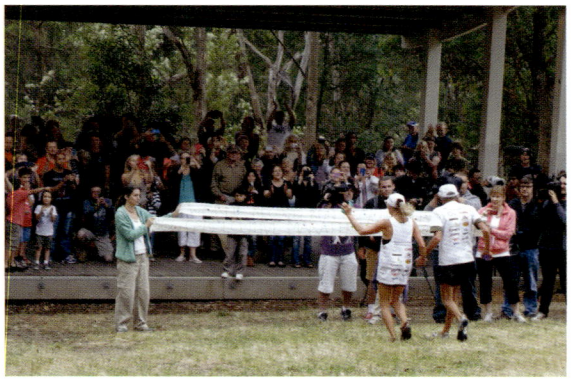
Step for step, stride for stride (Photo courtesy Rob Berry)

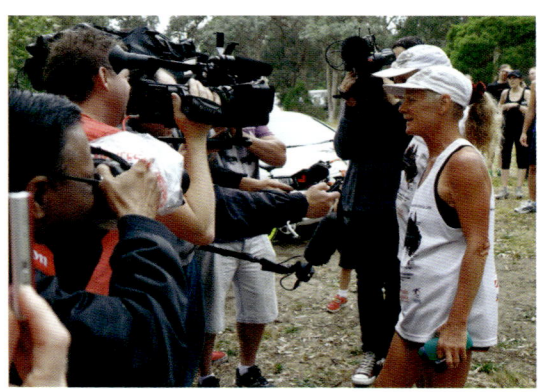
How do you feel? (Photo courtesy Rob Berry)

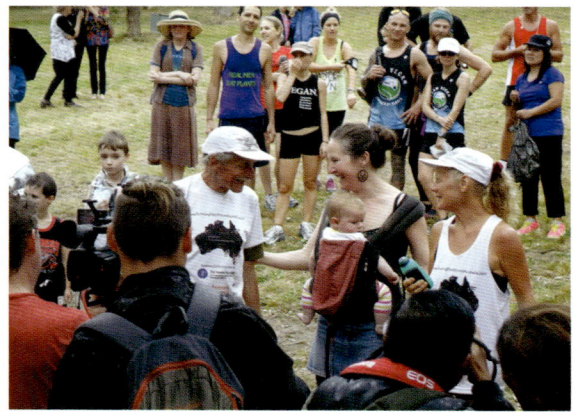
Happy to see our family (Photo courtesy Rob Berry)

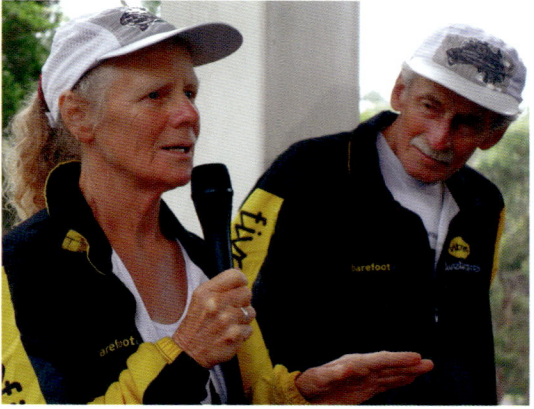
An emotional speech (Photo courtesy Rob Berry)

After the Run (Photo courtesy Cecil Bodnar)

RECIPE PHOTOS

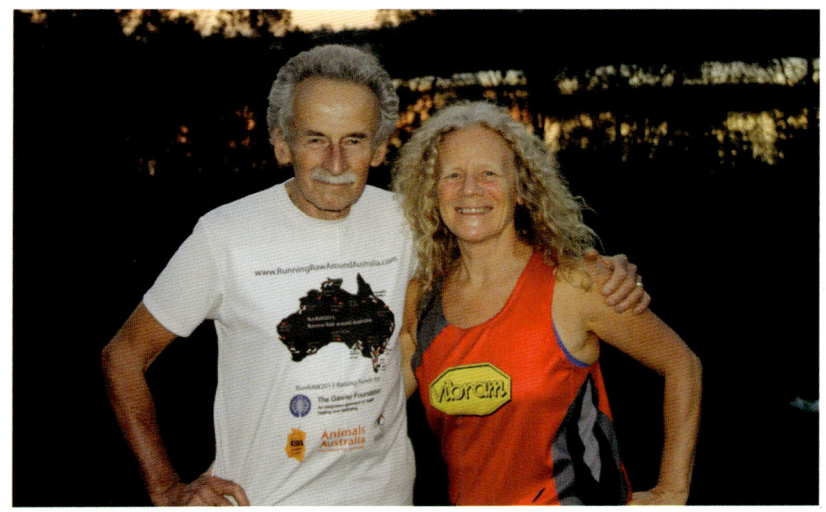

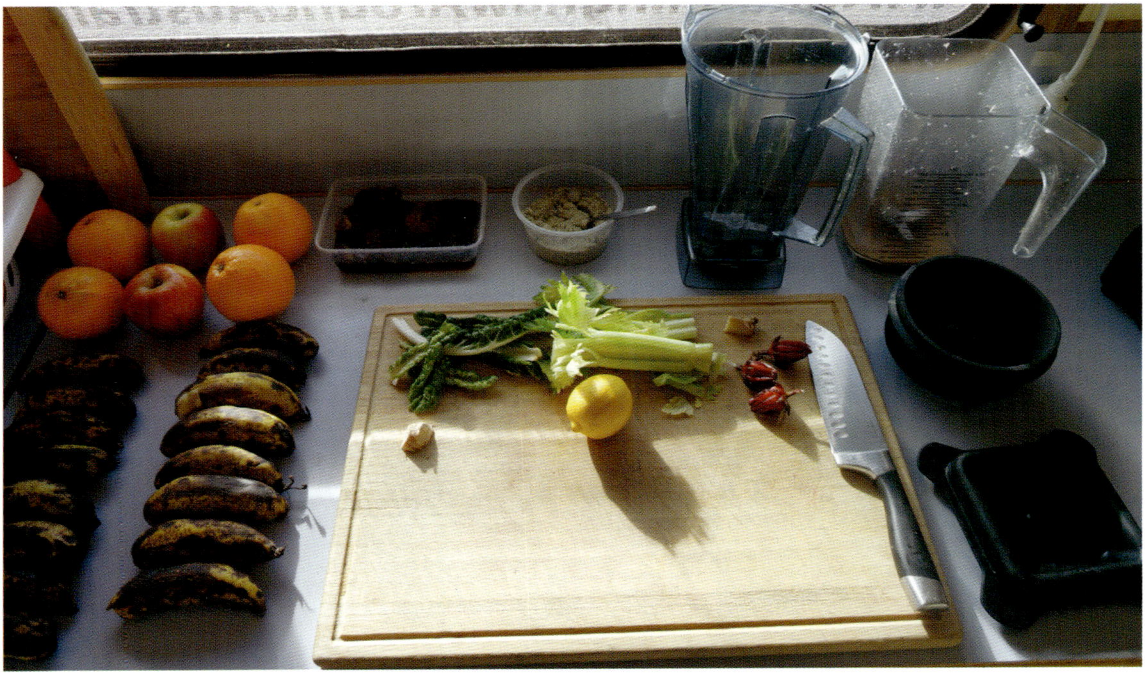

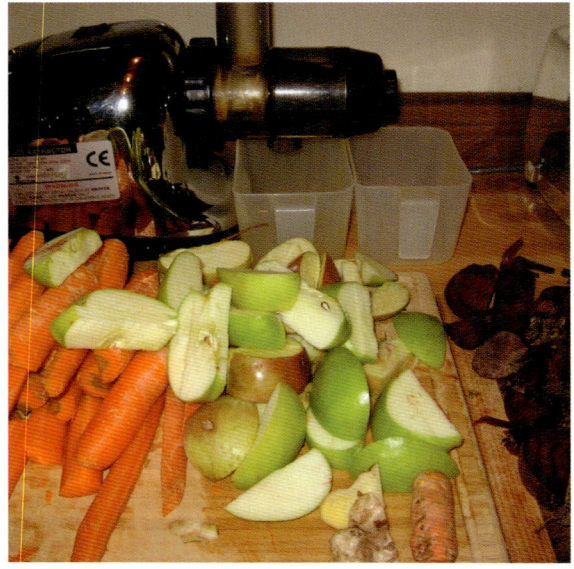

Beet Treat Juice Ingredients

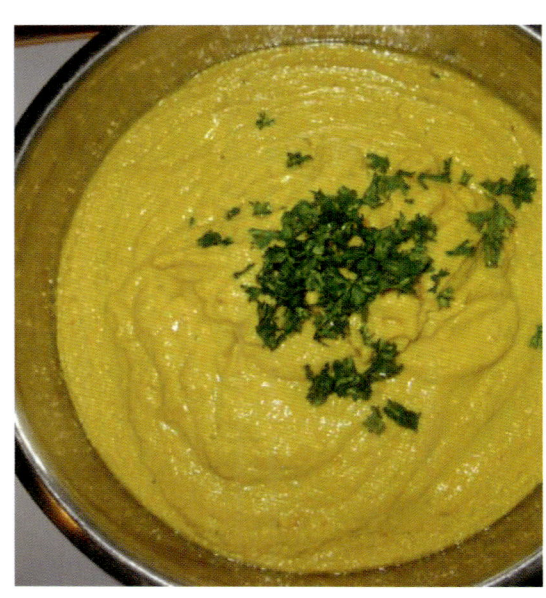

Dillicious Carrot Soup

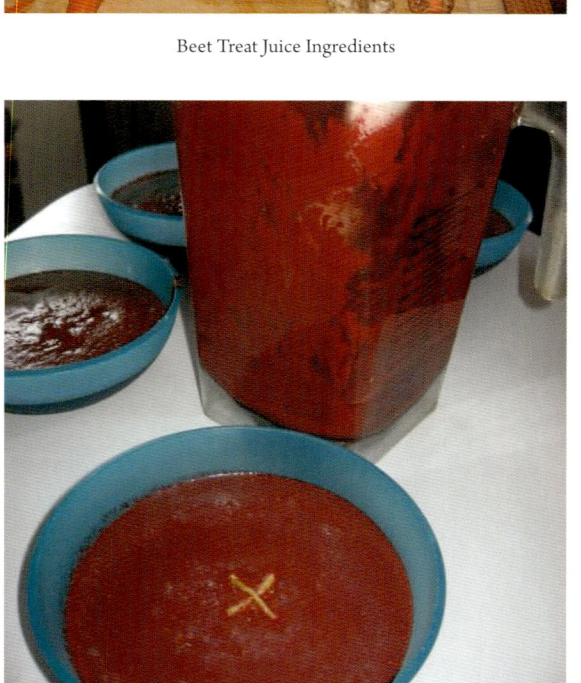

Beautiful Beetroot Soup

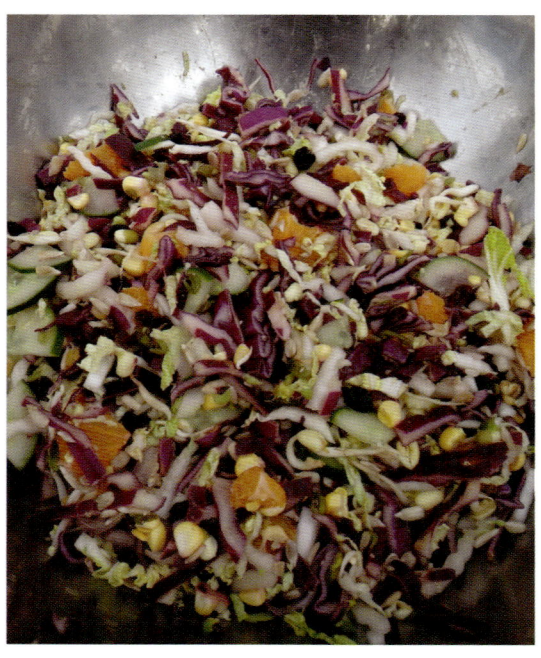

Down-Under Outback Coleslaw (Photo courtesy Ping Chan)

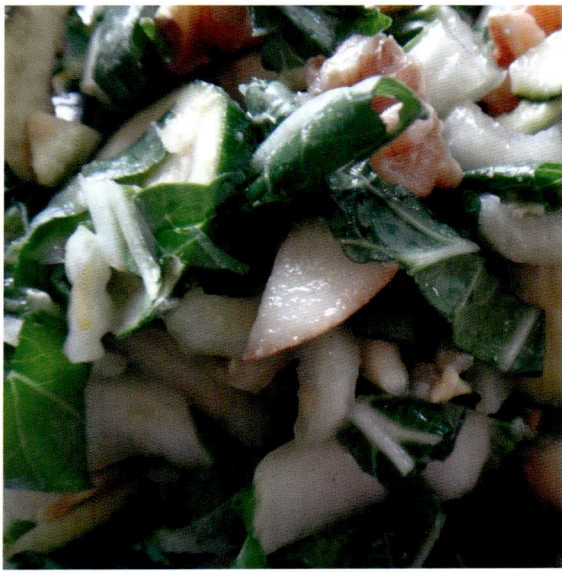
Spicy Greens Salad (Photo courtesy Ping Chan)

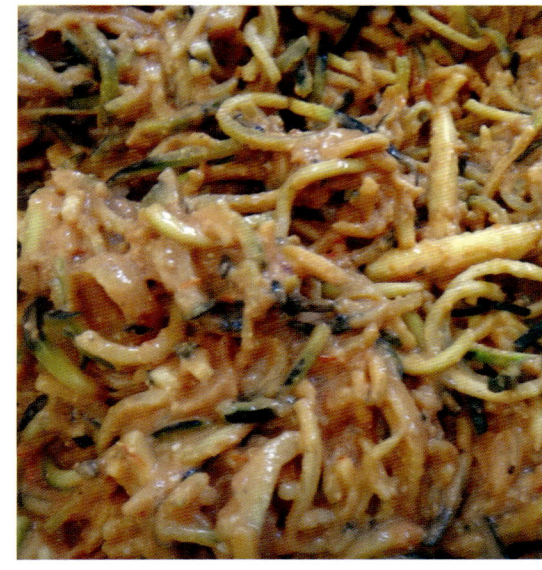
Dressed Naked Noodles (Photo courtesy Ping Chan)

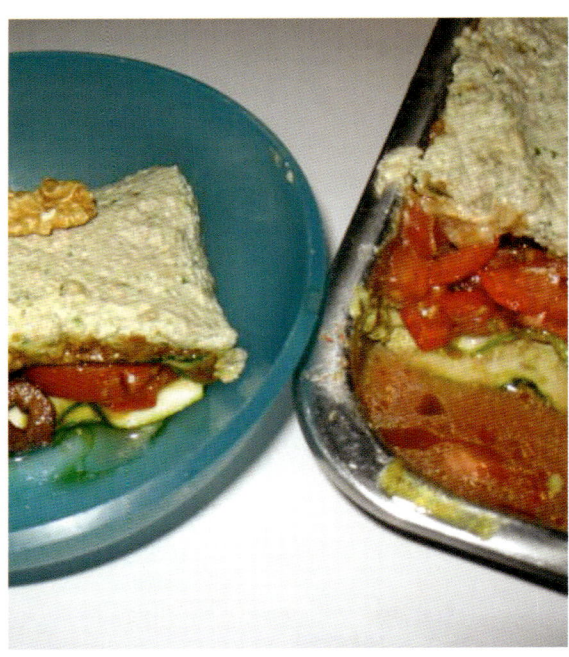
Living Lasagne

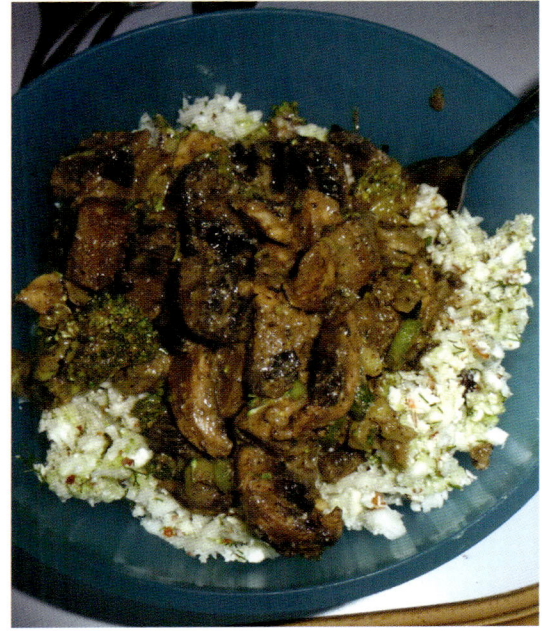
Curried Mushroom Rice

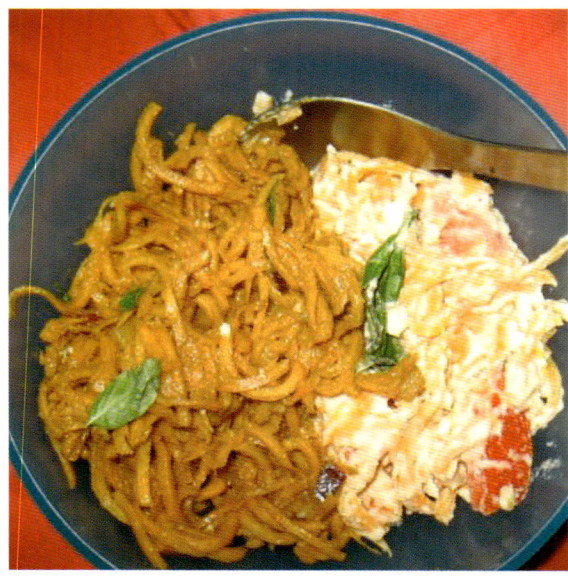

Pumpkin Fettuccini

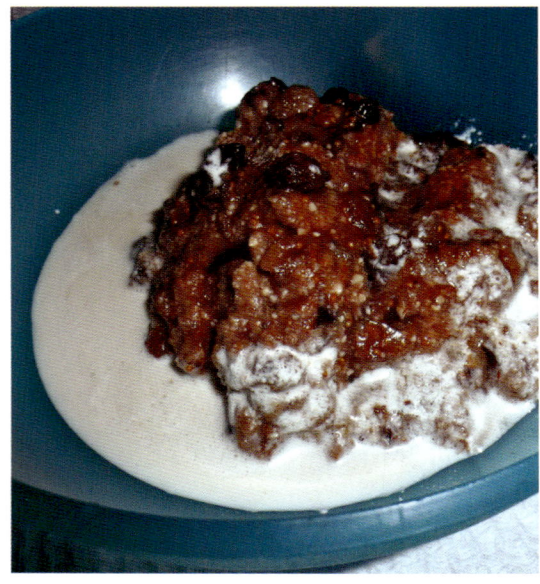

Three Chias Pudding with Almond Creme
(Photo courtesy Sylvia Pringle)

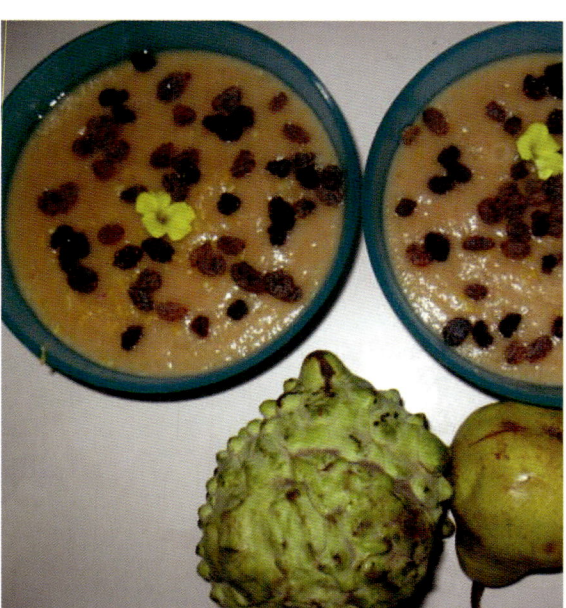

Pineapple or Custard Apple Pear Pudding

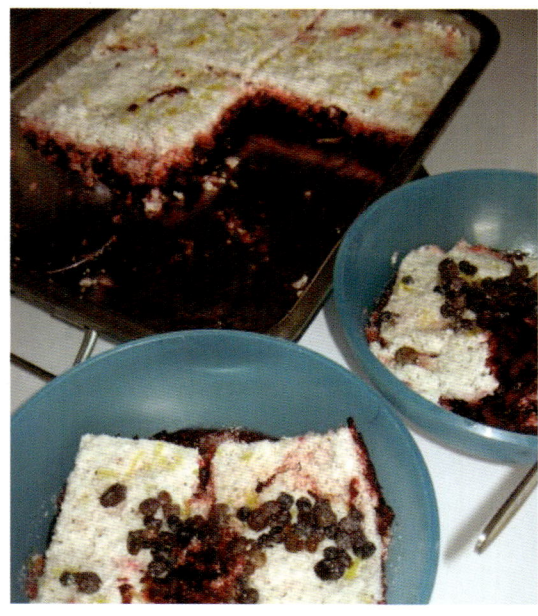

Beet Berry Slice

Here we go...*Downhill run through the countryside...*

Comments from Facebook/RunningRawAroundAustralia2013:
- *I am so inspired with your determination and energy!!* - **Patty**
- *Carnarvon bananas are the best...you guys are doing amazing.* - **Dianne**
- *You are wonderful!* - **Laura**
- *Nice trip!* - **Brian**
- *Wow still going* - **Heather**
- *Very inspiring, you are amazing!* - **Stephanie**
- *Great Menu sending Love and Energy from Germany.* - **Heike**
- *The change of scenery would be welcoming I would imagine? Keep up that energy!* - **Laurel**

Marathon #235.
August 23, 2013. 36 km north of Northampton to 40 km north of Geraldton. Started 5am, cold but no wind. (Temp 10-30 degrees) Running by the full moon till daybreak and beautiful sunrise. Great to be in the hills with lovely views across the green and yellow landscape. Still being accompanied occasionally by the yellow 'gyrocopter' beetle as we passed through stands of the olive gum trees. The road surface a mix of rough and smooth so easier underfoot. Stopped for a break in the middle of roadworks on top of one hill, thanks for the donation from Gary and the Boys from Central Earthmovers WA and for escorting us through the roadworks. Arrived in Northampton for midway break, quiet historic town with 3 antique shops, a grocery store, old original general store, hardware store (thanks for the donation), Post Office, stone church and schoolhouse. Stopped at the Carobbean Orchard just out of the township to buy some organic oranges, thanks for the really delicious, sweet and juicy fruit. Ran last 16km with a quick stop to eat some dates and watch the sunset as we climbed yet another hill to the roadside gravel pit where Myke and Melissa had set up camp for the night. Finished the Run at 46.24 km, another long day, but in bed by 8:30pm. Marathon Average 43.08 km. Total Km 10124.54.

Marathon #236.

August 24, 2013. 40 km north of Geraldton to The African Reef Tourist Park at Tacooma Beach, Geraldton. Started 5am in the dark and could see the lights of Geraldton 30 km away. Cold but no wind and downhill all the way. Landscape has changed to farmland with mostly wheat and canola, noticed that many of the farms are for sale. After being in the desert for the last few weeks the contrast is enormous, the lights have changed from red to green. Turned off onto the country road into Geraldton past old stone houses and small market garden stalls selling veges locally grown. Apparently the area used to be the tomato growing area for Australia before glasshouses were used, and some of the original growers still grow and sell tomatoes locally on the small stalls located around the area, complete with honesty box to pay for what you help yourself to. We bought several bags of tomatoes which are very sweet and juicy. Myke and Melissa stopped in the town to do the shopping while we ran through and followed the coast out to Tacooma Beach to the African Reef Tourist Park, a lovely caravan park right on the beach where we finished the Run at 42.61 km. Many thanks for the complimentary site (complete with shower and toilet en suite), what luxury! Thanks for your hospitality and support. Temp 13-30 degrees. Total Km 10,167.11. Marathon Average 43.08 km.

Marathon #237.

August 25, 2013. Tacooma Beach, Geraldton to roadside parking on side road 18 km north of Dongara. Started from campground 5am running by streetlights out of the built-tup area on the Brand Hwy. Following the Coast south with huge sand dunes on our right once we got out into the countryside, too big to see the Ocean. Stopped for our first break at 7:30am, very dark clouds gathering ahead and suddenly we had a torrential downpour, a real rain storm! We waited it out in the car then started out again as the rain eased, but it wasn't long before we were dumped on with more torrential rain, the road awash with running water, our clothes and shoes drenched and we were soaked to the skin. The rain had set in so there was no point in us changing our clothes or shoes, we plodded on through the water, getting off the road for the traffic, onto the shoulder with very course gravel and sharp stones. Made for a hard day's

Run, we were cold, wet and hungry when we finished at 42.47 km. Melissa picked us up and drove us to where she and Myke had everything ready for us, fresh juice and dinner which was very welcoming. Temp 16-18 degrees. Marathon Average 43.08 km. Total Km 10,209.58.

Marathon #238.

August 26, 2013. 18 km north of Dongara to off road parking spot opposite Mt. Adam turnoff. Melissa drove us back 3 km to where we had finished yesterday, started 5:15am with a clear sky, running by the light of the moon. Still water on the edge of the road from yesterday's storm, cloudy but no rain. Stopped for first break at the Dongara pioneer cemetery, a historic landmark where the early pioneers were buried, many in unmarked graves and many women and children, it must have been a hard life back in those days. Diverted off the Hwy to run through the village of Dongara, very quaint with historic buildings, then back onto Hwy following the huge sand dunes to finish at 43.78 km off the road opposite Mt Adam turnoff. Temp 16-24 degrees. Marathon Average 43.08 km. Total Km 10,253.36.

Marathon #239.

August 27, 2013. Mt Adam turnoff to 20 km north of Leeman. Started 5am, rain during the night but sky was clearing so we were hopeful that it was over. Ran 5 km on the Barand Hwy then turned off onto the Indian Ocean Drive, what a difference! The road surface was smooth, small shoulder with a soft edge and no more road trains! Aww, we'll miss you guys, but there will be the double trailers so keep in touch with our progress on the UHF. Road moving quite close to the coast, could finally see the Ocean beyond the sand dunes for part of the time. Quite a few holiday shacks amongst the sand dunes but no-one staying there in this weather, lots of water lying on the ground in driveways, dark clouds rolling in and strong wind blowing from off the ocean. Leaving our first break the rain set in and became torrential, we were soaked in seconds and with the strong wind we got very cold, even while running downhill. Had to change our clothes and warm up in the van after 10 km slogging into the wind and rain on undulating hills. Had some kiwifruit and felt revived, so back out on the road in the rain to the midway break for a yummy salad and to change shoes and jackets. Ran the last 12 km with no break in steady rain, up and down the sand dunes to finish at 42.73 km where Myke and Melissa had parked the vehicles on the side of the road for the night. Signs everywhere saying no camping, but we couldn't read them for the rain! Wet clothes and shoes off and hanging inside the caravan, not many changes of clothes left so hope the rain stops soon otherwise we will literally be Running Raw, now that ought to attract some attention! Temp 15-17 degrees. Marathon Average 43.08 km. Total Km 10,296.09.

Marathon #240.

August 28, 2013. 20 km north of Leeman to 7 km south of Green Head on the Indian Ocean Drive. Started at 5am after a stormy night of heavy rain and strong winds parked at the roadside, only one motorist stopped to ask if we were all right, no-one wanting to move us on during a night like that! Running in the moonlight till daybreak, cloudy sky with more rain to come during the day, running in misty showers on and off throughout the Run. More rolling dunes, narrow shoulders on the road, but surface not too rough. Had a good podcast interview with '100 not Out' by The Wellness Couch to be aired on Monday 2 September. Ran through Leeman, a little coastal village then on to Green Head another small coastal village for our last break, then ran on for another 7 km to finish at 43.86 km, where Melissa picked us up and drove back to the Campground where Myke had set up on a complimentary site, thanks to Wanda for your support and hospitality. Got all the laundry done, clothes and shoes dry and had very welcome hot showers. A very quiet spot, going to sleep to the sound of the ocean. Temp 14-23 degrees. Marathon Average 43.08. Total Km 10,339.95.

Marathon #241.

August 29, 2013. 7 km south of Green Head to 20 km north of Cervantes. Melissa drove us out to where we had finished yesterday, started 5:15am in the dark, running by the light of the moon till daybreak. Very black clouds rolling in again and looked like we'd get caught in a downpour several times during the day, but it moved away, so mostly running in misty rain showers. Had a sunny break around midway as we passed through Jurien Bay, stopping to stock up on produce and organise things for Perth via the internet and phone. Ran on up and over the dunes to finish at 43.06 km where Melissa picked us up and drove us on to where she and Myke had set up camp alongside the road. Off to sleep to the sound of rain on the roof. Temp 14-21 degrees. Marathon Average 43.08 km. Total Km 10,383.01. Three more marathons to go and we'll be two-thirds of the way Running Raw Around Australia!

Marathon #242.

August 30, 2013. 20 km north of Cervantes to Wanagarren Nature Reserve. Melissa drove us out 2 km to where we finished yesterday, started running 5am with the moon and some stars. Daybreak and the clouds started rolling in, cold wind getting stronger. Climbing uphill most of the day, a few showers before midway, just enough rain to soak us through, so changed clothes and shoes 3 times to stay semi dry and warm. Back on the road again after the midway break, sun shining and feeling good for a few minutes before the first shower rolled in from behind us drenching us to the skin, the wind pushing us along and then the rain turned to hail, little balls of ice coming at us horizontally and freezing us to the bones. Tried to phone the crew but couldn't get a signal, so decided to keep going as it was too cold to stop. It was all we could do to stay upright and keep moving, being thankful that the wind was coming from behind us, even though it was hard to keep our balance with it pushing us along faster than we could run! We were starting to feel like hyperthermia may set in when the crew vehicles went past us, unable to stop on the side of the road at that point. Watching them drive on was gut wrenching, but we knew they would stop as soon as they could so we slogged on through the surface water, keeping our focus on the road ahead. Through the driving rain we could see that they had pulled over about 1 km ahead, this was one of the hardest kilometers we've run. We eventually made it to the van, not able to speak and our fingers were too numb to pull our soggy clothes off, but with the help of our trusty crew we finally got changed into dry clothes and warmed up with some food. The sun came out so with only 4 km to go we set out again, only to get 1 km before another torrential downpour soaked us through. Finished at 42.38 km where Melissa picked us up and we drove on to find a side road with a parking area just 1 km ahead. Temp 14-21 degrees. Marathon Average 43.08 km. Total Km 10,425.39.

Marathon #243.

August 31, 2013. Wanagarren Nature Reserve to 3.7 km from Ledge Point on the Indian Ocean Drive. Very strong winds all night rocking the caravan so not much sleep. Melissa drove us back to where we had finished yesterday and we started running at 5:30am. Still wild weather most of the day, cold rain showers clearing to sunshine and blue sky, changing to rolling black clouds and more rain. The wind still behind us pushing us in gust from 30 to 50 km per hour. Myke and Melissa were able to find good spots to pull over where we needed them and providing food and water as we were feeling hungry all day because of the extra energy we are burning due to the weather. Landscape quite amazing with huge white sand dunes against a dark stormy sky. Only had half km to finish when a car pulled over, the driver calling out to say he'd seen us on the road earlier, they had been out kite surfing in the wind and wanted to know what we were doing running in the rain all day! Thanks for the donation guys, see you at the Perth Meet & Greet Evening on the September 5 at Cottosloe Civic Centre, 6:30pm. Finished the run at 44.42 km, adjusted the Garmin time because we forgot to turn the watch off when Melissa picked us up and drove us on to the campground at Ledge Point. Thanks for the complimentary site Wendy and Ken at Ledge Point Tourist Park, and for your support and hospitality. The laundry and hot showers are much appreciated. Temp 14-24 degrees. Total Km 10469.81. Marathon Average 43.08 km.

September 2013

MARATHONS #244-273

Marathon #244. September 1, 2013. Two thirds of the way Running Raw Around Australia! Ledge Point turnoff to Metro Rd clearcut 11 km south of GinGin turnoff on the Indian Ocean Drive. Today's Run is dedicated to all the Dads out there on Father's Day. Melissa drove us back to the main road where we finished yesterday. Warm this morning and no wind, seemed eerie running in the dark with no howling wind behind us. Did not rain all day, nice hilly run with 66 metre gain. Both feeling a bit slow today, most likely as a result of the last three days of being cold and running with a strong wind behind us, also not enough sleep. Did a newspaper interview on the phone with The Western Australian, photographer drove out to meet us and had photos taken on the road, should be in tomorrow's paper. The landscape is changing again, we've left the sand dunes behind and running through cultivated fields and hobby farms, also stalls on the side of the road selling produce. Bought some strawberries and fresh peas that were being grown outside under cloches, no doubt to protect them from the wind and rain! Decided to run the minimum and found a clear cut forest with a place to park away from the road at 42.59 km. Going to have an early night to the sound of light rain on the roof as darkness settles around us... Temp 16-24 degrees. Marathon Average 43.08 km. Total Km 10,512.40.

Marathon #245.
September 2, 2013. Metro Rd Clearcut to Quinns Beach 43 km north of Perth. Started 4:45am in the dark with the moon setting. Running through a pine forest and back into the sand dunes. Turned left onto Breakwater Drive heading down to the coast at Two Rocks, then left again following the coast. Met Amy as we ran past her house, lovely to meet you, see you on fifth at Cottosloe for our Meet & Greet Event. Continued on through 'sand suburbs', lifestyle

villages being built on the flattened dunes. Stopped in one of the new subdivisions for a break where Myke & Melissa had met Marama who lives nearby and offered showers or a bath, very tempting, but we had to run on further. Thanks for the offer and for the gift of bottled water. Finished the run 43.97 km at Quinns Beach, on the start of Ocean Drive. Parked in a parking lot overlooking the beach and Alice arrived half an hour after we finished. We all had dinner together, Melissa had made zucchini noodles with tomato sauce, Alice had made the same but with an avocado sauce, delicious dinner, thanks girls. Tonight is Melissa and Myke's last night with us, after being on board as support crew for 3 months they will be leaving us in Perth. Many thanks for all your help, we really appreciate all that you have done. Now it's just one more day together as we run into Perth. Off to sleep to the sound of surf rolling in... Temp 17-25 degrees. Total Km10556.37. Marathon Average 43.09 km.

Marathon #246.

September 3, 2013. Quinns Beach to Cottosloe Golf Course, Perth. Started at 5am running alongside the coast most of the day. With the wind behind us we ran into Perth in a storm, torrential rain soaking us to the skin, our shoes sodden as we ran through surface water on the road. Myke & Melissa managed to find a place to park the vehicles so we could refuel on fruit and change our wet clothes several times. Their friend Laksmi meet us all partway through the run to cheer us on and our friend Graeme (who is joining us as support crew again) arrived to encourage us through the last 10 km to finish at 42.57 km in the Cottosloe Golf Course Members Park. Driving back to drop off M & M at Laksmi's house, it seemed a long way to have run in the storm. Arrived at our host's store, Alive Organics, where John & Jill welcomed us with freshly made juice and bananas, then we drove to their home where we parked the van next to their house for the next 3 days while in Perth. Thank you so much for the warm welcome and for sharing your home and food with us. Temp 16-24 degrees. Total Km 10,598.96. Marathon Average 43.08 km.

Hey Everybody, we're back on the road after a wonderful 3 days in Perth, many thanks to Jazz, Kim, Melanie and the Perth Team for putting on a great event, to John and Jill for hosting and feeding us in their home and for sponsoring our fresh organic fruits and veg from Alive Organics, we are so grateful for your hospitality, support and friendship We've just finished Marathon #251 and are now camping overnight at Dawesville just south of Mandura heading towards Bunbury, will arrive there in 2 days. Our friends Graeme and Margit have joined us as support crew and are currently sleeping in their tents on the beach, we're about to hit the sack too. We'll post the updates and pics over the next couple of days, just need to catch up on some sleep... Many thanks to Myke & Melissa, our support crew for 3 months, have fun in Perth, see you in Melbourne.

Comments from Facebook/RunningRawAroundAustralia2013:

- *Saw you on the Sunrise program last week. ...awesome! About time the rest of the nation knows how inspiring you two are as well as those who support you. You are a continual inspiration to me and scanning the many comments are inspiring others the same.* - **Jamie**
- *Good luck & safe journeys. It was great to hear you speak on Thursday night & have read your book from cover to cover. it was so inspirational.* - **Felicity xxx**
- *I am in Bunbury, and would love to cheer you on, say hello...* - **Sharon**
- *What a beautiful picture! What a wonderful example! I'm Brazilian and, despite the distance, follow your steps with admiration and wishing the best to you!* - **Lara**
- *You guys are awesome! So I find out about your journey.. and that you are arriving in Perth after you have already left. Keep up the good work!* - **Reinbow**
- *You guys are amazing!* - **Betsy**
- *I'm on day 5 of mainly fruit..some greens and cashews but mainly bananas, dates, apples and oranges..I am doing good so far.* - **Kias**
- *Nice work guys! Keep it up.* - **Sally**
- *It may be a long home strait but you are on to it and heading home, great work...* - **Barbara**
- *Wow! To be past Perth! Such an amazing feat so far..Best wishes for the next stretch of your adventure...* - **Laurel**
- *Bye Byyee happy trails!* - **Kyah xxx**
- *It was just amazing to see you both in Perth. So inspiring. Good luck with the rest of your journey.* - **Dawn Xx**
- *Keep up the great work, you are an inspiration to us all!* - **metalroofingonline**
- *Thinking of you all!!!!* - **Melissa xx**

Marathon #247.

September 4, 2013. Perth, WA. Drove the two vehicles to the garage for their 10,000 km check and started running at 6:30am into Perth CBD to meet up with the crew from Channel 7 TV to do an interview for the Today Tonight Show, but found that they wanted to have the vehicles and crew there as well which wasn't a possibility for us, so called it off. Ran on to the South side along the river where we spent a couple of hours doing interview and filming to be aired internationally in Chinese and Portuguese speaking countries as well as in America. We split up for the rest of the run with Alan running back to pick up one of the vehicles and Janette running further south to the Radio Station for Sonrise 98.8fm to do an interview there. John drove in to pick up Janette where she finished the run and drove back to his house, meeting up with Alan who had finished. Margit our other support crew who is joining us and had flown in and arrived with Graeme arriving a little later and we all had dinner together in John and Jill's house. Today's run 45.86 km. Marathon Average 43.09 km. Temp 10-23 degrees. Total Km 10,644.80.

Marathon #248.

September 5, 2013. Perth, WA. Drove to the TV Studio for Channel 7 at 5:45am and did an interview for the Sunrise Show being aired live on the East Coast and 2 hours later in the West. Drove back to the van and posted the live show on FB. Spent the rest of the day running around the neighbourhood of Morley, stopping in at Alive Organics for a fresh juice or fruit every 10 km. Finished at 42.28 km back at the van and got ready to go to the Evening Event. Arrived at the Cottosloe Civic Centre around 6pm for the Meet, Greet & Eat, a wonderful evening meeting so many wonderful people, many thanks for the fantastic effort by Jazz, Kim, Melanie, Jodie for organising the event and everyone else who participated, supported and donated during the evening. Final amount fundraised is yet to be confirmed but it is over $6000.00, so thanks again Perth! Marathon Average 43.09 km. Total Km 10,687.08.

Marathon #249.

September 6, 2013. Perth, WA. Started at 5:30am, ran from Morley to Balcatta to do a photo shoot at Orbital, our autogas sponsors. Margit and Graeme drove to meet us and drive back to continue the run around Morley, stopping in at Alive Organics for juice. John joined us for the last leg, we stopped where we stopped at Healthy Valley Organics to pick up some food for the trip, then back to Alive organics to pick up the fresh produce. Thanks for coming on board as Sponsors John & Jill and providing us with all the organic food we need for the trip around the SW Coast and up to Norseman. We finished the run 43.05 km, (adjusted from Garmin 37 km as we forgot to start the Garmin watch partway through the run) back at J & J's house where we were joined by Jazz from Revital Health for a delicious organic rawsome dinner. Finished our last day in Perth with a hot bath and off to bed with the sound of rain on the roof... Temp 10-24 degrees. Marathon Average 43.09 km. Total Km 10,730.58.

Marathon #250.

September 7, 2013. Perth to Rockingham. Thunder and lightening and torrential rain overnight. Farewell to John & Jill at 6am then drove to where we had finished Marathon #246 coming into Perth at the Cottosloe Golf Club. Started running at 6:30am with Marlene who joined us for the marathon, great to have company on the Run and thanks for the delicious raw carrot cake you made that we shared for lunch. Good luck at the Ocean Road 100 km! Finished the run 42.67 km at the Rockingham train station car park, nowhere to camp the night so Margit drove to pick us up and drove back to the last break stop in the car park of a chemical factory, not an ideal spot, but it was too late to start searching for somewhere better. Marlene caught the bus back to Perth from just 1 km down the road from where we were set up. The factory security person came to say that we couldn't park there the night but after hearing about the Run, decided it would be okay, thanks. Marathon Ave 43.09 km. Total Km 10,773.25.

Marathon #251.

September 8, 2013. Rockingham to Dawesville Beach. Graeme drove us to where we'd finished yesterday started running 5am, good running on service roads and bike trails alongside the Hwy. Ran through the township of Mandura, lovely waterfront with lots of people out picnicking. Through Dawesville and on the last 10 km to finish 44.42 km on the Hwy where Graeme picked us up and drove back to a beautiful spot by the beach to camp for the night where Graeme and Margit pitched their tents right on the beach. Marathon Average 43.1 km. Total Km 10,817.67.

Marathon #252.

September 9, 2013. Beach to Hazlett Rd 50 km Nth of Bunbury Graeme drove us back to the main road to start at 5:15am A day of no towns running along cycle paths and the road, nice to run in the cool weather and smooth road with wide shoulders. All the motorists are waving and tooting and giving us the thumbs up. Graeme found a great side road to park for the night, we finished 44.01 km at the caravan just as the local farmer drove by. He stopped to see if we were OK and we got chatting about RunRAW2013. Anthony is a horticultural farmer growing plant crops, at the moment he has potatoes, cauliflower and olives. He was very interested in what we're doing and why and said he would come back later to chat some more. Sure enough, Anthony arrived during dinner and stayed for a long chat about organic farming. He gave us some olive oil pressed from his own olive trees. Thanks Anthony, it was a pleasure meeting you and spending time together. Temp 16-21 degrees. Marathon Average 43.1 km. Total Km 10, 861.68.

Marathon #253.

September 10, 2013. 50 to 6 km Nth of Bunbury. Graeme drove us back to the main road, started running at 5:30am on wide shoulder but rough stones. Got caught in huge downpour between the first and second breaks, then the sun came out and another downpour had us steam drying as we ran. Ran through Australind and met the school crossing supervisor as we crossed the road with the school kids. Had a few kids run with us for a short distance, but they couldn't keep up the pace! Ran on to finish 42.61 km, just 6km short of Bunbury where Margit was waiting to drive us on to the campground where Graeme was set up for the night. Late dinner, showers, laundry and bed. Temp 16-18 degrees. Marathon Average 43.1 km. Total Km 10,904.29.

Marathon #254.

September 11, 2013. 6 km north of Bunbury to 49 km north of Bridgetown. Graeme drove us back 6.2 km to where we finished yesterday. Started running in a heavy rain shower, continued raining on and off all day, but the road was smooth with wide shoulders and the scenery beautiful, farmland with cows grazing and some cropping. Mostly uphill, gained 189 meters on the run. Stopped at the Boyup General Store and they gave us a bunch of asparagus, grown locally and freshly picked this morning. We ate it as we continued on to Donnybrook where we stopped to shop for fruit and veg then on to finish 42.86 km where Graeme had set up camp in a sandy clearing in the pine forest. Very heavy rain so no tents tonights, Margit slept in the caravan with us and Graeme in the SuperRoo. Temp 12-18 degrees. Marathon Average 43.1km. Total Km 10,947.15.

Marathon #255.

September 12, 2013. 49 to 9 km north of Bridgetown. Started running 5am in the dark and rain. Stopped at Kirrup where Graeme met us, but no sign of Margit. With no phone reception Graeme hitched a ride back to find Margit did not have the car keys and Graeme had not taken a set with him! Luckily he was able to send a text message to us, so Alan hitchhiked with the keys and they all arrived back safe and sound! Running on into a changed scenery of orchards with the trees in bloom, looks like spring has sprung! Running on the edge when traffic was passing, Alan tripped on a piece of wire and landed on his hip scrapping his knee, foot and elbow. He continued running and everything seemed to be okay, tomorrow will tell. Finished in the dark 42.48 km at roadside camp. Temp 10-18 degrees. Marathon Average 43.1 km. Total Km 10,987.63.

Marathon #256.

September 13, 2013. 9 km north of Bridgetown to Manjimup. Started at 5am and noticed that the mornings are getting lighter earlier now. Alan's hip hurting, but he says it's only when he runs. Ran into Bridgetown, a very quaint town with historic buildings and landscaped gardens and parks. Ran on to 11 km for the first banana break then on through picturesque countryside of mostly hobby farms with sheep, goats, horses and donkeys with chickens running free range amongst the animals. Seems like most of the farms and houses are for sale in the area, the land is very wet with surface water in the fields and full dams providing great habitat for the waterbirds. Continued to rain on and off throughout the day, stopped at Balingup, a small very charming hamlet with interesting boutique shops and gardens with citrus trees laden with fruit. Ran on towards Manjimup and met local organic grower and avocado orchardist Anita, who stopped on the road as she passed us to offer fresh fruit from her orchard. Ran on through Manjimup and finished at 42.64 km where Margit picked us up and drove us to Lucinda's place just out of town. Graeme had already arrived and set up the caravan beside the house and his tent in the grass just before another downpour! We arrived in the rain to be greeted by Lucinda in her cosy home with the fire roaring. Thank you so much for your warm hospitality, sorry we arrived on a night when you were going out, but we'll catch up again when we return next year. Anita and Wayne arrived shortly after us and stayed to share a delicious meal and gift us some fresh produce from their garden and avocados from their orchard, thank you so much. We had a delightful evening eating by the fire and soaking in a hot bath before going to bed in the caravan to the sound of more rain on the roof...Temp 10-18 degrees. Marathon Average 43.09 km. Total Km 11,032.27.

Marathon #257.

September 14, 2013. Manjimup to 80km Nth of Walpole. Graeme drove us back to where we finished yesterday and we started running in the rain at 6am, ran back to Lucinda's house to say goodbye then on for 10 km before Graeme and Margit caught up with us. A beautiful run in the forest, tall trees glistening in the rain. Met a garlic farmer (who is originally from NZ) when we stopped outside his house for a break and he offered for us to take on water from his place, thanks for the water and interesting chat. Very quiet on the road and the rain kept coming down with at least 2 hours of torrential rain we got completely drenched and cold. We kept thinking of last night sitting by the fire all warm and cosy, eating and chatting with our new friends Anita (also a Kiwi) and Wayne, and that kept us going. We were having our midway break, eating a delicious cauliflower soup when Lucinda arrived. She had driven out to bring one of our water bottles we had left behind so joined us for lunch while the rain just kept coming down. Lucinda said, "I don't know what you two are made of to be running in this weather," sitting amongst wet clothes and shoes hanging up in the caravan. We said we were running on the warmth of her hospitality and the memory of sitting by her fire eating delicious fresh produce with Anita and Wayne from their orchard and afterwards soaking in her lovely hot bath. It's all about meeting beautiful people and sharing nourishing food and running in an enchanted forest in the rain...Finished the run 47.89 km. Temp 9-13 degrees. Marathon Average 43.1 km. Total Km 11,080.16.

Marathon #258.
September 15, 2013. 80 to 37 km north of Walpole. *Running in the rain in an enchanted forest... the giant trees towering above us forming a green canopy over our heads, water running down the trunks in glistening riverlets forming pools of white foaming bubbles at the giant base. The sun breaks through the canopy while the rain keeps falling, shards of light striking the wet leaves and turning them silver. The wind rustling through the leaves sending raindrops falling from the canopy, lighting up like diamonds and sending tiny rainbows in the air. The sound of water rushing along the roadside, lapping in pools beneath the trees and splashing beneath our feet. The sweet fragrance of vanilla permeates the air and star shaped white flowers cascade down the branches, vivid against the bright green vine trailing through the trees...and the rain keeps falling and we keep running, on a magical day in an enchanted forest.* Finished 42.57 km, the last 5 km with the sun filtering through the trees, creating tiny sparkles on the wet leaves. Margit drove us to where Graeme had set up camp on a side road. While we had our fresh juice they drove down the side road to find the elusive waterfall that we've been looking for since Townsville! Temp 9-17 degrees. Marathon Average 43.1 km. Total Km 11,122.73.

Marathon #259.

September 16, 2013. 37 km north of Walpole Sth Western Hwy to Coleman Beach Motor Camp Sth Coast Hwy. Walked back 1 km from caravan to where we finished yesterday and started running at 5:15am in the rain. First 11 km was through swampy area then back into the forest of huge giant karri (eucalyptus) trees with massive girths, the largest reported to be 22 metres around, but the side road that led to it was under water so we didn't see it. The trees alongside the Hwy were very impressive though and beautiful to run amongst them again, especially in the rain. Stopped at Walpole at the end of the South Western Hwy for our last break then continued onto the South Coast Hwy heading East. Finished 42.64 km where Margit picked us up and drove back to the Coleman Beach Motor Camp to a complimentary caravan site, thanks for your support. The campground was flooded and it was still raining, so we got a cabin for Margit and Graeme and we all hit the sack early. Temp 9-13 degrees. Marathon Average 43.1 km.   Total Km 11,165.37.

Marathon #260.

September 17, 2013. Coleman Beach to 15 km west of Denmark. Rained most of the night with two very heavy hail showers while we were getting ready to leave around 4:30am. Graeme drove us 7km past Walpole to where we finished yesterday and we started running in light showers at 6am through more giant trees and bush. Finished the run 42.46 km and Margit drove us into Denmark to our hosts Basil & Nikki's place. Shared a delicious meal in their cosy house beside a roaring fire then soaked in their enormous bath before going to bed. Thank you so much for your warm hospitality and new friendship Basil & Nikki. Temp 7-13 degrees. Marathon Average 43.1 km.   Total Km 11,207.83.

Marathon #261.

September 18, 2013. 15 km west to 37 km east of Denmark. Graeme drove us back to where we finished yesterday and we started running in the early daybreak 6.5 km back into Denmark, stopped for bananas with Basil and Margit then continued on through a sleepy town and out onto the Hwy. Had a few rain showers as we ran past small hobby farms and cottage industry for honeymead, toffee, chocolate woodturning, B & Bs, chalets etc. Heavy rain set in after 20 km with lightening and serious thunder claps. A herd of cows watched us go by with looks of astonishment on their faces, as if wondering what we would be doing out there running in the rain. Finished the run 42.32 km in a small community forest just off the Hwy as a heavy thunder storm set in for the night. We set up camp next to the community hall, pitched the tents under cover of the hall and had the composting toilets all to ourselves! Temp 10-15 degrees. Total Km 11,250.15.

Marathon #262.

September 19, 2013. 37 km east of Denmark to Albany. Graeme drove us out to the Hwy and we started running in the heavy rain and we were drenched within minutes. A few km out of town there was a sign for a fruit & veg shop, so we ran in to see if they had any bananas and met Mario who offered to give us a box for free and some ripe pineapples. Thanks so much for your support at Mario's Fruit & Veg. Caught up with Margit for a quick banana break then she drove back to pick up from Mario's while we ran on into town to meet up with Graeme at Organic Fruit & Veg in Albany, where he had picked up a delivery of fresh organic produce and dry foods from Alive Organics in Perth. Thanks again to John & Jill from Healthy Valley & Alive Organics for their generous sponsorship of keeping us stocked up with delicious nutritious fruit & veg, nuts and seeds. Thanks also to Albany Organics for their support in receiving the delivery and gifting some extra goodies. Continued on to finish at 43.15 km where Margit drove us to our host's home in Albany. Hayley, Kevin and son Archie welcomed us to their home, Hayley had prepared a delicious raw meal that we shared by the roaring fire, then into the hot bath before bed. A much appreciated welcome, thanks for your hospitality and friendship.   Temp 14-21 degrees. Marathon Average 43.1 km. Total Km 11,292.50.

Archie's Donation

When Archie's parents told him what we are doing and why, six-year-old Archie sat down and thought about it for a minute. Then, without saying a word, Archie went to his bedroom, found a piece of paper and a bright yellow pencil and started colouring. Onto the yellow page he carefully wrote these words: 'From Archie, I wil giv uo money.' Then he went to his drawer and took out his wallet, opened it up and took out all the money, four 5c pieces, one 10c piece and a twenty dollar note. Reaching for a roll of sticky tape he held the money in place, and with his tongue held out in concentration, he carefully attached the note and 10c piece to the bright yellow page. Then he picked up the four 5c pieces, put them in his pocket and went to find his father. "Can you take me to them?" he asked, "I want to give them some money." His father picked Archie up and gave him a hug. "That's very kind of you," he said and carried his son outside and down to the caravan. Archie knocked on the caravan door, "I want to give you some money because you are running so far," he said, holding out his hand with the four 5c pieces. "That's very thoughtful and kind, thank you Archie," we said and put the 20c into our donations jar. "I'm going to bed now," Archie said, "will you come up to say goodnight?" So we walked back to the house with them and into their cosy warm home. Archie raced over to the table and picked up the yellow piece of paper. "Here you are," he said handing it to us, "I did it by myself, I coloured it bright yellow like the sun to make you feel happy after running in the rain all day and I am giving you the pocket money in my wallet I got for this week because you need it to help other people and animals." His face shone with pride as we looked at the beautiful gift he had created. "Wow, thank you Archie," we said, "that is so kind and thoughtful of you." "Well," Archie replied, "I think if everyone would give one week of their pocket money, that would make a lot of money for other people and animals that need help." A conscious thought from a 6 year old who put his thought into action and gave what he could to help others. How much pocket money can you share this week? Please share this post from Archie.

Marathon #263.

September 20, 2013. Albany to 126 km west of Jerramungup. Last night we said goodbye to Margit who has been with us as support crew for the past two weeks. Thank you for all your help. After only 4 hours sleep we got up at 4am and sorted out the SuperRoo as we don't have a replacement crew, we're leaving the car with Kevin & Hayley in Albany and continuing with only the Ute and caravan and Graeme, our one SuperCrew. Said goodbye to Kev, Hayley and Archie and drove out to where we had finished the run yesterday. Graeme drove back into town to get a gas bottle while we started the run at 6:30am, just got to the van for the first break as a heavy thunder storm started, so waited it out for an hour. Ran on good smooth road all day, Graeme was able to find good stopping places despite the ground being very wet and soggy from the last 3 week's rain. Temp 15-23 degrees. Finished in dark 42.32 km. Marathon Average 43.1 km. Total Km 11,334.82.

Marathon #264.
September 21, 2013. 126 km to 82 km west of Jerramungup. Started running 5:30am, quiet traffic so ran in the middle of the road for most of the day through Bluegum plantations. Had a heavy downpour during first break so waited it out, catching up on the internet. Cold with a few sunny breaks throughout the day, finished in the dark again at 42.45 km only 4km short of Wellstead. Parked on a side road and met the farmer who lives there, thank you for your donation. Temp 7-18 degrees. Marathon Average 43.1 km. Total Km 11,377.27.

Marathon #265.
September 22, 2013. 82 km to 43 km west of Jerramungup. Started at 5am, very windy and overcast, building up to more thunderstorms. Just made it to Wellstead before a very heavy downpour, waited it out for 30 mins then out on the road again, Graeme taking on water from the town water tank. The weather changed every couple of hours from sunny to showers to sunny to heavy rain, jackets on, jackets off, but keep plugging into the strong head winds. Landscape changed to wheat fields and sheep country, very hilly rocky road. Graeme found a good parking spot for the night where we finished 43.91 km, exactly 43 km from Jerramungup, too windy to pitch the tent so we're all in the caravan together listening to the wind howling... Temp 9-18 degrees. Marathon Average 43.1 km. Total Km 11,421.18.

Marathon #266.
September 23, 2013. From 43 km west to Jerramungup. Started at 5am after very wild night with rain and the strong wind rocking the caravan. Had the wind behind us but it was so strong that it was pushing us out of control, picking one foot up and wrapping it around the other, took a lot of concentration to stop from tripping ourselves up. Only had one rain

shower, but gray and black clouds and wind very cold, estimated wind speed 60 km per hour and very gusty. We both got wind burnt on our faces and hands. Hilly terrain with 187-315 altitude gain and the last 5 km seemed to take forever. Finished 42.99 km at Jerramungup Caravan Park where Graeme had set up camp in our complimentary site, thanks so much for your hospitality and support. Temp 13-18 degrees. Marathon Average 43.1 km. Total Km 11,464.87.

Marathon #267.

September 24, 2013. Jerramungup to 70 km west of Ravensthorpe. Started 5:15am, still very windy pushing us along too fast! Undulating hills all day, caught up by Kay, the Adventure Runner from Japan, who is running around the world on his own, completely unassisted. He will be running 40,000 km on 5 continents, currently running across Australia from Perth to Sydney, pushing a jogging chariot with all his gear in it. We gave him some bananas and he continued on ahead of us as we've slowed down with the wind causing pain in our ankles and feet. Finished 43.88 km in farm driveway, early night with the wind still howling around the caravan rocking us to sleep... Temp 9-18 degrees. Marathon Average 43.1 km. Total Km 11,508.75.

Marathon #268.

September 25, 2013. 70 km to 27 km west of Ravensthorpe. Started at 5:20am after sitting inside caravan waiting for the heavy rain and strong wind to stop. The rain did stop, but not the wind, pushing us along at break neck speed again. Seemed like we were in a screaming hurry going nowhere, up and down the hills through bush and wheat fields, our feet pounding the rough stones, the road going ever on, but by mid afternoon the clouds rolled away and the wind dropped to nothing leaving us in an eerie calm to finish at 42.66 km. Temp 10-20 degrees. Marathon Average 43.1 km. Total Km 11,551.41.

Marathon #269.

September 26, 2013. 27 km west to 15 km east of Ravensthorpe. Started 5am in a clear, cool morning, but the wind soon got up again, pushing us forward as if there was no tomorrow. Rushed into Ravensthorpe to do a Skype interview but it was postponed, so did some food shopping and continued on with 15 km to go. Had a few birds (that looked like magpies but smaller) swooping down over our heads, doing some amazing acrobatics in the air, all in aid of moving us on past their nests. After a brief rain shower, the sky cleared and the wind dropped so we had a comfortable last leg to run through the wheat fields to finish at 42.27 km in a farmer's gateway. The farmer told us that he had 8000 acres of wheat, 2000 acres of canola, 2000 acres of rye and oats, that's a lot of grain that we wont be eating! Temp 10-18 degrees. Marathon Average 43.1 km. Total Km 11,593.68.

Marathon #270.

September 27, 2013. 15 km east of Ravensthorpe to 130 km west of Esperance. Very cold in the van this morning 4.7 degrees, coldest so far but no rain. Beautiful daybreak and sunrise as we ran past the 8000 acres of wheat and rolling hills. Spent 2 hours catching up on the internet at the first break, Kay caught up with us at the smoothie break and we ran together for the rest of the day pushing his chariot of 55kg. A swarm of wild bees surrounded the van so we left Graeme to it, but we were swarmed on the road twice as well, luckily no stings though. In our rush to leave, we didn't turn the Garmin on and only noticed 7 km down the road when a motorist stopped on her way to the Esperance Half Marathon to say hello and give us a donation, thanks so much Robyn for your support, hope you had a great run. Finished at 42.74 km (adjusted from Garmin data 34.92 km + 7.82 km) at a roadside parking area. Graeme and Kat pitched their tents under the picnic shelter and we shared dinner and a few stories from the road. Temp 4.7-22 degrees. Marathon Average 43.1 km. Total Km 11,636.42.

Marathon #271.

September 28, 2013. 130 km to 84 km west of Esperance. Kay still asleep when we started running at 5am, ran an easy 10 km to the first break through pleasant landscape of farms and bush. Stopped for an hour as we had internet coverage, Kay caught up but went on ahead as he wanted to do 60 km today. We continued on at a slower pace as we were still having some foot pain from running with the wind for the past few days. Later found Kay had stopped at 42 km as he felt dehydrated so we all ended up at the same spot again for the night. Hayley whom we left SuperRoo with in Albany decided to drive SR to Esperance for us and caught up with us a few km before we finished, having driven nonstop all the way. We had a quick hug on the side of the road as we were being swarmed by mosquitoes, so she continued on to Esperance while we finished the run at 42.60 km, just 95 km from Esperance and 95 marathons to go! Now what would you rather be doing on your sixty-fourth birthday? Temp 8-20 degrees. Total Km 11,679.02.

Marathon #272.

September 29, 2013. 84 km to 44 km west of Esperance. Started 5am, Kay and Graeme still asleep. Starry morning in a cloudless sky. Graeme met us at 10 km with bananas and at 17 km with green smoothies. Kay caught us up, had a smoothie and went on ahead. At 24 km we had apples and at 32 km homemade hummus with veg sticks. Last 7 km was flat and straight, surrounded by flies and mosquitoes. Almost dark when we finished 43.32 km at a farm gate, had marinated kale and cabbage for dinner and off to bed. Temp 14-23 degrees. Marathon Average 43.1 km. Total Km 11,722.34.

Marathon #273.

September 30, 2013. 44 km west to Esperance. Rained most of the night and we stepped out of the van into 2" of water, great start! Very uncomfortable heavy rain for the first 2 hours. Kay caught us up around 9am, stopped to say hello then continued on into Esperance where he will take a couple of recovery days. We told him he needs to eat more bananas and less cookies! Enjoy the rest Kay and we'll see you up the track. Hayley and Nicola stopped as they drove back to Albany while we were having our last break, having left SuperRoo for us to pick up at the campground in Esperance. Thank you so much for driving SR down for us Hayley, we really appreciate it. We all waited for the rain to stop before they left and Graeme drove ahead into town to do some food shopping, while we ran to the Bather's Paradise Campground to find SuperRoo. Thanks for your support and for letting SR wait for us on the front lawn!

SEPTEMBER 2013

We finished the run there at 47.09 km after having run along the waterfront for the extra km before realising we had passed the campground! Drove out 11 km north of Esperance to our hosts farm where Graeme had already arrived and parked the van for the night. Our hosts, Claire and David welcomed us to their home, Claire had made a delicious raw dinner which we shared with their family. Thank you so much for your hospitality, it was lovely to meet you all, and thank you for the wonderful spa bath! Although we were late to bed, we slept well after the soak in the tub! Temp 14-24 degrees. Marathon Average 43.1 km. Total Km 11,769.43.

October 2013

MARATHONS #274-304

Marathon #274. October 1, 2013. Esperance to 42.5 km north of Esperance on the Coolgardie-Esperance Hwy. Graeme drove us back 10.5km to where we had finished yesterday and we started 6am running back to the farm to say goodbye. Claire offered to go into town to pick up our mail from the Post Office and bring it out to us on the road and she also offered to bring SuperRoo up to a friend's farm just south of Norseman where we will be in a couple of days. We are so blessed to meet such kind and generous people along the way who are happy to help us out with the car and mail, host us in their home and give us fresh produce from their gardens. Thank you so much Claire, David and family. A long day on the road with starting late we finished late in the dark 42.51 km running the last 14 km without a break so Graeme could drive ahead to set up camp before it got too dark. Another late night, bed at 10pm. Temp 10-21 degrees. Marathon Average 43.11 km. Total Km 11,811.94.

Marathon #275.
October 2, 2013. 42 km north of Esperance to 115 km south of Norseman. Started 5am, both feeling weary with lack of sleep. Running alongside railway track most of the day with salt lakes and marshland on either side of the road. Long flat straights and more wheat fields, almost ready to harvest. Finished run 42.97 km where Graeme had set up camp right in a wheat field! Early night. Marathon Average 43.11 km. Total Km 11,854.91.

Marathon #276.
October 3, 2013. 115 km to 72 km south of Norseman. Started 5am after 9 hours sleep, had a good run to first break at 10 km. Wheat fields for as far as we could see either side of the road and huge harvesting machinery driving past getting ready for the harvest. Met with Claire as

we passed through Salmon Gums (named for the beautiful gum trees with salmon pink and olive coloured trunks) who was delivering SuperRoo to her friends farm where we will stay the night. Thanks again Claire! The last 15 km was all uphill, very hot (Temp 10-34 degrees) and into a strong head wind. Finished at 42.31 km where we were picked up by our host Andrew and Graeme. Drove back 5km to Andrew's farm where the caravan was parked by a guest room with a bath and a bed for Graeme, SuperRoo was tucked up in the shed and we were ready for a good night's sleep. Thank you Andrew for your hospitality. Marathon Average 43.10 km. Total Km 11,897.22.

Marathon #277.

October 4, 2013. 72 km to 25 km south of Norseman. All up with the swallows at 4am, ready to pull out with the ute and van 4.45am. Andrew offered to drive SuperRoo to Norseman on Saturday to meet us when we arrive there. Graeme dropped us off where we finished yesterday and continued on to the 10 km break. We started running at 5:15am, past more salt lakes with the salt crystals sparkling in the early morning sun. Both running well all day. Greg met us at 32 km with a van load of fresh organic produce from John and Jill at Alive Organics in Perth. Thank you so much for your sponsorship and support in providing us with the best fruit and veg since we've arrived in Perth and many thanks to Greg for his 700 km drive to make sure that we have food to get us across the Nullarbor. With everything loaded into the ute and van, Graeme drove slowly on the last 5 km to set up camp for the night in the woods, while we finished the run 43.62 km. Greg stayed for dinner and then left to return to Perth. How good a friend is that! Temp 16-30 degrees. Marathon Average 43.10 km. Total Km 11,940.84.

Marathon #278.

October 5, 2013. 25 km south to 10 km east of Norseman. Started 4:45am running in the dark. Starry sky and beautiful daybreak, misty morning running through the Great Western Forest, the largest Mediterranean Forest on Earth, covering an area larger than England! We will be in the Forest for the next two weeks, no more wheat fields, Andrew's was the last farm until we get to South Australia! The mist cleared by 10am and it became warm with a gentle breeze, perfect running conditions on a smooth road. Arrived in Norseman late morning at the same time as Andrew delivering SuperRoo. We went to the local shop to do last minute shopping while Graeme took Andrew home and drove back (saved Alan driving with Graeme in the Ute to get SR). We arranged with the Norseman Campground to leave SR there as our dear friend and SuperCrew Narelle will be arriving in Norseman in 4 days, so can stay the night then drive out to meet us on the road. We ran up to the Eyre Hwy turnoff where the Nullarbor starts, took photos and continued the run with only 10 km to go. Finished at 42.75 km and built a small rock cairn to honour the indigenous peoples of the Sacred Land that we were entering. Graeme had set up camp in the woods beside the road. Caught up on all the FB updates as we may not have internet again until we get to Eucla which is halfway across the Nullarbor and two weeks out. Temp 16-34 degrees. Marathon Average 43.10 km. Total Km 11,983.59.

Marathon #279.

October 6, 2013. Broke the 12,000 km mark today! 10 km east to 55 km from Norseman on the Eyre Hwy. Finished posting FB updates at 4:30am, started running 5:30am with the sunrising through the early morning mist on the Great Nullarbor Plain. We both felt quite emotional as we've been looking forward to this moment when we know we're on the way home, heading east at last. The road is smooth with wide shoulder and undulating hills along the edge of the Great Western Forest on one side and Salmon Gums amongst sage bush on the other. Very different to any landscape we've seen so far with a mystical feel about it. Noticed evidence of different wildlife as well, camel droppings and (sadly) bones on the side of the road, really hope we see some alive and well; emu droppings and feathers; wombat scratchings and reptiles; lizards and snakes. We saw a very live snake crossing the road, there was no traffic when we came across it, but it was moving quite slowly and had only made it to the middle of the road when two trucks approached. Janette walked out onto the road to slow the trucks down, signaled for them to go on ether side of the snake, which they did with a toot and thumbs up, and the snake continued crossing and slithered off into the grass on the other side. Not long afterwards, Janette noticed a thorny lizard standing up on it's back legs in the middle of one lane, standing his ground to the oncoming traffic! She shooed him off the road as a camper-van went by, tooting and waving. Yay, another save! By midway through the run the temperature had risen from 15 to 34 degrees, we had fruit at our breaks to keep up the energy; bananas, custard apple, oranges, grapefruit, 2 drinking coconuts (a treat from Greg who delivered our organic food from Alive Organics in Perth) and of course a green smoothie. Finished at 43.63 km had fresh carrot, beetroot, apple & ginger juice and a tomato salad for dinner. Total Km 12,027.22.

Marathon #280.

October 7, 2013. Another 10 Marathons down, only 86 to go! 55 km from Norseman to Fraser Range Caravan Park on the Eyre Hwy. Started 5am very cold (5 degrees) and a starry sky. Ran into the rising sun at 5:30am, so good to be heading east! Second day of smooth road and no traffic to speak of. Beautiful eucalyptus trees and shrubs in flower, light red sandy soil and birds flying through the bush, their bright green, red and blue feathers shining in the sunlight and their calls and birdsong filling the morning air. Today we met two spiders, one very black and well camouflaged against the road, the other had bright red legs and black body, we stopped to watch it cross the road and when it came close to Alan's red and black Vibram toe shoes it changed course and raced across towards the shoes! Must have thought it was the biggest spider, kept trying to get on his shoe even when he moved it away, obviously could recognise the colours! The temperature rose quickly reaching 34 degrees and with it came the flies! For the first time we had the large flies that really bite, even while we are running, so it became a race against the flies for the rest of the run! Finished at 42.37 km where Graeme was waiting for us and we drove ahead to the Fraser Range Caravan Park, thanks so much for the complimentary campsite. Did laundry, had showers, dinner and bed. Total Km 12,069.59.

Marathon #281.

October 8, 2013. Fraser Range Caravan Park to 50 km west of Balladonia on Eyre Hwy. Graeme drove us back to where we had finished yesterday, started running 5:15am into a beautiful sunrise. Long straight smooth road, only two corners today. Temperature rose very quickly again and reached 41.7 degrees, the hottest day we have had since January 18, when it was 44 degrees. We seem to be able to handle the heat really well, considering the sudden change from freezing cold and rain last week. Quite a few motorists slowed or stopped to ask if we were OK or needed water, met Robert who is volunteering for Australian Wildlife, thanks for stopping folks. We also met a woman who was waiting on the side of the road with her car. She had lost control of her car and veered off the road, peeling two tyres to the rims, luckily no one was hurt. A kind truckie had taken her children to Balladonia and a passing motorist had taken the tyres to be changed. We stopped to see if there was anything we could do, but she had water and shade to wait, so we gave her a hug and continued on our run. We later saw her again as she passed us with brand new tyres and the kids safely strapped in the back as they continued on their journey. It was the first accident we have come upon during 12,000 km. We finished the run at 42.61 km in a roadside parking spot. Total Km 12,112.20.

Marathon #282.

October 9, 2013. Only 84 Marathons to go! 50 km to 6 km west of Balladonia. Warm during the night and 14 degrees when we started at 5am. Nice sunrise, but clouds building from the south east. Temperature rose quickly to 30 degrees, but suddenly dropped to 20 degrees around midday when the clouds became black and thunderous, rolling in and bringing a sudden down-pour just as we made it to the van for our last break. Started out again and a camper stopped, Dave and Jenny from Heathmont VIC checking to see that we were OK and gave us a donation, thanks so much. A cold southerly wind and rain pushed us on to finish at 43.81 km where Graeme was waiting to drive us on to Balladonia Campground so we could fuel up, take on water and use the phone and internet. Phoned Narelle who has arrived in Norseman and will be driving out in SuperRoo to join us tomorrow, oh yay! Then we'll all be off together into the Great Unknown, will we be able to get water and food on the way across the Nullarbor? As the rain pours down and the tanks in the campground are overflowing, we are told that there is a drought here and we cannot take on water. We're also told that there is nowhere between here and Ceduna to buy food, so what to do? Stay tuned for the next exciting episode of Running Raw Across the Nullarbor... Marathon Average 43.10 km. Total Km 12,156.01.

Marathon #283.

October 10, 2013. 6km West of Balladonia to 4 km east of the sign for the Longest Straight Road. Graeme drove us back to where we finished yesterday and we started running at 5am daybreak. Road still smooth with wide shoulders, landscape changing to low scrub and smaller trees. Narelle left Norseman in the SuperRoo with more fresh produce and caught up with us at the midway break in time to share a delicious pear salad that Graeme had made. Great to have Narelle back on board, having been with us on the Barkly Hwy in April. Now we have two support crew who have been with us before so we can all relax and take each day as it comes, four friends together on the Nullarbor. Met up with Jazz's (Perth Event Organiser) parents Murray and Helen Dillon who were driving from SA. They had stopped at a roadside parking area so Graeme set up camp beside them. We stopped to take photos with Narelle at the road sign that marks the start of the longest straight stretch of road in Australia (146.6 km without a corner), then ran to the campsite with only 2.8 km to go, said a quick hello and ran on with the sun setting behind us. Narelle drove out to pick us up where we finished at 42.32 km. Drove back to the campsite and chatted with Murray & Helen who had brought us some food goodies and offered us a hot shower in their caravan. Narelle had made a delicious salad using some of the fresh produce she had brought from Norseman and Graeme had made fresh carrot and beetroot juice, so we ate before going over for a quick shower, thanks so much Murray & Helen. It was lovely to meet you and we'll see you again when we come back to Perth on our 'Running Out of Time' Book Tour. Temp 11-26 degrees. Marathon Average 43.10 km. Total Km 12,198.33.

Marathon #284.

October 11, 2013. Only 2 months till we arrive in Melbourne! 4 km east of Sign for Longest Straight Road to 98 km west of Caiguna on the Eyre Hwy, Nullabor. Had half an hour sleep in, Narelle drove us forward to where we had finished yesterday and we started running at

5:30am, heading East on the Longest Straight stretch of road in Australia. The road had been recently resurfaced so is a bit rougher than we've had the last couple of days, but no problems running on it. It was a bit undulating so we could only see about 7 km in either direction, but certainly very straight! Landscape continually changing from low scrub and tall salmon gums to grassy plains, no animals but plenty of birds especially the green and blue parrots. We got back into our old routine with the two vehicles, Narelle in SuperRoo meeting us at the first 10 km break while Graeme drove on to 17 km to make the green smoothies. Then we all met up together for the 24km and 32 km breaks after which Graeme drove on to find a good camping spot off the road in the trees while Narelle met us at 37 km with oranges and water. The temperature had risen from 10 to 33 degrees so we needed more water stops, but a following wind kept us cool enough to have a good day's run, finishing at 43.32 km. Marathon Average 43.10 km. Total Km 12,241.

Marathon #285.
October 12, 2013. 98 km to 56 km west of Caiguna. Set the alarm half hour early and the clock half hour forward to get ready for the time change in 2 days. So affectively we were up at 3:15am and started running at 4:30am in the dark for half hour, cloudy daybreak and weather got colder (from 15 to 23 and back to 15 degrees) and very windy from the SW throughout the day. Terrain much the same as yesterday the road straight but undulating so slow going. Traffic mostly big trucks in both directions and some caravans and campers, word has got around on the UHF radio about us so everyone waving and tooting and thumbs up, which really kept us going. Finished at 43.25 km camped on the roadside, Narelle made a delicious raw lasagne for dinner and we all had an early night, in bed by 7pm. Total Km 12,284.90.

Marathon #286.
October 13, 2013. 56 km to 11 km west of Caiguna. Started 4:25am after a good 9 hrs sleep last night. Another day with no corners, long straight road, smooth surface but windy and cold all day. Landscape ever changing, beautiful wattle trees in full bloom and full scent permeating the air. Narelle & Graeme had birthday surprises for Alan (68 today) at the 10

km break and continued to spoilt him all day with balloons and his favourite meals of chia pudding for lunch and cauliflower rice with marinated mushrooms for dinner. Finished the run at 43.14 km, Narelle waiting to drive us to Caiguna Campground where Graeme had set up for the night, taken on water and fueled the ute. Narelle put the laundry on while we had hot showers then we all enjoyed Alan's birthday dinner together. A special day for a special guy with special friends in a special place, how special was that! Temp 7-20 degrees. Total Km 12,328.04.

Marathon #287.

October 14, 2013. 11km west of Caiguna to 34 km west of Cocklebiddy. Stayed up late last night trying to catch up on phone calls and internet, only had 3 hours sleep before getting up at 3:30am, very cold and windy during the night. Graeme drove us back 11.5 km to where we finished yesterday. Started running 4:30am at daybreak, back to the campground where we stopped for 3 hours to finish posting updates on Facebook as the internet crashed last night. Back out on the road, both tired and running slow, Narelle staying with us in SuperRoo to watch out for us. For midway break Narelle made a delicious beetroot slice that looked and tasted like mulberry, yum! Passed the sign for Western Central Time Zone so put the clocks forward 45 mins, which really made us late! Finished the run 43.28 km in the dark, Graeme coming out to show us where he had set up camp about 100 metres down a track off the road, no traffic noise tonight! Temp 6-26 degrees. Total Km 12371.32.

Marathon #288.

October 15, 2013. 34 km west to 11 km east of Cocklebiddy. Cold start at 4:30am, couldn't feel our feet and hands until an hour after sunrise. Landscape becoming more sparse with fewer trees. Saw a very large mama emu with 4 little ones and found a tiny mama lizard, her belly full of eggs, slowly crossing the road. Janette carefully picked her up and put her safely into the scrub. She may have been a chameleon as she was perfectly camouflaged with the ground, black stripes and orange spots and the cutest little face. By midday the temperature had risen to 35 degrees, huge contrast to this morning. Continued running into Cocklebiddy with great expectations of finding a town, but only a roadhouse with no phone or internet, so we had a delicious fruit salad and continued on into the sunset for the last 10 km. Graeme had found a great spot in a field of grass to set up camp for the night. Finished the run 43.06km. Temp 7-35 degrees. Total Km 12,414.38.

Marathon #289.

October 16, 2013. 11 km east of Cocklebiddy to 35 km west of Madura. Stayed very warm throughout the night, 14 degrees at 3:30am when we got up and it had risen to 17 by 4:30am when we started to run. Stayed warm and windy all day, but the road smooth so a good run through a landscape of scrubby desert. Our food stores are being monitored by Graeme and Narelle is preparing delicious and nourishing meals with only a few ingredients for each meal so that we don't run out of food before we get to Ceduna in about 15 days. We left Norseman fully stocked, but as there is nowhere to get more on the way, it is crucial that we manage it carefully. Today we had our last green smoothie as there are no more fresh greens, so it will be fruit smoothies from now on. Will be interesting to see if it will effect our running. Meanwhile we have plenty of bananas, oranges, grapefruit, lemons, apples, pears, papaya and kiwifruit, tomatoes, zucchini, avocado, carrot, beetroot and cabbage, so menu planning will be fun. Finished the run at 44 km down a side road away from the Hwy but very exposed to the strong gusts of wind that are going to rock us to sleep tonight... Temp 14-31 degrees. Total Km 12,458.38.

Marathon #290.

October 17, 2013. 35 km west to 9 km east of Madura. Cold early morning start at 4:30am in the dark. Janette had a spectacular fall on the rough edge as a road train went past, rolling to the right away from the wheels. Seems like the only damage is two skinned knees, but hands okay as she had gloves on inside her jacket sleeve. She continued running until Narelle arrived for the first break and was a bit slow for the rest of the day. Temperature got hot and wind dropped as we ran down the Madura Pass, an incredible view of vast open plains sparsely dotted with trees. Stopped at the Madura Campground to set up for the night and for our midway break. We ran on the last 9 km to finish the run at 43.36 km and Narelle came out to pick us up and drive back. Hot showers but no internet tonight. Temp 4-30 degrees. Total Km 12,502.68.

"It's a long and...(not so)....winding road, thaaaaaaat leads, to Fed Square...". Eileen here, reporting on behalf of our intrepid duo who seem to be in and out of reception at the oddest times! They are both fit and well and about half way across The Nullarbor, with barely any trees and a temperature range between 4 and 42 deg C! Running in calm conditions one minute and gale force winds the next. I don't know about you, but I can't wait for the book!

Marathon #291.

*October 18, 2013. In memory of our dear Mum and SuperNana on the 90th anniversary of her day of birth, feeling her presence as the eagles fly above us and we run through this spirit land....*9 km to 53 km east of Madura. Got up at 3:15am and tried to connect to internet which had crashed last night, but no go so Narelle drove us 9 km from the campground at Madura to where we had finished the run yesterday. Started running at 6am just before sunrise on a long straight road, scrubby dessert on either side dotted with tall myall trees. Stopped for an interview with journalist Brianna who is writing an article on us for the Warrandyte Diary, our home newspaper. Sad moments on the roadside today as we removed several very large red kangas that had been hit and one wedge tailed eagle, almost too big and heavy to lift. There were many eagles flying and some perched in the myall trees, such beautiful birds, so sad and ironic to see them lying on the side of the road along with the kangaroos. Very few cars and trucks on the road so we ran in the middle for most of the time, temperature rose from 14 to 39 degrees, but no humidity so the heat wasn't too bad. Narelle stayed with us to give us water every 5 km, finding a single tree to park under for the shade. Flies were bad today, probably numerous because of all the roadkill, it's the worst we've seen so far. Graeme made yellow smoothies with oranges and bananas and a delicious fruit salad for midway break. Narelle prepared Raw Vegan Shepherd's Pie for dinner using mashed cauliflower for the topping and a lemon banana pie for desert. Even though we don't have many ingredients, we're being treated to some delicious meals, all raw vegan and beautifully presented. We finished the run at 44.02 km where Graeme had set up camp on the side of the road in amongst the scrub and grass. Wind is getting up and cooling things off, so we're off to bed for an early night. Total Km 12,546.70.

Marathon #292.
October 19, 2013. 53 km east of Madura to 18 km west of Mundrabilla. Very warm throughout the night, 24 degrees when we started running at 4:40am. Cloudy with a few drops of rain and strong head wind which slowed us down, until the wind changed direction 360 degrees and we were being pushed along from behind! Janette's knees are causing a bit of discomfort from the fall two days ago, but are healing well. Interesting terrain where we are running alongside an escarpment which used to be the land edge millions of years ago, beside the road there are thousands of fossilized shells where it was the sea, so effectively we're running on the Bight rather than beside it! This must have been the Land Before Time as there are many prehistoric looking critters as well, today we were confronted by a scaled Blue Tongue Lizard who clearly thought he was in another era, stopping in his tracks to hiss at us then turned when he heard a road train coming and hissed at that too! We tried to shoo him away from the road but he was having none of that, turned back and hissed at us then took off, shuffling and wriggling across the road to disappear on the other side. Rather comical but dangerous practice! The temperature continued to rise and reached 38 degrees by midway where we stopped for an hour to avoid the heat then continued to finished at 43.03 km at a roadside camp amongst the only trees for as far as we could see. Marathon Average 43.12 km. Total Km 12,598.73.

Marathon #293.
October 20, 2013. 18 km west of Mundrabilla to 40 km west of Eucla. Started at 4:25am, terrain much the same as yesterday, the road mostly smooth and traffic light. Had first break of bananas with Narelle while Graeme drove straight to Mundrabilla Roadhouse to get water. There were two large water tanks just off the road with a sign for drinking water so Alan ran in to check it out, plenty of clean rain water which Graeme went back to fill our tanks. Most of the roadhouses have not had drinking water available so we were pleased to find the tanks full. Finished the run 44.12 km at our camp site by 5:30pm after battling strong head winds most

of the second half of the run. Narelle had made a delicious dinner of coleslaw and we had an early night, in bed by 7:30pm. Total Km 12,633.85.

Marathon #294.

October 21, 2013. 40 km west to 3 km east of Eucla. Started at 4:15am, nice daybreak on a long straight road heading east into the sunrise. Came across a young Joey not long out of the pouch who had very recently been hit on the road, his little body still soft and warm. Janette picked him up and carried him into the scrub placing him in the shade under a bush, tucking his tail around him and his sweet face under his paws, he looked for all the world to be asleep. Sad enough to see the adult kangaroos on the side of the road, but to see such a young one is heart-wrenching. As I returned to the road, tears still streaming down my face, I noticed a car had pulled up and the driver was coming over. "He said you'd give me a flyer," he called out, referring to Alan whom he had stopped to talk to before driving ahead to where I was. I handed him a flyer and he looked at me sympathetically saying, "Are you doing this too love?" "Yes," I replied, not wanting to elaborate in case my emotions let me down. "Well, I'll make a donation through the website, keep it up," he said waving the flyer as he got back in his car and drove off. I wondered if he had seen me carrying the little Joey off the road... The wind picked up, strong head winds for a couple of hours then it swung around to a strong following wind, gusty at times making it hard to stay on the ground. A real blast running into Eucla, blown along the straights, almost took off on the RFDS emergency airstrip, then pushed up the Pass at a great rate of knots! The Nullarbor Nymph has nothing on us! Narelle met us with SuperRoo and gave us a tour of Eucla looking out at the view of the Great Southern Ocean and the long straight road we had run. We could see the migrating sand dunes that had covered the old Telegraph Station, the wind still whipping sand across the top of the dunes. A quick visit to the museum which was fascinating to see the old pictures before and after the sand had covered the Station. With only 3 km to go we ran out of Eucla in a wind storm, horizontal rain and sand pushing us to finish at 42.67 km, Narelle was there in SuperRoo to pick us up and drive to the WA/SA border, where Graeme had set up camp on a complimentary site in the Border Village Campground, thanks for your hospitality and support. Laundry, showers, dinner and catching up on the internet, as the wind howls around the caravan hopefully off to bed soon... Temp 14-29 degrees. Marathon Average 43.12 km. Total Km 12,676.52.

Marathon #295.

October 22, 2013. 3 km east of Eucla, WA to 35 km east of Border Village, SA. Graeme drove us back 8 km through the Border to where we finished yesterday. Started running at 4:25am back through the WA/SA Border and into the campground to use the internet for 2 hours before heading out into a cold, rainy and windy day on the road. Narelle stayed with us throughout the day as we were taking our jackets off and putting them back on with the rain squalls. Stopped at a lookout to see the spectacular view of the ocean and high cliffs (80-90 metres high). Not much traffic on the road except quite a few motorbikes, everyone waving and tooting as they passed us and some taking photos and videos. Guess it must be a surprise to see people running along the Nullarbor! Although our food supply is going down we're having great meals; 2 fruit smoothies, pear salad and sprouted chickpea hummus with vege sticks with bananas and dates at the breaks. Finished the run 43.02 km 2 km past a roadside truck parking area where Graeme had set up camp amongst the scrub. Temp 12-18 degrees. Average Marathon 43.12 km. Total Km 12,719.54.

Marathon #296.

October 23, 2013. 53 km to 80 km east of Border Village. Narelle drove us forward 2 km to where we finished yesterday. Started running 4:15am in the dark for an hour before daybreak. Cool morning with a strong easterly head wind which changed later to a gusty southerly. All much the same landscape with the occasional view of the ocean, stopped at the second viewpoint with great views of the cliffs in both directions, very windy onshore wind, but the ocean relatively calm. No sign of any sea life not even any birds. Met a couple of guys from South Africa cycling from Sydney to Perth (against the wind!) on their journey of 7 continents. Great to meet you both and good luck with your trip, may the wind be at your back for the next one! Finished the run 44.47 km at roadside picnic area. Food today included 2 fruit smoothies, fruit salad (kiwifruit, pear, apple, orange & banana), pumpkin and tomato fettucini with Botanical Cuisine pesto sauce for dinner. Put the clocks forward 2 hours to SA time and went to bed for an 8 hour sleep. Temp 14-19 degrees. Average Marathon 43.12km. Total Km 12,764.01.

Marathon #297.

October 24, 2013. 80 km east of Border Village to 61 km west of Nullarbor. Started the run at 6am (SA time) in dark for one hour with a gradual daybreak, cloudy sky, cold strong head wind all day. The wind is starting to wear us out and peel the skin off our faces. It's coming from the South off the Ocean and will not stop, can someone please turn off the wind machine? The road is smooth, flat and straight following the coast of the Great Australian Bight. When the traffic passes we have to step off the road and wait till they pass before continuing on the road, the edge is too stony to run on. The landscape is changing slightly with the shrubs getting more dense. We have not seen any wildlife for a couple of days apart from hundreds of bunnies scampering about amongst the scrub, diving down their bunny holes when we pass and another encounter with a blue tongue lizard on his way across the road. The Nullarbor belongs to the bunnies, the lizards and the ants. Narelle did some filming of us running down the straight road through a landscape all the same, but ever changing. It's a special place this Land With No Trees. Stopped at a lookout to view the Great Southern Ocean and seven headlands still to run, beautiful view even with the wind. Finished the run 43.16 km at a spot on the cliffs where Graeme had set up camp for the night. Food today 2 orange and banana smoothies, papaya and kiwifruit salad, raw lasagne made with zucchini, tomatoes and 3 sauces; Botanical Cuisine Pesto and Walnut Bolognese, and a sunflower seed cheese - delicious! Our food supply is going down, but we're eating well with only a few ingredients to make each meal. One day and 18 km to get to Nullarbor Roadhouse where we'll hopefully have internet. Only 68 Marathons to go to finish the Run, 69 to break the World Record for most consecutive marathons Running Raw Around Australia, who is going to join us? Temp 14-19 degrees. Average Marathon 43.12km. Total Km 12,807.17 km.

Marathon #298.

October 25, 2013. 61 km to 14 km west of Nullabor. Started running at 5:55am in the dark for an hour before daybreak. Cold morning until sun broke through the clouds and warmed up the day, apart from the cold strong head winds really giving us wind burn on the face and cracking our lips. Tried wearing a scarf but it was too hot and hard to breath, so put the fly net on which does cut down the wind on the face a bit. Saw a dingo cross the road ahead of us and run out into the grass, stopping to watch us a few times, then a few kilometres on we saw another one, also running away and stopping to watch us. Maybe we will hear them tonight when the moon comes up. Good to see them again, we've missed them. Finished the run 44 km where Graeme had set up camp amongst the grass off the road. Narelle and Graeme had made a delicious dinner of pumpkin fettucini with a jar of Botanical Cuisine Mushroom & Pepperberry Sauce mixed into fresh almond creme. Dinner at sunset, catching up on the internet (signal has come in because we're close to Nullarbor) and hopefully not too late to bed. Temp 7-31 degrees. Marathon Average 43.12 km. Total Km 12,851.41.

Just went outside to check the sky, it's full of stars and on the horizon I see the lights of Nullarbor, can't contain my excitement so better go to bed! We're running Marathon #299 through Nullarbor tomorrow, then will lose phone & internet signal for 3 days until we reach Nundroo. So Marathon #300 will be on the Nullarbor marking another major milestone on the Run. Running the Nullarbor is without a doubt the biggest challenge we have faced in the entire Run, we have been in training for this for the past 9 months and 12,000 km around Australia, but we had no idea until we got here how challenging it would be. The Nullarbor is 1181 km long (approximately same distance as Melbourne to Coffs Harbour) of mostly straight road through sparse landscape (nullarbor is Latin for no trees) and will take us 27 days to run, with nowhere to buy fresh fruit and veg. A quote from explorer Eyre who first walked across the Nullarbor and whom the Eyre Hwy is named after; "The Nullarbor is the sort of place that creeps into bad dreams." However, in it's own special way, the Nullarbor is a beautiful place, indeed a spiritual place in this sacred land and it will have a special place in our dreams for years to come. Meanwhile, with 300 km still to go, we couldn't be doing this without our Super Support Crew, Graeme and Narelle who are keeping us on the straight and narrow day after day. Thanks you two for being here on this special part of the journey, and a big thanks to everyone for your encouragement and support and a special thanks again to Rob and all those who have made donations towards the Run and the Charities. See you down the track...

Marathon #299.

October 26, 2013. 14 km west to 30 km east of Nullarbor. Started running 6am, following the lights of Nullarbor in the distance. Stopped at Nullarbor Roadhouse, crew did laundry and had showers while Janette caught up on the internet and Alan did some filming. Continued on the run after 3 hours. Landscape very strange, low salt bushes and no trees in all directions. Saw three different dingoes wandering along not far from the road, they all seemed indifferent to our presence. Struggled with a hot head wind for the rest of the run with the temperature rising to 37 degrees. Narelle stayed with us to give us water and a few moments out of the wind every 2 km, this was one of our hardest stretches so far. Finished just on sunset at 43.35 km, dinner of coleslaw and hummus and into bed as a storm started brewing in the West... Total Km 12,894.76.

Marathon #300.

October 27, 2013. 30 km east of Nullarbor to 14 km west of Yalata. Thunder and lightening storms and strong winds during the night, started running at 6am with incredible lightening show in the western sky. The dark storm clouds were building fast and heading in our direction, the thunder getting louder and lightening brighter. The storm eventually caught us up with a light rain shower as it passed over. By daybreak the sky had cleared and we had a beautiful sunrise. The landscape changed dramatically from treeless plain to thick forest of salmon gums and native shrubs, with the salt bushes giving off a distinct salty smell in the air. The terrain also became more hilly, we gained 60 metres today. The wind had shifted to the West and eased off so we had a light following wind with a temperature rising to 32 degrees. Reasonable running conditions with Narelle stopping every 4 km for water and dates. Saw a young monitor lizard crossing the road ahead of us, luckily no traffic so he made it safely to the other side. Not so lucky was a brown snake and a frog-mouthed owl, both of whom we moved off the roadside and into the forest. We've seen some strange things on the Run, but today was a classic, a man sitting in a tree smoking a cigarette and drinking a beer! Not sure how long he's been there, but he's starting to look a bit worse for wear! Narelle made a special effort today to celebrate our three-hundredth marathon with balloons and a delicious dessert. Finished the run at 44.44 km at the entrance to Yalata Community Land where we set up camp and had a delicious meal of zucchini and pumpkin spaghetti with tomato sauce. Another major milestone! Three hundred marathons and only 65 to finish the Run, 66 to the World Record! We're on count down now! Total Km 12,939.20.

Marathon #301.

October 28, 2013. 14 km west of Yalata to 23 km west of Nandroo. Started at 6am. Undulating hills and corners all day with a 60 metre loss. Good running conditions with a cool breeze, cloudy with some sunny breaks. Went through Yalata, where everything was closed down except the police station. Met a family travelling around Australia in their converted bus, brought back memories of when we travelled with our kids in a bus through Europe. Thanks Molly for writing in our guest book and for your kind donation. Have fun on the rest of your trip. Had our last smoothie today, no fresh bananas left. Dates for breaks, chia pudding (with dates, sultanas, currants, grated apple, soaked almonds with almond creme), sprouted chickpea hummus with tomatoes and carrot sticks. Interesting how well we are running on less food as our stocks are dwindling. Two more days and we'll be able to buy enough food to get us to Ceduna where our next delivery will be. Finished the run at 43.56 km camping by the roadside. Temp 15-24 degrees. Total Km 12,982.76.

Marathon #302.

October 29, 2013. 23 km west of Nundroo to 58 km west of Penong. Started at 5:30am, cool 10 degrees. Landscape much the same to start but changed dramatically later in the run, out of the dessert, through the forest and into the wheat fields. The wheat is being harvested and there is a lot of dust in the air, many trucks and equipment on the roads so we're having to get off every time they pass because there is no shoulder for us to run on. The temperature warmed to 24 degrees but we've had a strong head wind all day that is causing wind burn to our faces and cracked lips. Interesting eating program today: dates at 4:30am, dates at 7:30am, chia pudding with dates, sultanas and grated apple at 9am and 11am, 1 apple with tahini at 3:30pm, dates at 5pm and large coleslaw at 7:30pm. Finished the run at 43.40 km camped in a field off the road. Broke the 13,000 km mark with a Total Km 13,026.16. Marathon Average 43.13 km.

Marathon #303.

October 30, 2013. 58 km to 12 km west of Penong. Started at 5:30am, came across 3 wombats on the road that had recently been hit. We removed them to the side and were saddened that the first we have seen of them was this way. Ran 10 km and had dates with Narelle who then left to drive into Ceduna to pick up Michael who will be crewing for us to Melbourne as Graeme is leaving from Ceduna in two days time. Narelle is also on a mercy mission to bring back fresh fruit and veg for the next two days until we get to the quarantine border where we cannot bring any fresh produce through. Today we had chia pudding twice, dates and kiwifruit before Narelle and Michael arrived back with fresh food. We had been missing our greens so really enjoyed a delicious salad dinner. Although it was clear and sunny, the day's run was slow as we had very strong head winds again and it was quite hilly....pass the violin! Michael and Graeme went ahead with the ute and van to set up camp at Penong and we finished the run at 44.87 km where Narelle was waiting for us to drove in to stay the night, have hot showers and do the laundry. A long day for everyone but we're well fed and watered so all is good. Temp 10-26 degrees. Marathon Average 43.14 km. Total Km 13,071.03.

Marathon #304.

October 31, 2013. 12 km west of Penong to 42 km west of Ceduna. Narelle drove us back 12 km to where we finished yesterday and we ran back to campground to spend 3 hours on the internet which was very slow and eventually gave up on it and continued the run through wheat fields all day. So many trucks on the road today with wide and oversized loads, mostly huge mining vehicles and buildings or harvesting equipment that take up most of the road. We're having to get off each time, so we're thinking we should use the oversize sign to make sure they see us! Another long day on the road, 15 hrs from start to finish, 5am-8pm. Crew did a great job, Narelle staying with us for water breaks and preparing meals in between, Graeme co-driving with Michael as he gets used to the Ute towing the caravan. Finished the run 42.57km where they had set up camp, three tents and a caravan, and a delicious dinner using up the last of the food. Everyone in bed by 9:30pm under a starry sky... Temp 14-36 degrees. Marathon Average 43.14 km. Total Km 13,113

November 2013

MARATHONS #305-334

Marathon #305. November 1, 2013. From 42 km west to Ceduna. Started 4:30am in the dark on a long straight road running down the middle under the stars. We could see the lights of oncoming traffic about 10 km away so had plenty of time to get off the road before they passed us. Temperature was 14 degrees with a warm breeze, rising through the day to 37 degrees and the breeze became a very hot strong head wind, the heat rising from the road around 50 degrees. The Nullarbor still had a challenge to throw at us on the last day. Running through wheat fields on either side of the road, thousands of acres of yellow wheat waving in the breeze or cut short where it had been harvested. The air is filled with dust and it smells like bread cooking. We had to eat all the rest of the produce before going through the SA quarantine border so running on a big salad through the border and officially finishing our run across the Nullarbor. Felt really good to have achieved the crossing, but couldn't have done it so well without the constant support of our SuperCrew Narelle and Graeme. Also without a doubt, the organic food made a huge difference, we didn't have to eat as much as if it had been non organic and it lasted the whole trip across as well. Graeme and Michael drove into Ceduna to have new tyres put on the ute and Narelle went ahead to take SuperRoo in to have the battery checked and a new one installed if needed. We ran into Ceduna town where the local newspaper reporter met us and did an interview on the run, the article will appear in next week's issue. We had arranged to meet Narelle in the shop to buy some fresh produce but found that she was still at the garage where the new battery had been fitted but the car would not start. So a long night ensued with mechanics trying for four hours to start the car and not knowing why it would not start, eventually they towed it over the road to the campground where we had the ute and caravan and we called the RACV who sent their mechanic out. Unfortunately he did not know what the problem was and suggested we have his off-sider look at it in the morning since by then it was already 9pm. Meanwhile, we met up with our friends Greg and Hanneke from The Flight Centre in Perth who had flown from Perth to Adelaide, arranged to pick up an order of fresh fruit and vege from an organic supplier in Adelaide, drove 850 km to deliver the produce to us, and they sponsored the order! How incredible is that! Thanks so much you two for your kindness and generosity. We really appreciate what you have done to supply us with enough organic fruit and veg to get to the Victoria border, it really does make a difference. After dinner we finished the last 3 km of the run at 42.75 km. Total Km 13,156.35.

Marathon #306.

November 2, 2013. Ceduna to 43.87 km east of Ceduna. Started at 5am and ran out of Ceduna on the Eyre Hwy east towards Port Augusta. Got to 11 km when Greg and Hanneke stopped in their car to bring us a banana and say goodbye. Thanks again, we'll see you in Melbourne for the finish. Graeme arrived in the ute to pick us up and take us back to the campground to meet the mechanic and check on SuperRoo. He eventually came and started the car which went first go. He had an inspection of everything and couldn't find any reason why it would not start last night, took it for a drive and pronounced SuperRoo fit and able to keep going! This has put us 4 hours behind schedule. We said goodbye to Graeme who had been with us since leaving Perth and had done a Supercrew job with Narelle of taking care of our needs all the way across the Nullarbor. Michael has taken over driving the Ute and Van and we jumped in with him to drive out the 11 km we had already done this morning. Narelle did some last minute shopping and caught us up at 17 km where we continued with our routine running and stopping for water as the temperature had risen to 41 degrees. A long slow day in the heat and strong head winds, finished the run at 43.87 km. Temp 14-41 degrees. Marathon Average 43.14 km. Total Km 13,200.22.

Marathon #307.

November 3, 2013. 43.87 east of Ceduna to 3 km west of Wirrulla. Started at 5:20am in the dark, already 17 degrees, but a cold head wind made us very cold. Janette found it hard to stay awake on her feet, Alan also weary as we had only had 9 hours sleep the last two nights. Made it OK to the 10 km mark where Narelle was waiting with water and a warm blanket. Stopped till we were warm enough to continue on to the 17 km mark and had green smoothies and a longer rest in the van. Felt less tired and carried on with very strong head winds making for a slow day. Found a baby fox lying dead on the side of the road, so perfect, so soft, so tiny, so sad. Janette laid him beneath a tree and cried for his loss. We also found 3 birds who had been killed by the updraft from the trucks, so a sad day on the road. Michael found a spot to camp off the road that was further than we could run so finished the run at 44.01 km and Narelle picked us up and drove us on. Had a delicious kale salad for dinner, so good to have fresh greens again. In bed by 8pm so we'll get 8 hours sleep tonight. Temp 17-26 degrees. Total Km 13,244.23 km.

Marathon #308.

November 4, 2013. 3 km west of Wirrulla to 4 km west of Poocheera. Narelle drove us back to where we had finished yesterday and we started the run at 5:30am, running back past the van and past the village of Wirrulla without stopping. Michael and Narelle stopped in Wirrulla to top up with water at caught us up at the 10 km mark. Running much better today after a good sleep, started out at 10 degrees and got hotter 30 degrees with the wind coming from the North East early in the run and changing to South East, dropping in strength. Met Sam on a solar powered electric tricycle he had built himself and has also been circumnavigating Australia. Such a breath of fresh Eyre to see a young man out on the road, just doing it. Keep following your dreams Sam and they will lead you to the next adventure, we'll see you in Melbourne. Finished the run at 43.24 km where Michael had set up camp on a slip road off the Hwy. Average Marathon 43.14 km. Total Km 13,287.47.

Marathon #309.

November 5, 2013. Today's run is dedicated to all the horses who should be running free....4 km west of Poocheera to 5 km east of Minnipa. Started at 5am, both of us weary through lack of sleep, so running slow and feeling the heat as the temperature rose from 14 to 33 degrees.

Ran past Poocheera and on to Minnipa, Narelle staying with us for water and stopping at the van twice for food. We're having to eat the kale as it will spoil in this heat, so it's going in the green smoothies and we're making wilted kale salads. Also having more avocados than we would normally because they are all ripening at once, doesn't seem to be having an adverse affect on our running. Finished the run at 42.99 km where Narelle picked us up and drove on to where Michael had set up camp off the road. Had a bush shower pouring cold water from a bucket over us to cool down before dinner and bed by 8pm. Marathon Average 43.14 km. Total Km 13,330.46.

Marathon #310.

November 6, 2013. 5 km east of Minnipa to 12 km east of Wudinna. Michael drove us back 2 km to where we finished yesterday and we started running at 5am, both overdressed as the temperature was 24 degrees already. Stopped at the van as we passed to change into less clothes and continued on into a vivid red sunrise, red sky in the morning, runners take warning! It was almost 30 degrees by 7:30am, Narelle stopping to give us more water and oranges. By midday it was 43.8 degrees with a strong hot wind and we were slowing considerably by the time we reached Wudinna, the heat was rising off the road and burning our faces. Some of the locals told us that they could not harvest the wheat because of the fire risk. We decided to stop in town and have some food, had a delicious beetroot soup then continued on out of town while Narelle stayed behind to do laundry and Michael took on water. The day was declared catastrophic fire rating and kids were sent home from school, the heat was quite oppressive as we left the town but we continued on with Narelle staying close to replenish water for us. Finished at 43.64 km where Narelle had hung the laundry out on a line between the trees, looked like a gypsy camp, very inviting! Made curried veges and cauliflower rice for dinner, a cold bush shower and off to bed 9pm. Total Km 13,344.10.

Marathon #311.

November 7, 2013. 12 km east of Wudinna to 47 km east of Kimba. Temperature dropped during the night and clouds rolled in. Started running 5am in the dark, weather forecast for showers then rain later, cold in contrast to yesterday. Wheat fields on either side, some already harvested, others rushing to get done before the rain comes, so a lot of dust in the air and the smell of bread baking. Maybe the wheat got cooked yesterday in the heat! Had bananas at first break, then smoothie at 17 km, bananas again at 24 km, then pineapple, banana and avocado pudding at 32 km. Started to rain steadily during the last 13 km, Michael had driven ahead to set up camp, Narelle was with us but we hadn't put a change of clothes in the car, so decided to run it out with Narelle staying close. Janette put on a thin plastic hoodie poncho which kept some warmth in and Alan put on an extra jacket, but we were both drenched through and very cold when we finished at 42.53. Narelle was there to wrap us in sleeping bags in the car and drive us on to where Michael had set up camp in a parking area off the road 3 km further on. Our clothes and shoes were soaked through, we got dried off and into warm clothes with a blanket around us while we drank fresh juice that Michael had made, then had a delicious salad dinner and climbed into bed by 8pm. Off to sleep with the sound of rain on the roof... Temp 11-20 degrees. Total Km 13, 386.63.

Marathon #312.

November 8, 2013. From 47 km to 5 km east of Kimba. Narelle drove us back 3 km to where we had finished yesterday, started running 5:15am in the dark, some stars but dark clouds still on the horizon. Stopped at the van to drop off torch and put on an extra vest as there is a cold head wind. Ran on to 11km for first break amongst the wheat fields, the wheat heavy with water from last night's rain. Continued on with an easy run on smooth road surrounded by wheat for as far as the eye could see, one field we estimated was 10 km square. Temperature rose throughout the day as the skies cleared and sun warmed us, running well to finish at 42.95 km, just 5 km short of Kimba. Narelle drove us in to the Kimba Roadhouse Campground where Michael had set up in a complimentary site, thank you for your support and kind hospitality. Narelle drove into town to shop for more bananas and greens and picked up a copy of the West Coast Sentinel newspaper which had a good article about us from the interview we had when we arrived in Ceduna. Hot showers, laundry and dinner of sprouted chickpea hummus and veg sticks before catching up on the internet. Temp 14-30 degrees. Total Km 13,429.58.

Marathon #313.

November 9, 2013. 5 km to 38 km east of Kimba. Michael drove us back 5 km to where we finished yesterday, started running 5:30am back to the campground along a horse trail, nice and soft underfoot. Stopped at the van to do some more catchup on the internet for 2+1/2 hours so a late finish coming up today after only 4 hours sleep last night for Janette. Continued the run out of Kimba and past the biggest Galah we've ever seen! Apparently Kimba is half way across Australia from west to east, so we're now officially heading for home! Slow going on long straight road. Met Trilby and her children Harry and Annie and their rescued kangaroo, Rattieroo on the last 5 km, they stopped to ask where we were running to as they had seen us several hours earlier. They were very interested and invited us to meet Rattieroo who was in a shopping bag in the car. The cutest little kangaroo joey, rescued from his Mama's pouch when they were found on the side of the road, poor Mama had to be put down as she was too badly injured. So, little Ratteroo took up residence in the shopping bag and has been taken care of since, he will grow to be a big male with the freedom of living on a 40,000 sq km station. So if you are traveling on country roads, please keep a warm bag or box with towel in the car to wrap any rescued little one if you ever see any wildlife lying on the side of the road, please stop and check to see if they are injured and if there is any little one tucked away inside a Mama's pouch and phone the Wildlife Rescue for that area… We reluctantly said goodbye to this lovely family who clearly love animals and the land and left with the soft touch of Rattiroo's ears on our fingers. Finished the run 42.55 km 2.8 km past a roadside parking area where Michael had set up camp. Narelle drove us back and we had a delicious dinner of zucchini noodles with Botanical Cuisine Walnut Bolognese Sauce, then off to bed for an early night. Temp 9-20 degrees. Total Km 13,472.13.

Marathon #314.

November 10, 2013. 38 km east of Kimba to 5km west of Iron Knob. Narelle drove us forward to where we finished yesterday and we started running at 5:30am as the first light brought daybreak and a promise of a good day. Cool windy start, but warmed up after sunrise. An uneventful day with very little traffic and the landscape changing from wheat fields to desert scrub. We did see four emus prancing off into the distance, looking like men in tights embarrassed about how their tutus swayed from side to side. Got phone coverage at the top of a hilly stretch of the road so stopped to catch up on messages and make a few calls. Heard from Karen who was planning to join us next week as support crew but had a sudden change of plans, so called Eileen to put the word out on Facebook. Had a great response and now have Sylvia joining us to do the Adelaide to Melbourne leg, many thanks to Sylvia and everyone else who offered to help. Continued on to finish the run 43.89 km just 5 km short of the town of Iron Knob, Michael had set up camp off the road with a view of the Iron Knob. Dinner at sunset and tents flapping in the wind...Temp 14-24 degrees. Total Km 13,516.02. Only 52 Marathons to go!

Marathon #315.

November 11, 2013. *Today's Run dedicated to our parents and grandparents who experienced the longest days during the First and Second World Wars.* 5 km west of Iron Knob to 28 km west of Port Augusta. Started 5am in the dark, both a bit tired with only a few hours sleep again, catching up on the internet when we can. Landscape is now like the Nullarbor again, low scrub and no trees. Coming into a range of hills at the end of the run, finished 42.54 km and Narelle drove us on 2.5 km to where Michael had set up camp in a rest area at the junction of Port Lincoln and Port Augusta. Heading for an early night in bed before sunset 7pm. Temp 11-27 degrees. Total Km 13,558.56.

Marathon #316.

November 12, 2013. 28 km west of Port Augusta to Stirling North. Michael drove us back 2.7 km to where we had finished yesterday. Started running at 5am Michael filming us in the dark and at daybreak as we arrived back at the van. We were greeted at the park by a small fox who was climbing out of the rubbish bin, then he ran off into the scrub. We continued on towards Port Augusta, the landscape bare of trees with low salt bushes and several flocks of sheep walking slowly in a single line along a ridge towards us. When they saw us coming they turned around and walked back the way we were running, then broke into a run as we came alongside, the lambs kicking their heels in the air and their little tails wagging behind them! Stopped for the second break at the van where Michael had parked beside another field of salt bush. We had our green smoothies and left to run into the town, glancing behind we noticed something floating in the air above the van then realised that it was Michael's tent! He had put it up beside the van to dry off the morning dew and a sudden gust of wind had picked it up and taken it off, spiraling upwards into the sky. Then we saw Michael, running for all he was worth jumping over salt bushes across the field, chasing after his tent. It looked like a scene out of a Month Python movie! As he caught up and was below the tent it suddenly dropped back down to the ground, bowling over and over with Michael trying to tackle it, but another gust of wind whipped it up into the air again and off it went again, flying like a kite over the salt bushes spiraling up and down above Michael who had taken up running after it again. The tent was getting higher and further away, heading up into the sky and although Michael was still running he was losing ground. It appeared that all was lost and the tent would take off on a flightpath to Darwin, Michael last seen running into the outback, leaping over salt bushes and waving his arms wildly in the air....but suddenly the wind dropped and so did the tent, coming down like a deflated balloon it crashed into the only tree on the landscape! Michael kept running until he reached the tree, pulled the tent out of the branches, turned around and marched back to the van, dragging the tent behind him like a scolded puppy. Meanwhile, we were cracking up on the side of the road, having had the best piece of comic entertainment for the whole trip! Unfortunately, none of it was caught on film and for some reason Michael refused to reenact it! We left the performance and continued running into Port Augusta, called into the Trans Continental Newspaper office to do an interview while Narelle did the food shopping. Then we heading out of town across the Salt Lakes to Stirling North where we finished the run 42.41 km and set up camp behind the local garage/store/post office, thank you for your hospitality and support. Temp 15-27 degrees. Total Km 13,600.97.

Marathon #317.

November 13, 2013. Stirling North to Spring Creek. Narelle drove us out to the Hwy to start at 5am. The lights of the huge power plant looked like it was Christmas. A strong wind coming off the water made it very cold and the road has become very busy with traffic, which will eventually turn into freeway closer to Adelaide, so we decided to take an alternate route that will be quieter, less traffic pollution and more scenic. Turning left onto the B83 route to Wilmington we approached the lower Flinders Range, Mount Remarkable and the Horrocks Pass. A great run up through the Pass, felt good to be running hills again, up the winding road through stands of huge River Gums to the summit, over the top and down into the beautiful valley to Wilmington. Coming into the town the road was being resealed and the wet tar stuck to our shoes, making a snapping sound as we ran through the sleepy town which appeared to be all for sale. We turned south onto the B82 Horrocks Hwy and ran out into a landscape of wheat and barley fields, small stone cottages standing amongst the golden sheafs swaying in the wind. With only 8 km to go, we could feel the difference being off the main Hwy and in the countryside, the fresh air made us light on our feet and we finished at 44.14 km with no affects from running the hills. Michael had set up camp by Spring Creek, a dry stoney creek bed with huge River Gums towering above us. Narelle had prepared a delicious raw lasagne and we had a quiet night with no traffic noise, the only sound a cuckoo calling in the distance.... Temp 13-24 degrees.Total Km 13,645.11.

Marathon #318.

November 14, 2013. Spring Creek to Wirrabara. Started running 5am in the dark heading due south with the Southern Cross in the sky directly in front of us. A cool and clear morning and brilliant sunrise. Stopped in the very quaint town of Melrose for our green smoothie break which we had in the rose garden. The town is at the base of Mount Remarkable and is popular for it's biking trails. As we left we saw a bird hanging upside down (like a bat) in a tree and noticed that it appeared to only have one leg and it was caught in the branches. We tried to encourage the bird to keep struggling to get free by jumping up and down underneath it, but it was still stuck and we were debating whether we would climb the tree to release the bird or phone Narelle to alert the fire brigade to come and rescue it, when suddenly it dropped out of the branches and flew to the ground. Immediately another bird, presumably it's mother, flew over to it, hopping around and chirping happily. Then she flew off, the smaller bird following her, flying free again...We continued on through Murray Town, Alan stopping in at the Pub to check if there were any long lost relatives at the bar and finished the run 42.67 km at the Wirrabara General Store, thanks to the proprietors for their donation and support. Michael had set up camp next to the town oval and we have hot showers and toilets, and our very own grandstand to watch the night sky. Narelle pitched her tent on the oval, outstanding in her field as always! Temp 12-29 degrees. Total Km 13,687.78.

Marathon #319.

November 15, 2013. Wirrabara to Georgetown. Started running 5am from the van, through the park and onto Horrocks Hwy in the centre of Wirrabara. Today was a 4 town day, running through history in each town. First was Stone Hut, named after a stone hut still outstanding in it's field, renowned for it's bakery cafe and wine tasting, unfortunately we were there too early at 6:30am; next was Laura, renowned for it's ice-cream, which of course we did not taste, but a resident next to where we were parked offered for us to pick fresh oranges from their tree, thank you so much and for the donation. The town is very quaint but most of the buildings including the bank are for sale. Thanks also to the newsagent who helped us with info on our phones, cameras and computers and who had the right size memory card for our camera, so we're back filming again. The third was Gladstone, renowned for the largest grain storage in inland Australia and there was a good supermarket where we were able to stock up on bananas again. We finished the run 42.43 km in Georgetown, where we set up camp in a free site in the centre of town next to the Memorial Park and Narelle pitched her tent between the swings and roundabouts in the children's playground. She had made another delicious dinner of Zucchini Noodles with Mushroom Pepperberry Sauce (thanks botanical cuisine), another great day on the road. Temp 15-29 degrees. Total Km 13,730.21.

Marathon #320.

November 16, 2013. Georgetown to 20 km north of Clare. Started 4:55am in the dark, running well despite the strong head wind. Sunny but windy all day, running amongst fields of mature beans, peas and oats, and harvesting of the wheat. Went through one town today, we had read that it was a town where you get to talk with the locals, but all was quiet when we went through, it was hard to find anyone to yack to in Yacka! Met Rusty the dog on the bike with his farmer friend whose wheat field we stopped alongside for midway break of our favourite beetroot dessert. Rusty was perfectly balanced on the back of the bike, licking our hands while we chatted, then leaning out with his ears back as the farmer took off on the bike. Finished the run 43.59 km at roadside gravel pit where Michael had set up camp for the night. Narelle made another delicious zucchini and broccoli dish for dinner, her last night with us as she leaves tomorrow. We will miss her wonderful attention, her happy smile and infectious laugh, and of course her yummy meals. Thank you Narelle, for joining us on the Nullarbor to Adelaide journey, it has been a treat to have you with us again. Tomorrow we will be joined by Sylvia who will be with us, along with Michael from here to Melbourne. Only 46 marathons to go! Temp 12-29 degrees. Total Km 13,773.80.

Marathon #321.

November 17, 2013. 20 km north of Clare to Auburn. Out of the wheat fields and into the vineyards. Started 5am running by the light of the setting full moon. Very cold head winds going up the hill to the summit then the wind dropped as we started down the other side. Stopped at 12 km for first break then continued on, phoned ABC Radio to talk with Macca on the Sunday morning show, on hold in the queue for almost an hour then had about 1 minute on air as we came into the town of Clare. Had our green smoothies while catching up on the internet then continued on out of town, heading south on the B82 Horrocks Hwy towards Auburn, surrounded by vineyards, lovely to be amongst the lush green of the grapevines. Meanwhile Sylvia was on her way being driven by friends from Adelaide to come and find us on the road. Narelle made lunch and dinner ahead and she was packed ready to leave when Sylvia arrived, meeting up just 4 km Nth of Auburn. Had a quick break and chat with Sylvia's friends, then they were off taking Narelle with them. With only 4 km to Auburn, Michael and Sylvia drove ahead and we ran in to finish the run 43.60 km at the town recreation park where

Michael had set up camp for the night. Had a delicious meal of raw lasagne made and left for us by Narelle, thank you again:) then off to bed by 8:30pm. Only 45 marathons to go! Temp 12-30 degrees. Total Km 13816.84.

Marathon #322.

November 18, 2013. Auburn to Green Rd, Mornhill on the B32 Main North Rd, 25 km north of Gawler. From vineyards to wheat fields again! Started 5am in the dark by the street lights through town and out into the countryside by the light of the setting moon. The familiar sound of laughter from kookaburras welcomed the break of dawn and made us feel right at home. Cool morning, not too windy, climbing a gentle slope for 2 km to look back at the view of rolling hills, vineyards and wheat fields. Sylvia's first morning went well, first stop at 11 km then on to green smoothie break at 18 km. Road is smoother, safer with wide flat shoulders, but busy with wheat trucks and other double carriers. Finished the run in heat (temp 10-37 degrees) at 42.40 km where Sylvia picked us up and drove to where Michael was waiting with the van to follow us to a good camping spot on a side road that Sylvia had found earlier. Set up camp outside a wheat farm, had fresh carrot and beet juice that Michael had made, and Sylvia made a fresh green salad with asian greens, corn, tomato, and cucumber with orange tahini dressing for dinner. Very warm evening, still 34 degrees at 6pm. Only 44 marathons to go! Total Km 13,859.24.

Marathon #323.

November 19, 2013. Mornhill to Elizabeth on the A32 Main North Rd, 21 km Nth of Adelaide. Sylvia drove us back 3.7 km to where we had finished yesterday and we started the run 5am by the light of the moon. Warm breeze and red sunrise bringing a very hot and humid day. Sylvia was waiting outside Dino's Fresh Fruit & Veg shop in Roseworthy so we stocked up while we were there and had a banana break in the car, thanks for your support Dino. Finished the run 44.44 km in suburb of Elizabeth where Sylvia picked us up and drove us back to where Michael was waiting and then on to Dalkeith Camping Ground, 11 km north of where we finished the run. Set up camp and had dinner, storm brewing with very strong winds rocking the caravan, hope the tents stay on the ground tonight! Hot showers and off to bed. Temp 16-37 degrees. Only 43 marathons to go! Total Km 13903.44.

Marathon #324.

November 20, 2013. Elizabeth to Eagle on the Hill Bike Parking. We all drove out of the caravan park towards Adelaide and stopping where we had finished yesterday. The wind had dropped but evidence of the storm was everywhere with branches all over the road. Started running 5:30am on the Main North Rd into Adelaide, not used to all the traffic finding it very noisy and breathing in the fumes was very different to the quiet we have experienced over the last six months. Met up with Channel 7 News and did some filming and interviews. Anna our friend who is hosting us drove to meet us and Michael and Sylvia followed her back to her place while we ran into Adelaide CBD and met up with Narelle for lunch at Bliss Organic Cafe. Met Pip And Grace from Bliss and discussed the set up for tomorrow night's event there. Had a delicious lunch and said goodbye to Narelle who is flying home tomorrow, thanks again to Narelle for the wonderful support and friendship given us during the 66 days spent with us on the road. Left Bliss and met up with Channel 7 News again to do some more filming which will be shown tonight and tomorrow night on the 6-6:30 news. Ran out of the CBD to pick up the bike trail towards Mt Barker and ran uphill, a very steep climb to finish the run 42.93 km at the bike parking near Eagle On The Hill. Sylvia drove up to meet us and take us back to Anna's place where everyone had dinner together, then a lovely hot bath before bed. A long day but great to be in Adelaide at last. Temp 16-21 degrees. Only 42 marathons to go! Total Km 13.946.37.

Marathon #325.

November 21, 2013. Adelaide. Drove with Michael and Sylvia to Torrens Weir in the city to meet up with the Adelaide runners. Started running 6:30am with 30 runners around a 10 km loop along the river trail. Nice run and chat afterwards, thanks Neil for organising that for us, it was great to meet everyone and have company during our run. Had a radio interview before continuing on our own along the river trail out to the beach and joined by endurance cyclist Kay on the way back. Our friend Harley joined us for a smoothie break at Bliss then we continued the run down to the river. On the way back we ran through a park and noticed a young rainbow lorikeet on the ground nibbling at the grass and falling asleep on his feet. Looking closer he appeared to be too young to fly as his tail feathers were not fully developed so we figured he must have fallen out of the tree. Janette put her finger out in front of him and he climber on and let out a loud "peep!" Immediately he was answered (presumably by his mother) with what sounded like "get yourself back up the tree!" so he hopped off his finger perch, gave it a nip with his little beak and marched over to the tree, hopped onto the base and proceeded to walk up the trunk, hanging onto the bark with his claws and beak! He walked out on the first branch, gave another "peep" and was answered with an approving "peep, peep" from up above, then promptly closed his eyes. Perhaps that was how he fell out of the tree in the first place, literally falling asleep! Very cute little fella. Ran back to finish at Bliss 42.45 km and helped set up for the event at 6:30pm. A wonderful evening with 50 people all bringing potluck raw vegan food to share after we spoke about RunRaw2013. Many thanks to Grace, Pip and all the staff of Bliss Organic Cafe for sponsoring the venue and helping during the evening, and a big thanks to Nicole for all her hard work organising the event and to those who helped her. Thanks to Freelee and Harley for welcoming us to Adelaide, and to everyone for your donations and support, it was great to meet you all. Temp 15-29 degrees. Only 41 marathons to go! Total Km 13,989.30.

Marathon #326.

November 22, 2013. Broke the 14,000 mark today. Eagle on the Hill Bike Parking to 4 km west of Strathalbyn. Harley arrived with his bike which we put in the van, Michael drove on to Stirling and Sylvia drove us all up to Eagle On The Hill to start the day's run at the bike parking where we had finished the day before yesterday. Started running on the bike trail 6am, Harley showing us the way through a beautiful area of Adelaide Hills. Running well on very steep hilly terrain, through lovely little hamlets tucked in the hills, the trees lush green and glistening wet in the rain. Stopped midway for a delicious fruit salad, Harley said it was the best he'd ever had! Continued through farmlets in light misty rain, stopped to talk to some horses with two very cute and curious foals who came up to the fence and nibbled our fingers. Is there anything softer than a horses nose? Finished the run on a downhill at 42.66 km Sylvia coming to pick us up and drive us into Strathalbyn. It was great to have Harley along for company on the run through some of his favourite biking area, thanks for the magical mystery tour Harley, hope you stayed awake for the ride home! We drove to the Campground and set up in a complimentary site, thanks for your support and hospitality. Temp 11-20 degrees. Only 40 marathons to go! Total Km 14,031.96.

Marathon #327.
November 23, 2013. 4 km west of Strathalbyn to Wellington. Sylvia drove us back 3.5km to whee we had finished yesterday and we started running in the cool rain at 5am, downhill back through Strathalbyn and on towards Wellington via Langhorne Creek. Landscape has changed back to dessert scrub interspersed with dairy farms and wheat fields. Busy on the road with traffic, getting lots of toots and waves, motorists most likely having seen the coverage on Chanel 7 TV. A mother and daughter in Langhorne Creek stopped us to give a donation, thanks so much for your kindness. Continued on to finish the run 44.50 km about 5 km west of Wellington. Sylvia picked us up and drove us back to the campground where Michael was set up in a discounted site, thanks for your support and hospitality. Sylvia made green wraps with sprouted chickpea hummus and salad for dinner, off to bed when the internet dropped out at 10pm. Temp 12-22 degrees. Only 39 marathons to go! Total Km 14,076.46.

Marathon #328.
November 24, 2013. Wellington to Coomandook. Michael drove us back 5 km to where we had finished yesterday, started running 5am with Michael filming, back to campground and all headed for the ferry that crosses the Murray River, a punt that is an extension of the road. We ran on and about the ferry while it crossed and ran off heading East to Tailem Bend then south on the Dukes Hwy towards Keith, where we will turn off towards Mt Gambier on the Riddoch Hwy. Smooth roads with wide shoulders, not too much traffic on a Sunday. Finished the run 45.09 km 2.3 km short of the small village of Coomandook, Sylvia picked us up and drove us

on to where Michael had parked for the night in a rest area between road and rail...everyone loves the sound of a train in the distance, everyone thinks it's true...Temp 16-27 degrees. Only 38 marathons to go! Total Km 14,121.55.

Marathon #329.

November 25, 2013. Coomandook to 15 km west of Tintinara. Michael drove us back 2.3 km to where we had finished yesterday. Started running 5am just twilight and half moon. Ran back to the van, dropped off jackets and on to 11 km banana break and a green smoothie break at 18 km. Road is smooth with wide shoulder and terrain flat for easy running. A sad moment when we came across a young fox lying on the side of the road, his neck broken. His eyes wide open and a shocked look on his face, he must have been hit only minutes before. His body still warm and fur so soft as we closed his eyes, picked him up and laid him to rest under a nearby tree. We had only run on for a few minutes when a rabbit was running across the road in front of a car which did not hit him but he must have died of fright. His little nose still twitching as his eyes glazed over and closed, we took him off the road and found a patch of soft grass to lay him down. The road has been kind to us but it is a death trap for the animals. The most roadkill we have seen are the Stumpy Tailed Lizard, who ironically have been around since the Land Before Time, but unfortunately have not adapted to the danger of crossing the road. We have seen them stop in the middle of the road, turn around and face oncoming traffic, even a road train, baring their purple tongue in a standoff attempt to scare the oncoming monster. Progress is not a part of their understanding and they are being left behind, literally on the side of the road...Today our support crew Sylvia and her husband Keith decided they would like to stay on with us to do Tasmania, so that will be great. Food today included bananas, green smoothies, melon and vege curry with cauliflower rice, we're happy to have Raw Chef Sylvia stay on:) Finished the run 44.83 km at roadside parking area where Michael had set up camp and made fresh juice. Temp 12-34 degrees. Only 37 marathons to go! Total Km 14,166.38.

Marathon #330.

November 26, 2013. 15 km west of Tintinara to 5 km west of Keith. Started 5am almost daybreak, feeling a bit tired as we still need to catch up on sleep. Stopped in Tintinara to buy some fruit and veg at the general store, thanks for the discount on the bananas! Temperature rising throughout the run and the road getting hotter underfoot, the tar melting and sticking to our shoes. Sylvia and Michael are doing a great job of looking after us in the heat, plenty of food and water and moral support. Temp reached from 12 to 38 degrees in the morning. Finished the run 44.44 km where Sylvia picked us up and drove us on to where Michael had set up camp at a roadside spot for the night. Zucchini pasta for dinner and heading to bed. Only 36 marathons to go! Total Km 14,210.82.

Marathon #331.

November 27, 2013. 5 km west to 38 km south of Keith. Sylvia drove us back 3 km to where we had finished yesterday and we started running 5am back to the rest area. Very warm so discarded our jackets at the van and continued on 3 km to Keith and the turnoff to the Riddoch Hwy, heading Sth towards Mt Gambier. Temperature rising rapidly to a very hot day, staying well hydrated with water and a juicy fruit salad midway. Ran through Padthaway where there is a very nice park with toilets and free shower on one side of the road and a tavern with tearooms on the other. We had hoped for a store where we could buy some fruit & veg but no, our expectations deflated again. Finished the run 42.93 km at Anna's (our host in Adelaide) mother Elaine's place. A lovely old homestead on 10 acres set in amongst huge trees and a wonderful garden that Elaine tends with loving care, some chickens and ducks wandering about and a few sheep in the paddock. Elaine said she keeps the ducks because she likes them and the sheep are great lawn mowers. Michael was able to fill our water tanks from Elaine's rain water and Sylvia did the laundry and hung it out to dry in the heat while we were treated to an outside cold shower in the garden and all had dinner together on the patio beneath the shade of grapevines growing profusely. Thank you Elaine for your kind hospitality and for sharing your home with us. A long hot day ending in a beautiful setting with a lovely lady... Temp 20-40 degrees. Only 35 marathons to go! Total Km 14,253.25.

Marathon #332.

November 28, 2013. 38 km south of Keith to 25 km north of Naracoort. Started at 5am at daybreak and a very warm morning at 26 degrees. Ran well to 12 km for banana break, landscape is very lush green vineyards on both sides with a band of gum trees along the road. Feels like we're getting closer to home as a family of kookaburras laughed at us going by. A cloudy sky turned to cool showers and steady rain for a few hours, very slight breeze and easy running all day. Our food stores are getting low as we approach the Victorian border so it was chia pudding for midway break and pumpkin fettucini for dinner. Tomorrow will be our last shop as we pass through Naracoort with only two days to the border. Finished the run 44.89 km at a roadside parking and heading for bed as the sun sets at 9pm. Temp 26-30 degrees. Only 34 marathons to go! Total Km 14,298.64.

Marathon #333.

November 29, 2013. 25 km Nth of Naracoort to 32 km north of Penola. Started 5am, very cold and foggy, eerie landscape at daybreak with tops of trees ghosting through the fog. We could hear sheep and cows but couldn't see them until the sun rose and burnt off the fog. Banana break at 10 km with Sylvia then on through vineyards and gum trees, the strong smell of eucalyptus hanging heavy in the air. By the green smoothie break it was warm enough to take our jackets off, but the strong head wind still cold and tiring to beat into. Still feeling weary as we had not enough sleep again last night, busy posting daily updates on Facebook until 10:30pm but still had to get up at 3:45am as always. Ran through Naracoort and stopped at a fruit stall selling fresh ripe locally grown nectarines which were delicious. Sylvia had already stopped and bought more fruit and of course bananas and had told them all about RunRaw2013, so we were given free nectarines and oranges, thanks so much for your support. We had 5 km to go when a car stopped and a lady hopped out and invited all of us to stay the night at her place which is exactly the right distance for our marathon today. Sylvia and Michael drove ahead to Julie's place while we ran on finishing the run at 43.70 km right at Julie's driveway. Walked in to her beautiful garden where Michael & Sylvia had set up camp for the night. Met all the family (including the dogs) and took photos before they went out for dinner. We had a delicious meal of fresh salad greens from Elaine's garden, tomatoes and cucumber with an orange tahini dressing. Hot showers and off to bed early. Temp 6-23 degrees. Marathon average 43.07 km. Only 33 marathons to go! Total Km 14,342.34.

Comments from Facebook/RunningRawAroundAustralia2013:

- *Awesome.* - **Erica x**
- *You two make me feel inadequate. You are awesome!* - **Lindy**
- *Oh wow, nearly over, I wonder what on earth you will do when you have finished your last marathon?* - **Madeleine**

Marathon #334.

November 30, 2013. 32 km Nth to 12 km east of Penola. Started 5am, very clear and cool, almost frosty morning, running amongst hay fields and vineyards. Stopped at Father Woods Park for 12 km banana break, impressive tree carvings depicting the history of the area and how Father Woods preached under a huge red gum tree 1845-1889 and the tree is still standing. Sylvia left after the smoothie break to drive to Mt Gambier to visit her family while we continued on with Michael stopping every 8 km for our breaks. Hundreds of hectares of lush green vineyards stretch on either side of the road for as far as the eye can see and as we approached the town of Penola the road frontage was lined with a mass of red roses. We ran through the town, noting how pretty it was with many large trees, shrubs and more roses in all the gardens, and the grocery store had the most comprehensive fresh produce department we have seen since Perth. Turning left off the Riddoch Hwy we took the Casterton Rd and left Penola to run through pastoral countryside, cattle, sheep and goats grazing amongst the tall grass or lying in the shade of the huge red gums and river gum trees. The landscape changed again to pine and eucalyptus forest during the last 10 km of the run and we finished at 44.19 km where Michael had set up camp off the road next to the forest. Todays run has been one of the most beautiful for scenery and easy running. Temp 7-28 degrees. Only 32 marathons to go! Total Km 14,386.53.

December 2013

MARATHONS #335-365

Marathon #335. December 1, 2013. 12 km east of Penola, SA to Casterton, VIC. Started 5am with a brilliant red daybreak glowing like a fire through the forest. A momentous day as we crossed over the border into Victoria, the kookaburras call bringing us home and although there was no sign of an actual border we could feel that we were finally back in Victoria, the 'Welcome to Victoria' sign bringing tears to our eyes. It's been a long run since we left Melbourne on January 1 and started this epic journey around Australia. With a renewed spring in our step, we ran down the middle of the road, marveling at the huge gum trees lining the road and dotting the hay fields. Contented sheep lying at the base of the trees watched us go by, curious cows came to the fence while huge bulls stood stock still, staring at the spectacle of two humans running for no apparent reason. White cockatoos screeched overhead while the black cockatoos flew gracefully amongst the trees softening the sound of birdsong in the air, running through a picture postcard of pastoral beauty. Sylvia arrived mid morning with fresh produce and made a delicious fruit salad for midway break, then we had fresh watermelon and oranges at the last break, finishing the run at 47.17 km (longest run) so we could stay overnight with Sylvia's friend Molly who lives in Casterton. Set up camp outside her house, Molly invited us to have showers and do laundry, thank you so much for your hospitality and for the yummy fresh greens from the garden. Temp 10-31 degrees. Only 31 marathons to go! Total Km 14,433.70.

Marathon #336.
December 2, 2013. Casterton to Wannon, 19 km west of Hamilton. Started at 5am running downhill into Casterton township, through the sleepy hollow and out the other side without seeing a soul, the old houses picture perfect surrounded by roses in full bloom. The sun was

rising as we reached the top of the hill to look back at the view, rolling hills with hedgerows and large gum trees dotting the fields of green hay, painting a beautiful pastural scene with herds of black cattle with their calves, horses with their foals and flocks of sheep with their tiny lambs all grazing contentedly, their bodies partly hidden in the long grass. We could see the road winding through the hills ahead and in the distance the town of Coleraine nestled in a green valley. We stopped to buy ripe bananas at the store and had our midway break under the trees as it was getting too hot to be in the caravan. Another steep uphill climb after leaving Coleraine and for the rest of the run it was hot and humid, finishing at 46.12 km near the Wannon Falls. Drove down to the free camping area above the falls, a quiet bush camp ideal for an early night. Michael made fresh carrot and beetroot juice and Sylvia made a mixed salad with marinated mushrooms for dinner. Quick catchup on the internet and we're off to bed as the sun sets. Temp 18-37 degrees. Only 30 marathons to go! Total Km 14,479.82.

Marathon #337.

December 3, 2013. Wannon to 4 km west of Penshurst. Sylvia drove us 2.3 km back to where we finished yesterday and we started running at 5:15am under cloudy skies. Ran back past the campsite at daybreak and on for 10 km banana break, then Sylvia and Michael drove on to Hamilton to do a big shop of fresh fruit and veg to get us to Geelong. We stopped for a fruit salad break then ran out of town, still following the Hamilton Hwy along a bike trail from Hamilton to Tarrington, where there was hay bale art on the main street through the town. Caught up with Sylvia there as she was taking photos of all the art pieces which had been made to decorate the town for Christmas. Michael had gone ahead to find a spot to camp for the night and ended up in the town of Penshurst as there was nowhere to pull over on the side of the road, so he got set up in the Municipal campground at $10 for the night with free showers and laundry. We had a few raindrops as we ran the last 8 km to finish at 45.23 km, Michael arriving to pick us up and drive us 4 km on to the campground. Michael had made another great juice and Silvia created another great salad for dinner, hot showers all round, laundry done, tents up and we're off to bed to the sound of raindrops on the roof...Temp 15-35 degrees. Only 29 marathons to go! Total Km 14,525.05.

Comment from Facebook/RunningRawAroundAustralia2013:
- *Although I have been following your exploits for months I can still hardly believe what you two are doing. What an inspiration. Love and best wishes to you both, and to your support crew!* - **Tony**

Marathon #338.
December 4, 2013. 4 km west of Penshurst to Hexham. Michael drove us back 2.4km to where we finished yesterday, ran back through Penshurst and out into the countryside at daybreak. A cloudy sky with rain showers on and off during the run and a cold wind from the South, running through a green landscape of grassy fields, the road smooth but no shoulder at the edge so we were having to get off the road and stand in the long grass to wait for the traffic to pass. We finished the run 45.23 km in Hexham, a small historic settlement where we met Joe and Maria who live in one of the old houses which they are restoring and offered for us to set up camp outside, plug into their power and use their shower and toilet. Thank you so much for your hospitality and for the fresh greens and berries from your garden. It was lovely to meet you and your family of 9 cats and 5 horses! Silvia made a delicious lasagne using the Botanical Cuisine Pesto and Bolognese Sauce, very yummy! Off to bed by 8pm, oh yay 8 hours sleep tonight! Temp 16-23 degrees. Only 28 marathons to go! Total Km 14,570.28.

Marathon #339.
December 5, 2013. Hexham to 4 km east of Darlinghurst on the Hamilton Hwy. Started 5am, very cold, windy and raining. By 7 km into the run the rain became very heavy and cold so we took shelter under a wheat silo in a farmyard we were just passing. Stayed huddled up trying to keep out of the wind but eventually got too cold so phoned Sylvia and asked her to come and bring a change of clothes and shoes. Got warmed up in the SuperRoo, had some bananas and set off again into another rain squall which turned to hail. The day continued with rain squalls alternating with sunshine and the wind turned to the West, still strong and was pushing us along through the puddles on the road. We could hear the sheep bleating but couldn't see them as the grass was so tall, the cattle appeared to be floating on top of the grass as we

couldn't see their legs hidden by the grass. Most of them ignored us as we passed they were so busy eating the grass, but we came across one bull who was sitting under a tree and when we called to him "Where do you get your protein?" he stood up, rippled his muscles and gave us 'The Stare' he's obviously heard that one before! Stopped for the last break at the caravan and did a live interview on Geelong Radio (strangely enough got asked THE question, "Where do you get your protein?!" Same place the bull gets it from:) Ran through Darlinghurst (famous for it's speedway) and finished the run 44.10km at a truck parking where Michael had set up camp and made juice. Silvia made zucchini noodles with fresh tomato sauce for dinner and we're all off to bed for another early night. Temp 6-21 degrees. Only 27 marathons to go! Total Km 14,614.38.

Marathon # 340.

December 6, 2013. 4 km east of Darlinghurst to 73 km west of Geelong. Started 5am, cold and cloudy but no rain. Road smooth but no shoulder and long grass along the edge, had to get off into the grass as the traffic passed. Stopped at 12 km for banana break and ran on through farmland with stone walls for fences built around 1880, the land later given to returning soldiers after WW1 who received 300-400 acres each. Lots of very tall hay in the fields hiding the sheep and almost hiding the cattle, good to see so much green again. Stopped for a break in Berrybank near Mount Elephant an extinct volcano, then continued running the last 8 km well to finish at 46.47 km off the road on a mown grassy area where Michael and Sylvia had set up camp. Food consumed today included banana and grapefruit smoothie; 10 bananas each; green smoothie with bananas, orange and kale; watermelon and rock-melon; fruit salad with bananas, orange, apple, pear, kiwifruit, loganberries and red-currants; asian salad with greens, cucumber, tomatoes, carrot and curry dressing. Ready for bed before sunset, early night for a good sleep before tomorrow's run into Geelong. We've been increasing the distance averaging 45 km each day for the past two weeks to be on schedule for Geelong and Melbourne,. We have also been trying to get more sleep and eating more fruit now that it's more available, so are feeling strong and running really well. Looking forward to seeing everyone tomorrow in Geelong. Temp 7-19 degrees. Only 26 marathons to go! Total Km 14,660.85.

Marathon #341.

December 7, 2013. 73 to 30 km west of Geelong. Started 4:45am, cold until sunrise then warmed up quickly to become hot by afternoon. Ran at faster pace and took shorter breaks today, Eileen joining us when we had 15 km to go and we all ran together to finish at 42.48 km. Sylvia picked us up and drove into Geelong to Eileen's house, lovely to sit in the garden drinking fresh juice that Michael had made. Had showers and getting ready for tonights event when our son Kaje arrived, hadn't seen him since we left Melbourne January 1, the next few days are going to be an emotionally charged experience for us. Had a lovely evening with 40 people attending the Potluck Meet & Greet, thank you all for coming, for your donations and sharing your support with us, and many thanks to Eileen for organising the event and hosting us in Geelong and thanks to those who gave us fruit and veg fresh from their gardens and the organic stores. Temp 6-33 degrees. Only 25 marathons to go! Total Km 14,703.33.

Marathon #342.

December 8, 2013. 30 km west of Geelong to 20 km west of Queenscliff. Sylvia drove us back 30 km to where we had finished yesterday and we started at 6:30am, running with a warm wind from behind us heading towards Geelong and a beautiful sunrise. Joined by Eileen on the bike and Sylvia was waiting at 12 km for the first break of fruit salad and bananas. Eileen continued on her ride in training for the Ironman and we ran on towards Geelong, picking up the bike trail along the river to meet up with Sylvia at 32 km for the 2nd break of melon. Meanwhile Michael had driven on with the ute and van on the Bellerine Rd to Queenscliff, so we continued running along the rail trail to meet up at Eddy's Fresh Fruit & Vegies Store where Michael had a green smoothie ready for us. We all met Eddy, his mum Sev and grandfather Charlie who grow produce themselves to sell in their fruit and vege store which is right on the Bellerine Hwy about 8 km from Geelong. Thank you for your hospitality in allowing us to camp the night in your parking area and for the box of fresh fruit and veg, we appreciate your support and highly recommend anyone in the area to visit Eddy's Fresh Fruit & Veg Store to buy locally grown produce and get friendly service. Thanks again. We ran on along the trail for the remaining 6 km and finished at 42.67 km where Sylvia picked us up and drove us back to the van. Eileen arrived with fresh kale from her garden (yum! thanks) we made sprouted chickpea hummus and veg sticks for dinner, Michael and Sylvia pitched their tents in the orchard and we're all heading for bed and an early night. Temp 16-28 degrees. Only 24 marathons to go! Total Km 14,746.00.

Marathon #343.

December 9, 2013. 20 km west of Queenscliff to Dromana. *Today's run is dedicated to our daughter whose birthday it is today, Happy Birthday Sweetheart, with every step we send our love.* Michael drove us back 6.2 km to where we finished yesterday. Started 5am and ran back towards the Queenscliff-Sorrento ferry while Michael and Sylvia drove the vehicles to the ferry lineup. Boarded the 10am ferry in the rain, very low visibility so worked on the computer during the crossing, many thanks for your support in discounting the cost. The rain was getting heavier and wind stronger by the time we landed and started running, so a few more hours of being soaking wet as we passed through Rye and Rosebud. Running well despite the rain, stopped for a break and the rain finally stopped with the sun coming out to dry the road. We got changed into dry clothes and shoes and continued following the coast road and taking in the scenery of the seashore with coloured boathouses. We finished the run 45.49 km at Dromana, setting up in a campground so Sylvia and Michael could get a cabin since their tents were still wet from last night. Did the laundry and dried everything out, had dinner and into bed after a long, wet day. Temp 14-20 degrees. Only 23 marathons to go! Total Km 14,791.49.

Marathon #344.

December 10, 2013. Dromana to Edithvale on the Nepean Hwy. Wind got up during the night and was very strong coming offshore as we started out at 4:45am this morning amongst branches down on the road. We were being blown sideways as we ran up the cliff road, very steep climb and stopped at the top for a banana break then ran down into Mornington and through the town, feeling strange to be amongst shops after so many days of countryside. Running on past Mount Eliza and another hill climb to stop at the lookout above Frankston where we were met by Graeme, our friend who was with us twice as support crew, thanks for coming out great to see you, especially as we are so close to home. Continued on downhill and through Frankston and Chelsea and finished the run 42.92 km at Edithvale. Michael had made fresh juice so we drank the juice, took photos on the beach and drove on 10 km to where we are staying for the next few days until we take the ferry to Tasmania on Saturday 14. Had a delicious kale salad for dinner before saying goodbye to Michael who has been with us for 6 weeks as support crew, driving the ute towing the caravan, managing the food supplies, making juice and smoothies, shooting film and making us laugh. Thank you Michael for your support and friendship and for the great leg recovery therapy. Still windy at 10pm as we're off to bed to the sound of the surf crashing on the beach...Temp 15-28 degrees. Only 22 marathons to go! Total Km 14,834.41.

Marathon #345.
December 11, 2013. Edithvale to Picnic Point Sandringham, off the Nepean Hwy and onto Beach Rd. Started 5am running along the beach trail back to where we finished yesterday in Edithvale then turned around and ran back to the van for our first break at 21 km. Cloudy but not cold so good running on a mixture of concrete, sand, gravel and tar seal. Great to see so many people out on the trails running, walking and enjoying the morning air with quite a few recognising us as "the old couple running a marathon a day around Australia." Maria stopped to say how inspired she is to start running again and looking after herself, you go girl, remember you are worth it! Channel 7 arrived to do interview for 'Today Tonight' and to film us making a smoothie, then we went back on the trail with Ch 7 filming us running along Beach Rd through rain squalls and sunshine. (Channel 7 'Today Tonight' airing 6-6:30pm today (tonight)! We continued running out for 10 km and back to finish at the caravan 42.53 km. Felt good to be running by the ocean and to see familiar areas as we approach Melbourne. It will be hard to leave on Saturday to go to Tasmania and do the last leg as we're so close to home, but we're not finished yet and the folks in Tassie say we've left the best bit to last, so we're also looking forward to running from Devonport to Hobart and on to the southernmost point before returning to Melbourne and running the last two marathons on December 31,

2013 and January 1, 2014. We're also looking forward to seeing everyone at the Meet, Greet and Eat Event tomorrow night at Kindness House (Melbourne), see you there! Today's temp 17-25 degrees. Only 21 marathons to go! Total Km 14,876.94.

Marathon #346.

December 12, 2013. Picnic Point Sandringham to Port Melbourne and back and around Beaumaris neighbourhood. Drove to where we had finished the run yesterday, parked the SuperRoo at Train Station Sandringham and ran along the ocean trail towards Port Melbourne. Checked in at the ferry to find out when we need to arrive tomorrow then ran back to the car and drove to the van, meeting up with Channel 7 for 'Today Tonight' to do some filming along the trail. Finished the run 42.27 km back at the van and were greeted by our son and his family whom we haven't seen since we started the run on January 1 and our youngest grandchild whom we hadn't met at all, since she was born while we were on the Run. A very emotional and happy reunion, sharing a delicious raw dinner prepared by our crew Sylvia, our PR person Eileen and our friend and sponsor Chef Omid of Botanical Cuisine. It is going to be hard to leave in a couple of days when we are so close to home. Temp 16-30 degrees. Only 20 marathons to go! Total Km 14,919.21.

Marathon #347.

December 13, 2013. Beaumaris ocean-side trails. Ran 20 km along the trails and back to the van to meet up with NZTV crew for filming making our green smoothie and running along the trails. Met Andrew from 'Malt Cafe' in Beaumaris as we were running around the neighbourhood and he invited us to the Cafe for some delicious raw food (Highly recommend going there if you are in the area). Great to meet you and we'll keep in touch when we get back. Finished the run 44.52 km and drove both cars to Kindness House in Fitzroy for a great evening with about 100 friends and family, great to see so many familiar faces. Thanks to everyone for a delicious potluck meal, to Mark and the Veg Vic folks for organising the event, to Phil Wollen for his kind words and to everyone for the donations raised during the evening. Drove back to van in the Ute while our son took SuperRoo home as we're not taking both vehicles to Tasmania. Only 19 marathons to go! Total Km 14,963.73.

Marathon #348.

December 14, 2013. Broke the 15,000 Km mark today. Beaumaris, Beach Road ocean-side trails. Up at 4am with only 3 hours sleep, ran down the coast and back for 20 km and met up with NZTV crew to film a formal interview then drove with caravan to a spot along the coast to do some more filming and to finish the run at 43.12 km. Then we drove to the ferry terminal and met up with Sylvia and her husband Keith who had flown in from Brisbane to join us as support crew for the Tasmania leg of the Run. It took a couple of hours to get on the ferry and up into our cabins. We all had dinner in our cabin, a huge salad made from all the food we had left, as we cannot bring any fresh fruit and veg into Tasmania. Sylvia and Keith went off to explore the ship and we had a shower and collapsed into the bunks, the rolling of the ship sending us off to sleep... Temp 16-33 degrees. Only 18 marathons to go! Total Km 15,0006.51.

Marathon #349.

December 15, 2013. Devonport to Christmas Hills Raspberry Farm Tasmania. We slept soundly through the night, not hearing a thing until 5:45am when we were woken by the sound of an announcement over the intercom in the cabin telling passengers that they could go to their cars in half an hour to prepare for disembarking. Sylvia and Keith came to our cabin and we all ate what was left of the bananas then went down to the van, driving off the ferry immediately. We parked in the ferry carpark to show Keith around the ute and van for driving and Tim arrived with our order of organic fruit and veg (thanks to Joanna for organising and sponsoring that for us). Once restocked with food we were ready to go, Tim running with us out of Devonport on the road to Launceston staying with us for 12 km and then turning back, thanks Tim for picking up our food orders and bringing it to us and for accompanying us on the run out. We look forward to seeing you again on our way back through to the ferry for the return trip to Melbourne. Met up with Sylvia and Keith at 15 km for our smoothie break, running well up and down the rolling hills through the countryside so green and lush and the air so fresh and clean-What a welcome to Tasmania! Finished the run 44.68 km at Christmas

Hills Raspberry Farm, setting up camp in their carpark, thanks for your hospitality and for the delicious raspberries! Only 17 marathons to go! Total Km 15,051.19.

Marathon #350.

December 16, 2013. Christmas Hills Raspberry Farm to 2 km east of Carrick. Started 5am running through small villages of old stone houses, the landscape very beautiful and looking like the English countryside with hedgerows and trees dotted through the green fields, cattle and sheep grazing amongst the long grass. Continued through fields of daisies (grown for pyrethrum) and poppies (for medicinal opium) and finished the run 42.40 km just 2 km past the town of Carrick. Keith and Sylvia had parked in the grounds of the Town Hall and met local committee member Gillian who said it would be fine for us to camp overnight there. So while we finished the last 4 km out and back, K & S made fresh juice of carrots, beet and apple, and a carrot dill soup to go with a marinated kale salad for dinner. Heading for an early night as the sun sets...Temp 7-30 degrees. Only 16 marathons to go! Total Km 15,093.59.

Marathon #351.

December 17, 2013. 2 km east of Carrick to Epping Forest Roadhouse. Drove 2km to where we had finished yesterday started running at 5am to Longford where Sylvia and Keith had stopped to buy more local produce then on to Perth where we turned onto Hwy 1 again, heading South. The road was a bit rough with no shoulder and more traffic, so we're jumping off onto the stones to get out of the way. Landscape very picturesque, rolling green hills with trees and hedgerows, curious cattle and sleeping sheep. Finished the run 42.2 km at Epping Forest where we set up camp behind the Roadhouse overlooking an expansive view of the countryside, thanks for your hospitality and donation. Sylvia and Keith booked in to a local B&B Rose Cottage and we were invited to have a shower there, thanks for your hospitality. Temp 16-30 degrees. Only 15 marathons to go! Total Km 15,135.90.

Marathon #352.

December 18, 2013. Epping Forest Roadhouse to 7.4 km south of Ross on Hwy 1. Started at

5am running on rolling hills through more farming countryside with some fields of poppies, the flowers not yet opened as they close up for the night. Fascinating watching them open into full bloom as the sun rose and shone on the fields. Stopped in Campbell Town for midway break, a picturesque town with old stone houses and beautifully kept gardens, roses in full bloom giving the air an 'olde worlde' perfume. Ran on to small village of Ross, also very pretty with avenues of trees and an ancient bridge over the river, rose gardens a mass of colour creating a scene from one of Monet's paintings. We ran on to finish at 42.48 km where Keith and Sylvia picked us up, Keith jumped on the bike to ride back while we drove back to the Ross Campground for the night. Had several people stop on the road to give us donations, thank you all for your support. Temp 14-30 degrees. Only 14 marathons to go! Total Km 15,178.38.

Marathon #353.

December 19, 2013. 7.4 km south of Ross to Jericho. Drove forward 7.4 km to where we finished yesterday and started running 5:15am, fields of poppies on both sides of the road with stoney edge and long grass. Early in the run Janette was off to the side in the grass when she felt a sudden excruciating pain in her foot. Thinking she had stood on a thorn, she looked to see if the thorn was still imbedded in her foot to find nothing there but two puncture holes and the surrounding area an angry red. The sudden sharp pain had lessened to a dull numbing pain so we continued running to the first break at the van. By the time we got there, the pain had increased and had moved up the leg to the knee, causing her to limp. We took the shoe off and noticed that it was stained where the injury had occurred, the two puncture holes in the foot quite distinct and the area around the holes was red and inflamed. The pain was similar to that of a wasp or hornet sting, very intense but without the sting. It was about that time that we wondered if it was a snake bite not having seen the culprit, but with the two puncture holes it was highly possible. So we figured there was only one thing to do...run it out! So we put some vinegar on the injury and continued on the run, foot and leg feeling quite tight and still very painful. Now it may not have been a snake because we did not actually see one, but something sunk it's teeth into my foot and I'm sure it had every reason to get my attention if I was standing on it. So I just hope that the little critter is OK, by the end of the day the pain had subsided in my foot, only the punctures and redness around them to show for it. We reckon I must have good snake karma because of all the snakes I've rescued from the road as I have no ill effects from the experience. Back to the Run, we climbed 426 metres up St Peter Pass and into the rolling hills for the rest of the day. Keith and Sylvia found a parking spot outside a farmer's gate in the village of Jericho, so we went in and asked if we could stay the night. He said we were welcome to come inside the gate and park anywhere on the thousands of acres so long as we didn't party all night, thank you so much for your hospitality! Set up camp in the front field and tried to keep the noise down as we had a delicious dinner of zucchini noodles with fresh tomato sauce and so far as we know, no walls came tumbling down! Only 13 marathons to go! Total Km 15,220.78. Distance 42.40km.

Marathon #354.

December 20, 2013. Jericho to Pontville. At 4:45am our new friend Aaron arrived from Hobart to join us on today's run. There was thick fog hanging in the hills and as we climbed uphill to the summit of Spring Hill at an elevation of 488 metres and then up Constitution Hill at 462 metres, we were immersed in the dampness of the fog and although it was cool it was good to be running hills again. On the downhill run the fog lifted and by the time we arrived at the van we were warmed up and ready for a feed of bananas. Aaron was keeping us on our toes so our running time was good, one of the fastest we've done, especially the last 10 km that we ran with him downhill. We only had 10km to finish when Aaron had to leave, so we ran on at a slower pace through several historic towns with stone buildings and character houses and roses in bloom everywhere. Keith and Sylvia drove ahead to Pontville and set up camp in the oval grounds and we finished the run there at 42.31 km. A great run, always good to have company on the road, thanks Aaron for joining us and for the box of ripe bananas! Only 12 marathons to go! Total Km 15,263.09.

Marathon #355.

December 21, 2013. Pontville to Hobart. Started running at 5am with a brilliant red sunrise.

Ran on the Hwy through Brighton and picked up the bike trail after the first banana break at 12 km. Ran on the concrete trail all the way to Glenorchy where Keith and Sylvia had driven to our hosts Gozia and Luke live. We unhitched the ute from the caravan so Sylvia and Keith could drive to Salamanca market in the city, while we ran on the bike trail all the way into Hobart CBD to meet up with the Veg Tas group on the Parliament lawns. We had also arranged to meet our dear friend Ann who had flown in from Canada to join us for the last leg of the Run. Keith and Sylvia loaded up on fresh fruit and veg from the market while we went to the 'Running Edge' for Garmin promo photos before running 8 km back towards Glenorchy, where Keith picked us up at 44.52 km and drove back to Glenorchy for a wonderful potluck, meeting new friends and sharing delicious raw food, thank you all for your support and to Gozia and Luke for your hospitality and gift of delicious fruit. Only 11 marathons to go! Total Km 15,307.61.

Marathon #356.

December 22, 2013. Hobart to Huonville. Up at 4am and all in the ute to drive into Hobart to start the run at 6am on the A6 Hwy to Huonville. It was a cold rainy and windy day, climbing out of Hobart, the road rough with little or no shoulder and nowhere to get off on the corners. Luckily not much traffic early on as it is Sunday. Did a telephone interview for the Hobart Mercury Newspaper and stopped to do a photo shoot during the run in the rain. Despite the rain and wind, the landscape was very beautiful, lush and green and the last 10 km was either up or downhill running, the change of pace felt good. Finished the run 42.30 km at Huonville Campground, a great spot in a field amongst the geese, chickens, sheep and cows of their petting farm. Keith and Sylvia got a room in the hotel as it was still raining and their tent was already wet, while Ann bunked in the caravan with us, all off to sleep to the sound of more rain. Temp 11-13 degrees. Only 10 marathons to go, now we're on serious countdown! Total Km 15,349.91.

Marathon #357.

December 23, 2013. Huonville to Dover on the A6. Started 5am and ran to town of Franklin on the Huon River, very quaint small wooden boat building town, but everything was closed for Christmas so we continued on, following the river down the estuary to Port Huon, where there are colourful sail boats moored along the rivers edge. Took a very steep uphill 'short cut' to bypass Geeveston, up and down hills all day to Dover. The road became very narrow with no shoulder, the bank dropping away on our right side and a steep cliff on the other.

It seemed like we were running along the top of a very narrow wall that we could not get off, it just kept going on and on and we began to think we were running along the imaginary marathon 'Wall'. We could not get off and we could not run through it, we were trapped on a moving escalator going nowhere. Usually when you are depleted and 'run into the wall', there is no recovery, it's game over and you come crashing down...but we didn't feel depleted and were not in danger of crashing, we just could not get off the wall that went on forever, into a great void of nothingness with no purpose. Our legs keep going, our feet slapping the stones beneath, step after step, on and on the wall stretches out before us, when will it end?

Eventually the road widened as we entered Dover, a small fishing village with a campground on the beach where Keith and Sylvia and Ann had set up camp for the night and we finished the run at 42.50 km feeling drained and weary. Tomorrow Sylvia and Keith leave us when we reach the southernmost point in the sealed road at Southport, so as a special treat with a Christmas flavour, we made sticky fig pudding with fig sauce and almond creme, now it feels like Christmas. A special thanks to Sylvia and Keith for their attentive support and valued friendship that has developed during their time with us on the road. Temp 10-14 degrees. Only 9 marathons to go! Total Km 15,392.41.

Marathon #358.

December 24, 2013. Christmas Eve. Dover to Southport. Started running 5am as the daybreak burnt the sky a brilliant red. We ran along the C638 towards Huon Point for 5 km and then turned around and ran back to the campground for our 10 km banana break, giving the crew a chance for a sleep in. No sign of any movement so we ate our 10 bananas and quietly left to continue the run back to the A6 and south towards Strathblane another quaint boating village. Caught up with the crew on the way to Southport for a green smoothie, then continued on to Southport, where Keith parked the caravan in the Campground and disconnected the Ute so Alan could drive Keith and Sylvia back to Hobart. We arrived for a peach and mango break, Alan got changed for the drive and Janette continued on the run 10 km along the beach road in Southport to finish the run. A sad goodbye to Sylvia (who had been with us since Adelaide) and Keith who had joined us in Melbourne to make a great support team for the Tasmania leg. Thank you both for your much appreciated support and loving friendship. Alan ran 5km around the docks in Hobart after dropping Sylvia and Keith off, then drove back and ran another 5km to finish the run at 42.61km. Now we have our Canadian friend Ann with us for the next 4 days until we get to Launceston where she will leave to fly home. Tomorrow is Christmas Day and we'll be running to the southernmost point accessible in Australia, along the track to South Cape Bay. It's unlikely that we will have any phone or internet coverage so we wish everyone a happy and healthy Christmas Day and we'll be back online Boxing Day. Temp 14-20 degrees. Only 8 marathons to go! Total Km 15,435.02.

Marathon #359.

December 25, 2013. *Christmas Day, in memory of Janette's father, for whom it's always been a special day...Happy Birthday Dad, this one is for you.* Southport and South Cape Bay Trail to Ida Bay, Started at 5am from the Southernmost Pub in Australia, following the reindeer hoof prints along the beach to the end of the sealed road as the sun rose into a pink sky reflecting shards of sparkling light across the water. The turquoise blue of the sea, the deep green of the trees and the vivid red of the morning sky creating a kalaidescope of Christmas colour as we turned and ran back to the van. Drove to Ida Bay Heritage Railway Campground and unhitched the van leaving it set up for the night while we drove the gravel road to the southernmost point at Cockle Creek and the 'end of the road'. From there we took the 7.5 km trail to South Cape Bay, stopping at the lookout to view South Cape and the Great Southern Ocean below. Now we have been to all points of the compass on our route while Running Raw Around Australia. Had a banana break and returned to Cockle Creek along the trail then ran the gravel road to Ida Bay to finish the run at sunset 42.55 km. It was a long but beautiful sunny day with a gentle breeze running in a picture perfect landscape on hiking trails and gravel roads, spent with our friend Ann reminiscing about Christmas Days gone by. Temp 15-30 degrees. Only 7 marathons to go! Total Km 15,477.57.

Marathon #360.

December 26, 2013. Boxing Day Ida Bay, Hastings Caves and Thermal Springs. Started running 5:30am from Ida Bay to Southport turnoff and return to the van for 20 km. Mild morning with no wind and no traffic on the road, returned to the van for a green smoothie break then drove to Hastings Caves so Ann could visit the caves while we finish the run. Running up and down the gravel road lined with ferns and thick forest, the landscape is reminiscent of parts of New Zealand and of Vancouver Island Canada, so although we are about as far away as we can be, it still feels like home. We finished the run at 42.69 km and went for a dip in the Hastings Thermal pool near the Caves, the water was only tepid but refreshing after the run. Drove back up the A6 to Huonville stopping at the Huonville Caravan Park Campground where we had stayed on the way down. If you are ever passing through this area it's worth a stay, a self sufficient farm setting with orchard and animals wandering around, you get to feed the cows, pigs, chickens, ducks and geese and watch the dog round up the sheep to bring them into their enclosure for the night. We set up camp and had hot showers, a delicious salad for dinner and caught up on the internet before heading for bed, Ann strung her hammock between the trees under a starry sky and the platypus slipped quietly into the water gliding slowly downstream... Temp 14-25 degrees. Only 6 marathons to go! Total Km 15,520.06.

Marathon #361.

December 27, 2013. Huonville Campground to St Peter's Pass Picnic Area on the A1. Started 5am and ran from the campground into Huonville and along the Huon River for 10 km before turning around to run back. Found two Tasmanian animals on the side of the road, a Tassie Devil and a Quoll, both had recently been hit. We lifted them from the road and laid them to rest under a tree poor little guys. Back to the campground to finish Lap 1 at 21.02 km, packed up and drove north to St Peter's Pass Picnic Area where we set up camp for the night. While Ann made fresh carrot and beetroot juice and a salad for dinner, we ran down the Pass and took a side road off into farmland. The farmers were rounding up sheep for shearing, amid a chorus of bleating, hundreds of woolly faces watching us run by. Finished Lap 2 at 22.15 km for a total of 43.17 km for the run. Temp 15-28 km. Only 5 marathons to go! Total Km 15,563.21.

Marathon #362.

December 28, 2013. St Peter's Pass Picnic Area to Carrick. Started 5:15am running uphill and turned onto a side road that led out into farmland. Continued running for 11km before turning around and running back to finish Lap 1 at 20.11 km. Ann had made a delicious fruit salad which included fresh berries that we bought from the growers in Huonville yesterday, very yummy. Drove to Launceston Airport for Ann to catch her flight back to Canada. It's been great having her on board for the last few days of the Run, thanks Ann for joining us and helping out with support, especially making the delicious meals and treats over Christmas! Now there's just the two of us until we get to Melbourne where our friend Graeme will return for the third time, meeting us off the ferry and driving the support vehicle for the last two marathons. Meanwhile back in Tassie we drove to Carrick where we had stopped overnight on the way down, set up camp outside the Town Hall and ran out on a small country road to Bishopbourne and back to finish Lap 2 at 22.22 km for a total of 42.33 km for the Run. Ann had made zucchini noodles and tomato sauce for us which was a delicious dinner before heading off to bed for an early night since there is no internet in Carrick. Temp 12-19 degrees. Only 4 marathons to go! Total Km15,605.44.

Marathon #363.

December 29, 2013. Carrick to Devonport. Countdown 4 marathons to go! Started running 5:30am on the Tourist Drive to Bagley. Very quiet on the road, only had two cars pass us and the sheep were all asleep in the fields. Turned around just past the township and returned to Carrick along the same route to finish Lap 1 at 24.24 km. Drove to East Devonport and set up camp in Abel Tasman Campground on the river just behind the ferry dock. Had a green smoothie of orange, bananas and silverbeet greens, then ran over the bridge past the docks and into Devonport township along the waterfront then turned around and ran back to the van for another smoothie of watermelon and silvan berries fresh from Huonville yesterday. Ran out along the East Devonport foreshore trail and back in time to watch the ferry come in. A lovely sunny day's Run with a cool sea breeze to finish Lap 2 at 18.39 km for a total of 42.63 km for the Run. Temp 12-22 degrees. Only 3 marathons to go! Total Km 15,648.07.

Marathon #364.

December 30, 2013. Devonport. Started running 5am along the 3km foreshore trail, doing laps up and down and watching the ferry come in and a big freight boat being brought in with the little tug boats, good entertainment as we ran along the foreshore to put on the km. Stopped at the van for a banana or ten then ran over the bridge and along the town foreshore to meet up with The Advocate Newspaper reporter and photographer who was also doing photo shoot for The Age newspaper. Joined by Tim and his brother and sister to run back over the bridge with us, great to see you again for another short run together. Finished the run at the van 42.61 km and drove down to the ferry line up to wait for loading. Eventually drove on board and parked, went upstairs and found our cabin, showered and rolled into the bunks as the ferry hit the choppy sea, crossing Bass Straight and heading for home on a starry night. Temp 12-23 degrees. Only 2 marathons to go! Total Km 15,690.68.

A storm brewing for a rolling night on the Tassie ferry...

Comments from Facebook/RunningRawAroundAustralia2013:

- *Keep going. You must be rolling along on such a high. Amazing stuff!* - **Brian**
- *Congrats guys. Happy new year.* - **Christine xxx**
- *Yep. You two are pretty awesome.* - **Troy**
- *I ask myself: What will your legs do in 2 days? Is it possible to stop Running Raw?* - **Marco**
- *See you at the finish! Amazing effort.* - **Steve**
- *January 2nd is going to feel so strange! I'm so amazed and proud of you! Never doubted for a moment that you would do it!* - **Kim**

Marathon #365.

December 31, 2013. Melbourne. This is it! The last marathon of the year! Drove off the ferry and stopped in the carpark outside where Graeme was waiting to take over driving for today and tomorrow. Started running at 7am along the foreshore towards Black Rock. Stopped at Brighton Train Station for a green smoothie and banana break, thanks for the box of bananas Steven! Met up with TV crews and did interviews and filming as we continued running along Beach Rd to Black Rock. Stopped for a fruit salad break and more media interviews, TV and Radio. Turned onto Bluff Rd running all the way to Nepean Hwy where we were met by our son, daughter-in-law and 3 grandchildren. A very emotional moment and so wonderful to see them. Continued on to meet up with Martin from Kids Under Cover who joined us for the rest of the Run, also joined by other runners as we ran along St Kilda Rd. Finally arrived at Federation Square where we received a standing ovation as we ran past to finish at The Atrium amidst a crowd of about 200 well wishers and TV crews. We were quite overwhelmed with such a wonderful welcome, thank you all for your support in being there today, it was great to share the moment with our family and friends. Total Km 15,734.16. Only 1 marathon to go to set a new World Record! Distance 43.48km.

Comments from Facebook/RunningRawAroundAustralia2013:

- *Absolutely wonderful. Congratulations! A remarkable feat. I feel humbled and amazed. Sending love to you and a Happy New Year.* - **Stephen**
- *Congratulations, the world needs more people like you...have a happy and blessing New Year.* - **Haydee**
- *You two are amazing, well done! A happy healthy blesssed New Year to you!* - **Connie**

January 1 2014

MARATHON #366

Marathon #366. January 1, 2014. Melbourne to Warrandyte. This is it! The last consecutive marathon to set a new World Record for the most Consecutive Marathons, Running Raw Around Australia! Drove to Federation Square, Melbourne from Graeme's house where we had stayed the night. Met by three hardy souls Mark, Martin and Ben to join us on the Run. Started 5:45am running together along the Yarra River Trail out of Melbourne City towards Collingwood where we planned to meet other runners to join us, but we missed the trail turnoff, running around Studley Park Rd and adding a few extra km to the tally, we picked up the trail again about 8 km ahead at Burke St, so phoned Graeme who was waiting with several runners and cyclists. They moved on to meet us further on at the halfway point and were caught by the roaming police sitting in the car park drinking green smoothies and eating fruit deliciously ripe peaches kindly donated by ACN Orchards in Bunbartha, must have looked like the aftermath of a New Year's party, but they realised we were still going strong so left us to it! Our friend and past support crew Melissa joined us on her bike along with several local runners and two from Adelaide who had flown in especially to join us on the Run today. At the Westerfold Park stop we were joined by more runners and again at Beasleys Nursery stop for a total of 52 running behind us up the hill to Pound Rd and down into Warrandyte, the view of the village in the trees below bringing a wave of emotion as we ran together towards the finish line. Ahead we could see our son and two of our grandchildren waiting for us and with only 500 metres to go they joined us, running hand in hand in the rain into the park and down towards the stage, where hundreds of well-wishers were gathered to welcome us home. As we ran through the finish banner at 47.85 km, breaking the tape and setting a new world record, a rousing cheer came from the crowd and we could no longer hold back the tears. To be surrounded by our family and friends, members of our community as well as folks who had come from further afield was very humbling and we thank you so much for your support today. Many thanks also to those who helped to organise the 'Finish' and gathering in Warrandyte and a special thanks to our friend who flew in from Brisbane specially to help with selling Janette's book. After saying a few words and speaking to the media we were able to mingle with everyone and have some fruit before being driven to our home where the crew from Channel 7 had set up lights and cameras to do an interview for the 'Today, Tonight' program. After they left we were happy to head for a hot bath and into our own bed, done and dusted, no more consecutive marathons, sleep in tomorrow, then maybe we'll go for a run! Temp 20-25 degrees. Today's Distance 47.85 km. Marathon Average Km 43.12. Total Km 15,782.00.

Comments from Facebook/RunningRawAroundAustralia2013:

- *Happy New Year to two true Champions of Australia. What a huge achievement!* - **Bill**
- *E poi arrivi all'ultimo giorno del 2013 e scopri che due vecchietti hanno corso 365 maratone in 365 giorni. Simply Amazing... and then come the last day of 2013 and discover that two old have run over 365 marathons in 365 days. Simply Amazing ...Running Raw around Australia.* - **Simone (Translated by Bing)**
- *You're both amazing! Congrats!* - **Annia**
- *Champions!!!!!!!!* -**Chloe**
- *Wow. What a journey! Congratulations.* - **Jeannette**
- *Amazing effort, makes my effort on the fatmans great aussie trek pale into insignificance... hearty congratulations to you.* - **Brendon**
- *You both are incredible, thank you for sharing your journey, this last entry brought tears of joy:)* - **Katerina**
- *CONGRATULATIONS!! UNBELIEVABLE!! SUCH an inspiration!!* - **Sherry**
- *Congratulations!* - **Marta**
- *Well done xxxxxxx* - **Ginger**
- *Well done...simply amazing.* - **Rachael!**
- *Incredible! Congratulations.* - **Zoe x**

JANUARY 2014

- *So amazing. Thank you.* - **Michele**
- *Phenomenal effort!* - **Will**
- *Woo Hooooo!* - **Lee**
- *Congrats. An amazing effort at your age. Inspiration to many I am sure.* - **Stewart**
- *Incredible xxx congratulations an amazing, super human effort xxxx inspirational xxx RAWSOME xx* - **Kim**
- *Good work so awesome!* - **Jewel**
- *I have loved following your page, you are both inspirational. Congratulations!!* - **Bec**
- *Amazing and inspirational. Fantastic work guys!* - **James**
- *Well done, à great job, onya love from Holland.* - **Flip**
- *Huge Congratulations.* - **Leeanne**
- *Awesome achievement!* - **Elizabeth**
- *Congratulations guys! x) You really did it!* - **Tobi**
- *Fabulous effort guys, really well done!!Been great to follow!! What do we do now?* - **Brenda**
- *Congrats!!* - **Elik**
- *Simply brilliant. I have loved reading and following every post of yours over the past year. Inspiring to say the least.* - **Kimmie**
- *I agree with all the above posts!! Fantastic - have loved following you around Australia through Facebook!!!* - **Betty**
- *Congratulations! You are such an inspiration to so many people - wish there were more people like the two of you in the world who encourage us all to dream big & never give up believing in yourself, even when everyone else may seem to have given up. I have so much respect for you both. Congratulations.* - **Louise**
- *WONDERFUL! Congratulations! I wish i could have been there. With you in spirit. We're all SO proud of you. Thank you for blowing the socks off what we think we're capable. You both truly are an inspiration. And special thanks to your support team. Loved getting the updates.* - **Tathra**
- *A privilege to speak to you Janette. You and your husband are an inspiration. You will never fully know the impact your example has had on so many people. It's a huge ripple effect. Our*

- combined stories and lives will save human kind. Much love. - **Jeannee**
- Just loving, from the bottom of my heart, what you've achieved. I tell people, who question raw diets, all about you two. Hoping all the best for you in 2014.-Raw Galore xx You did it!!! WOWSA!! - **Monique**
- You have inspired me! Thank you! - **Meg**
- AMAZING PEOPLE!!!! Thank you for all your inspiration this past year. - **Laura**
- WOW WOW WOW! INSPIRATIONAL! Raw, healthy, fit and what an amazing achievement at any age! You show anything is possible if you set the intention and believe. - **Yvonne**
- Proud of you! - **Monica**
- Congratulations! We met you on the road south of Katherine NT and have been following you since. Well done. - **Vanessa**
- WEEELLLL DONE!!!! SO PROUD OF YOU GUYS!!! - **Michaela**
- Wonderful! Have enjoyed following your journey!! Congratulations. - **Elisha**
- Amazing! Congratulations!!! - **Rod**
- Well done you two amazing wonderful people wish we where there as well. Rest up and take care. - **Marleen**
- Brilliant! Congratulations on a determined, amazing effort. Enjoy being still! - **Deb**
- Amazing!!! - **Nuno**
- Thanks so much for letting us share this with you! I think that doing the last few km with you on New Year's Day will be the highlight of my year! You are both absolutely inspirational people of the human kind :)) - **Mandii**
- How moving well done what an excellent achievement. - **Kara**
- New you would make you tough buggers,Congratulations! - **Cameron**
- Congratulations from Spain. You amazed the world!! - **Nano**
- Well done!! Such an amazing achievement and a great job raising awareness on vegan & raw food. I for one never thought you could have achieved that (run 366 consecutive marathons!!) on a vegan diet. You have challenged everything I thought I knew about nutrition. - **Nikki**
- Well done from Scotland, you ARE amazing!! - **Jackie X**

JANUARY 2014

- *You two are amazing. Been following along from California and Canada all year... Congratulations!* - **Larry**
- *Congratulations on your achievement!* - **David**
- *Just awesome.* - **Maryanne**
- *Congratulations - enjoy time with family!* - **Peter**
- *You guys are so terribly amazing! Congratulations in this incredible achievement.* - **Anna**
- *Congratulations! You truly are an inspiration!* - **Stephanie**
- *Congratulations You guys are amazing!* - **Trina**
- *We'll done amazing feat take care put your feet up'* - **Craig**
- *Congratulations! Good for you.* - **Ania**
- *From Canada; been following your inspirational adventure all year and will miss reading your posts. Congratulations!* - **Roch**
- *Congratulations. What a great journey.* - **Tara**
- *Congratulation and WELL DONE to you both from UK.* - **Jackie**
- *Amazing and inspiring!* - **Jo**
- *SUPER! You're AMAZING and an INSPIRATION. I'm happy that you're completed this journey, though I'll miss your daily posts from the road. CONGRATULATIONS and THANK YOU!* - **Aldonio**
- *Wow - so inspired by you both.* - **Berenice**
- *You guys are an inspiration !!!!!* - **Jami**
- *I'm watching from Maine (US) and celebrating with you! Warm congratulations! (Brrrr, it's about -35 F here with the wind!)* - **Mary-Anne**
- *What an amazing year to show case both fitness and healthy eating! well done.* - **Stuart**
- *Amazing! Congratulations!* - **Tommy**
- *Congratulations what a completely inspiring journey, you guys are amazing!!!!* - **Jacinta**
- *F I N I S H WOHOO ! !* - **Marco**
- *Just amazing! Wonderful!! Thank you so much for your inspiring work, it has been heartwarming, astonishing, INSPIRING to watch your progress over the last year. I wish you all the best for many more wonderful things to come.* - **Clodia**

- *It was so great to see you run home congratulations Allen and Jeanette ,it was a thrill to meet you and see how happy you were to be home with your family. I hope I see you jogging around Warrandyte , I will try and catch up for a chat . Haha.* - **Debbie**
- *Congratulations, you guys are amazing. I'm going running now.* - **Nicolas**
- *Which one of you had the idea, and did the other think they were crazy? Congrats for an accomplishment surely not to be matched in a long, long time!* - **Hillary**
- *Congratulations! Now for a whole new year to do normal stuff.* - **Debbie**
- *It was beautiful to follow you in this amazing journey throughout the year and feel so inspired every day! Thank you! You are a true example and inspiration! Congratulations!* - **Christine**
- *Why am I not surprised that you like this?* - **Wally**
- *Wooohoooo!!!!* - **Marlea**
- *Banana Power.* - **Rob**
- *Big congrats and kudos from a cold & wet UK. I didn't think you would do it, but I was proven wrong. You are my heroes.* - **Demone xx**
- *You are a role model for others around the world. Congratulations!!!* - **Stephanie**
- *From Dallas, Texas: Cong.* - **Leah**
- *You are a wonderful inspiration. What wonderful news!* - **Charlene**
- *Absolutely amazing feats - well done for planning and executing for success in the way you have! It's been a huge privilege to read your daily updates, and I'll miss them for sure. And I just love your cause - what a fantastic advancement for veganism worldwide! You deserve all the accolades you get!* - **Norman**
- *Fantastic...what an achievement.* - **Karen**
- *Apologies for missing the grand finale but I'm pleased I ran the first 5km with you two. A brilliant shining achievement for you both to be very proud of for all time.* - **Alistair**
- *This is what I was telling you about, 365 marathons in one year!* - **Keshia**
- *Incredible!! You are both shining lights on this Planet!!* - **Hayley**
- *Totally amazing!! Congratulations from South Texas, USA!!* - **Diana**
- *Finally, someone on this planet that is showing us true compassion for life, unselfishness and humbleness, thank you immensely is not enough.* - **MJ**

JANUARY 2014

- *I have watched from the beginning, off and on, and have been beyond inspired!!! Abundant Blessings to you both!!* - **Karen**
- *Sooo Coool! Wow!!!* - **Brett**
- *I followed you for only a few weeks but you amazed me each day! CONGRATULATIONS to both of you from Blainville near Montréal.* - **Guy**
- *No words to describe your passion...YOOU SUCCEED ..lots of emotion in any sport women or men.* - **Marino**
- *You mean I'm going to have to do 367 now??? Well done, great achievement!* - **James**
- *Hi.. I've followed your journey online and through the stories of my friend Narelle who was part of your support crew. Congratulations on such an inspiring courageous and educational effort. Thank you for sharing your journey.* - **Laurel**
- *Congratulations! What an inspiration!* - **Wendy**
- *Congratulations!!!* - **Jonatan**
- *Congrats!! Well done!! Perfect!!!* - **Katsuhiko**
- *Truly inspirational!!* - **Marc**
- *What an amazing effort - congratulations.* - **Del**
- *Congratulations!* - **Deb**
- *I'm inspired! Congratulations!* - **Belinda**
- *Huge congrats . Amazing and Happy for you both...* - **Joy**
- *I'm in awe!* - **Kate**
- *Incredible.* - **Dave**
- *Compassion is the driving force here, congratulations to two very amazing, inspirational people.* - **Lisa**
- *Congratulations on an amazing feat of endurance, health and courage.* - **Eric**
- *So incredible and inspiring guys. Thank you.* - **Deb**
- *Mazal tov. Well done. Amazing. Love dxx* - **Doris**
- *Stupendously amazing effort! So very inspired.* - **Corinne**
- *Unbelievable! Inspirational! Awesome effort. Congratulations to you both, and all on raw power. Don't turn into sleeping beauties!* - **Stephen**

- *Amazing. Well done!* - **John**
- *You are so inspiring and every single day following you and your stories here helped a lot in every day life. Thank you so much.* -**Sabine**
- *Inspirational, congratulations!* - **Janine**
- *What a wonderful journey you have had, we have been following you, my husband has prostate cancer and has been fighting it for 5 years, in 2015 I have organised a few friends and we are walking around Australia to raise money for prostate & breast cancer we wish you both all the best.* - **Ian & Chris**
- *Annoyed I only just found out about you guys today, I would have come to cheer you on in Melb! Congrats for achieving your goal!* - **Candice**
- *Did you see this?? Amazing doesn't come close to describing them!!* - **Jo**
- *So beautiful to see how much community support Running Raw Around Australia 2013 has been getting!! One of the most beautiful stories *ever* and it is brilliant to see how it has brought so many people together! Keep spreading this story around. Infinite love and congratulations to Janette and Alan.* - **Jessie**

January 12, 2014. Warrandyte, Victoria, Australia

Well, folks, it's been 10 days since we stopped running a marathon every day around Australia, but we have started the marathon of media interviews worldwide! Our phone has been ringing constantly, we've done several interviews daily and the calendar is still filling up fast. We are turning the phone off during interviews, in the evenings and on the weekends just so we can catch up, so please send us a text or email if you need to get in touch. Meanwhile we're still running in the mornings (not so early as before)! It is such a delight to run along our river trail, the morning sun sparkling on the water and the kookaburras laughing in the old gum trees. As I sit in my studio at home, replying to the thousands of emails and Facebook messages, I reflect on the year of marathons and feel blessed to know that for many who have followed us online and through the media, it was a year of inspiration and motivation towards a more conscious lifestyle.

By running a marathon a day around Australia we have achieved worldwide acclaim, but for us the achievement means much more than that. Due to the massive media coverage since completing Marathon #366 on January 1, 2014, the positive message that we shared during RunRAW2013 has reached millions of people worldwide. So, as we run into the New Year, writing the book and making the documentary based on RunRAW2013, going on speaking tours around Australia and internationally, we know that together we have made a difference.

The best kept secret is out folks, and with many thanks to you all for your support and encouragement, we will continue to share it everywhere we go....and we believe if we and others continue do so, we will no longer be Running Out of Time.

Recipes from the Road

To run a marathon a day, every day for a year, the body requires low fat, high calorie, nutrient dense living food with enzymes intact, to be easily assimilated by the body into fuel burning energy. A low fat raw vegan diet consists of fresh, ripe, preferably locally grown organic fruits and vegetables. Having experienced increased energy and physical performance during ten years of eating 100% raw vegan food, we knew that so long as we could obtain enough fresh produce during the Run, it would be possible to sustain the endurance needed to achieve such a physically demanding goal. We were also aware that consuming 100% raw vegan food increases brain function, thereby providing clarity of mind to enable the focus, discipline and mental determination required to remain committed to the physical goal under all circumstances, adverse weather conditions and variable terrain.

During the year leading up to the Run, we experimented with eating while training, as we realised that to be continually running every day we would need to be continually eating in a way that would sustain us physically and mentally over the full year. After completing over 6000 km in training we developed a menu plan that was continually adjusted as we went along, depending on the availability of produce. In advance, we took the precaution of dehydrating 2000 bananas to use when ripe bananas were not available. We also carried 20 kg of fresh dates as a back up when fresh fruit was scarce. Through experimentation, we discovered that we would require 3000 to 4000 calories per day to sustain a level of peak physical performance required to run a marathon every day for 366 consecutive days. We knew that empty calories obtained from processed and cooked foods (such as grains and pasta) use stored energy from the body which creates a bodily letdown that would require extended recovery time. However, it would be crucial for us to recover quickly, so calories obtained from fresh, ripe, organic fruits and vegetables being fully usable immediately, provide instant energy and constant recovery while running. Knowing that (for instance) 1 banana or 1 kiwifruit provides 100 calories and 1 date provides 75 calories, it was not a matter of counting calories, but counting fruit!

To assist with recovery we estimated that a minimum of 9 hours sleep between marathons would be ideal, although it was not always possible and we did notice a marked difference in our ability to maintain a regular pace while running during those days when we did not get enough sleep.

Every morning when we got up at 3:45am we made an Alkaline Energiser Smoothie to drink while we were getting ready to hit the road around 5am. At 7am our crew would catch us up and give us bananas and replenish our water which we carried in two 300 ml bottles. They would continue on to approximately the 17 km mark and make a Green Goodness Smoothie which we all enjoyed together for 'breakfast.' We had one more banana break before stopping for 'lunch' at about the 32 km mark. Lunch usually consisted of any one large fruit, such as melon, papaya or pineapple, or we may have several smaller fruit such as 10 oranges or kiwifruit. Another option if we had enough ripe fruit was to make a fruit salad. We found fresh fruit to be the most easily digestible food while on the run. Within 20 minutes of completing each marathon we would have a freshly made juice of carrots, beetroot, apple, greens stalks and ginger to recharge the body. As the Run continued and we were progressively losing weight, we found that by the time we finished each marathon we were craving fat. The body was into fat burning mode, but we didn't have any excess by then! So we found that eating an avocado shortly after finishing the run each day satisfied the craving. Our dinners usually consisted of a large salad depending on the produce we had available or we would create a raw gourmet meal with whatever ingredients we did have that was ripe and needed to be eaten. Going up the East Coast in summer there was no shortage of fresh ripe seasonal fruit including tropical varieties, so our diet was predominantly fruit and greens. However, in the Northern Territory and across the Nullarbor in the South, there was no fresh produce available so we had to stock up with fruit and vegetables that would keep well, hence we developed some interesting recipes. The following recipes are a guideline for ideas on how to combine a few basic ingredients to create delicious and nutritious meals. With Raw dishes, you can add or change any ingredients with those you have available, thereby creating a new recipe anytime. Growing or buying fresh garden produce and preparing the ingredients is part of the fun. Adding colour and flavour is easy with fresh fruit and vegetables as your main ingredients, and being creative with presentation gives wonderful eye-appeal to the meal. The best part of preparing Raw meals, is that you don't have to wait for it to cook!

Smoothies:

Alkaline Energiser
1 lemon, 1 grapefruit, 10 bananas
Peel and place citrus in blender jug, add water to blade level.
Peel and add bananas.
Blend using the pulse button a few times first then medium blend to combine.
Drink before going for a run or any early morning exercise.

Green Goodness
Basic Ingredients: 2 oranges, 10 bananas, ginger root to taste, bunch green leaves (stalks removed and save for juicing) Add any other ripe seasonal fruit and/or berries as desired and alternate greens with silver-beet, spinach and kale.
Peel fruit and place juicy fruit in blender jug first, add water to blade level, add bananas and blend with pulse action until liquified.
Add greens into liquid and blend on medium until combined.
Drink for breakfast, part way through a long run and/or after finishing exercise.

Banana Break
2 oranges, 10-15 bananas, any one ripe fruit and/or berries
Peel oranges, place in blender jug with water to blade level.
Add bananas and other fruit as desired.
Drink anytime you feel hungry or just need a break.

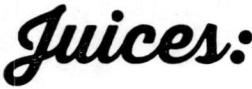

Beet Treat

1-2 kg carrots, 2-3 beetroot, 1-2 apples, ginger root to taste
Juice with cold press juicer.
Drink before lunch or dinner and/or after exercise.

Heart Beet

1-2 kg carrots, 2-3 beetroot, bunch of greens stalks (silver-beet, spinach, kale, soft stem herbs, broccoli stalk peeled), 2 stalks celery if desired, ginger root to taste, small piece turmeric root, 1 green apple, 1 lemon
Juice alternating ingredients to push the stalks, apple and lemon through with carrots and beets.
Drink immediately, in a heart beet.

Soups:

Dillicious Carrot Soup
2 kg carrots, 1 large bunch dill, 1 avocado
Juice the carrots, pour into blender jug, add other ingredients and blend till smooth. Serve in soup bowl, decorate with a sprig of dill.

Beautiful Beetroot Soup
2 kg carrots, 2-4 beetroot, 2 avocado, 1/2 orange
Juice carrots and beets, pour into blender jug, add one and a half avocado and juice of half orange, blend till smooth. Cut remaining half avocado into small pieces, sprinkle onto bowl of soup.

Salads:

Down-Under Outback Coleslaw

Any selection of root vegetables (carrots, beetroot, turnip, rutabaga, sweet potato etc), 1 green cabbage, half red cabbage, 2 red apples, 1 cup soaked currants, 1 fennel bulb and leaves (save stalks for juicing) or 1 small bunch fresh dill, 1 cup soaked and drained sunflower seeds or walnuts chopped; Grate vegetables and apples into large bowl. Cut cabbages into small strips, add to bowl. Finely chop fennel and leaves or fresh dill, mix into salad. Drain and add currants. Use soaking water in dressing.

Make dressing: 1 cup dry sunflower seeds, 1 tbsp un-hulled tahini, half cup pitted green olives, half cup sun-dried tomatoes, half avocado, half tsp ground cardamon, half tsp mixed spice, water from soaking currants, juice of 1 lime or lemon, juice of 2 oranges

Blend sunflower seeds to powder. Add all other ingredients and blend till smooth.

Pour dressing over salad and mix in thoroughly. Leave to stand 2 hours before serving.

Optional Ingredients: Add chopped cauliflower and/or celery

Spicy Greens Salad

Any selection Asian greens with juicy stalks, small bunch spinach, 1 bulb fennel and leaves (use stalks for juicing), 2 bulbs lemongrass, 2 bulbs green onions, 1 med carrot, 1 small beetroot, 1 cup grated daikon radish, cherry tomatoes, fresh Thai basil, chili optional

Chop greens stalks and tear leaves into bite size pieces. Finely chop fennel and leaves, finely slice lemongrass and onions, grate carrot, beetroot and radish, mix all together in a large bowl. Slice tomatoes in half, finely chop basil and chili if desired. Add to salad.

Make Dressing: juice 1 lemon and 1 lime, 1 avocado, small piece ginger root peeled, 2 tbsp black tahini, 1 tsp Malaysian curry powder, 1 tsp garam masala

Blend all ingredients until smooth and mix through salad.

Sprinkle finely chopped raw cashews on each serving.

Dinner:

Dressed Naked Noodles
1 kg zucchini, (optional additions - 1 small daikon radish,1 large carrot, and/or 1 medium beetroot). Strip peel the zucchini, (peel optional ingredients). Make into noodles using a spirooli, place in large serving bowl and mix in optional additions if used. Cut across noodles 4 ways to shorten the length. Make sauce and pour over noodles when ready to serve, mix thoroughly and decorate with complimentary herbs.
Dressing-Tomato Sauce: half cup soaked, rinsed and drained sunflower seeds or fresh walnuts, 2 tablespoons sultanas soaked in quarter cup water, 6-8 pitted olives, half chopped red onion, 2 cloves garlic crushed, 1 cup sun-dried tomatoes, small bunch fresh herbs (basil, oregano, marjoram, rosemary, or combination) or 2 tsp dried mixed Italian herbs, 1 kg chopped fresh tomatoes, 1 avocado.
Blend seeds or nuts until powdered. Add all other ingredients into the blender jug in order listed. Pulse a few times then blend on medium until smooth and creamy.
Pour over noodles in bowl, mix well, decorate with chopped herbs and serve immediately.

Living Lasagne
4-6 medium sized zucchini sliced thinly lengthwise, 6-8 med tomatoes sliced thinly, 2 large mushrooms chopped, 2 bunches spinach. Keep ingredients separate.
Make sauces separately to alternately spread between ingredient layers.
Tomato Sauce: Same as for Dressed Naked Noodles
Pesto Sauce: 1 cup soaked, rinsed and drained walnuts or pumpkin seeds, large bunch fresh basil. Blend with a little water if required.
In a medium sized casserole dish spread a small amount of Tomato Sauce on bottom of dish. Layer half or third (depending on size of dish and amount of ingredients) the zucchini strips, cover with a layer of spinach, sliced mushrooms and tomato slices, then spread a layer of pesto sauce and then tomato sauce, Continue to alternate layers until all ingredients and sauces are

used, keeping aside 2 tbsp of each sauce for decoration.
Cashew Creme Sauce: 2 cups soaked, rinsed and drained cashews, juice of half lemon or lime. Blend adding small amount of water until smooth and creamy. Spread over last layer of lasagne. Crunchy Cashew Topping: Roughly chop 2 cups dry cashews. Sprinkle onto Cashew Creme Sauce.
Cut and serve lasagne in square pieces on a flat plate, drizzle some of each sauce around on the plate to decorate. Place a spring of complimentary herb on top of serving.

Curried Mushroom Rice
Rice: 1 med cauliflower, half cup dessicated coconut, 1 avocado, one-third cup soaked currants, 1 tsp curry powder, juice half lime or lemon, 6 sprigs of parsley finely chopped.
Grate cauliflower into medium sized bowl, add and mix in coconut. Mash avocado, curry and lime juice and mix into cauliflower thoroughly. Stir in currants and parsley.
Mushroom Sauce: 6 portobello mushrooms chopped small, flowerets from 1 medium head broccoli each cut in half and mixed with mushroom.
Make Pesto Sauce same as for Living Lasagne. Make Almond Creme same method as for Three Chias Pudding. Pour Almond Creme into Pesto Sauce a small amount at a time stirring with a fork until thoroughly mixed. Add to mushrooms and broccoli stirring in to cover. Marinate 6 hours.
Serve Rice on plate and heap Mushroom Sauce on top. Spoon small amount of sauce liquid around rice to decorate plate, place small sprig of parsley on top of serving.

Pumpkin Fettuccini
1 large butternut pumpkin. Peel skin off whole pumpkin and discard. Continue to peel with wide blade peeler to the middle of pumpkin (discard seeds) until all flesh is peeled into thin wide lengths. Cut each piece lengthwise into quarter inch strips to resemble fettucini. (You can also make pumpkin noodles using a spirooli.) Place in large bowl.
Make sauce: 1 cup soaked and drained pumpkin seeds (pepitas), 1 cup pitted black olives, small bunch fresh rosemary or 2 tsp dried Italian herbs, half cup sundried tomatoes, juice of 1

lemon, juice of 1 orange, 2 tbsp unhulled tahini
Blend pumpkin seeds dry to make a powder. Add all other ingredients, blend until combined. Mix through pumpkin strips until thoroughly coated. Marinate 6-8 hours, stirring occasionally until pumpkin strips have softened.
Chop two medium tomatoes into small pieces, mix into the pumpkin fettucini. Serve in bowls with a sprinkling of whole pumpkin seeds on top.

Desserts:

Three Chias Pudding

3 heaped tbsp chia seeds, 1 tsp cinnamon, half tsp allspice, half tsp mixed spice, 1 cup soaked sultanas, half cup soaked currants, 2 cups water

Put chia seeds in a large deep bowl, add spices and mix in with fork. Add sultanas and currants with soaking water mixing with fork, add water. Leave to soak while you make Almond Creme. Add almond pulp to chia pudding, mix in well and add more water if required for consistency. Thinly slice three ripe bananas into chia pudding (or any other fresh fruit - pears are great) Serve chia pudding in small bowls with almond creme poured on top.

Almond Creme:

Soak 2 cups almonds in water overnight. Drain and rinse until water is clear, soak for a further 8 hours. Drain, rinse and drain again. Keep soaked almonds in fridge (keeps fresh 2 days) until ready for use. To make Almond Creme place soaked almonds in blender, add water to blade level, pulse a few times. Add small amounts of water while blending on medium until pulp and liquid is creamy (about 1 litre). Place a fine mesh sieve over a deep bowl and pour half the amount into sieve. Using a large spoon, gently push the creme liquid through the pulp and sieve into the bowl. Continue until no more creme comes through, do not stir or push too hard as some of the pulp will go through into the creme. Spoon the pulp out of the sieve into a separate bowl. Repeat with the remaining amount. Pour the Almond Creme into a covered container and keep in fridge until ready to serve. (You can cover the almond pulp and keep in fridge until ready to use in recipe, or keep in freezer if not using immediately)

Pineapple or Custard Apple Pear Pudding

1 ripe pineapple or custard apple, 1 avocado, 2 bananas, 2 pears, 1/2 tsp allspice

Peel, core and chop fruit, blend all ingredients and spice until smooth and creamy. Serve in small bowl decorated with pinch of allspice on top.

Beet Berry Slice

Base: 2 cups macadamia nuts, 3/4 cup soaked dates (saving 4 dates for topping)

Drain dates and blend with macadamia nuts until sticky (add small amount of date water if necessary). Mix well and press into shallow casserole dish.

Filling: 3 medium beetroot, 1 apple, 2 cups soaked sultanas, half cup soaked currants, quarter tsp mixed spice, 2 tbsp chia seeds.

Peel beetroot and discard. Grate beetroot into medium size bowl with small gauge grater or chop smaller after grating on large gauge. Peel and grate apple and mix into beetroot. Add mixed spice, mixing well with a fork. Drain sultanas and currants (keep drained water in fridge for making 3 Chia Pudding or adding to smoothies). Add fruit to beetroot and mix in well. Add 2 tbsp chia seeds. Let stand 20 minutes to thicken (while making Almond Creme) then spread beetroot filling on top of base in casserole.

Topping: Make Almond Creme. Put creme in fridge until serving. Mash 4 soaked dates into almond pulp, mix well and spread on top of beetroot filling. Sprinkle finely chopped macadamia nuts and a few soaked currants over top.

Cut and spoon portions into small bowls and serve with Almond Creme.

These are a few of our favourite recipes that were created with the ingredients we had available while on the Road. However, there are many more simply delicious raw vegan recipes that I have created over the years which will be included in my next book: *'Raw Can Cure - Recipes for a Raw Lifestyle.'*

   Enjoy!

Janette Murray-Wakelin
www.RawCanCure.com
www.RunningRawAroundAustralia.com

Author's Bio

Janette Murray-Wakelin is the author of the highly acclaimed book 'Raw Can Cure Cancer' and is an inspirational and motivational speaker who lives in Australia. On January 1, 2014, Janette together with her husband Alan Murray, acquired world acclaim by setting a new World Record for running the most consecutive marathons, as the only couple over the age of 60, fueled entirely on raw fruit and veg, wearing barefoot shoes. During 2013 they ran a marathon every day, 366 marathons in 366 days an average of 43.12km per marathon, covering a distance of 15,782 km while running together around Australia. As veteran ultra endurance runners, Janette and Alan have proved beyond any doubt that living a raw, vegan conscious lifestyle results in optimal health where physically, mentally and emotionally, anything is achievable. Janette is currently writing her third book, 'Raw Can Cure - Recipes for a Raw Lifestyle.'

www.RunningRawAroundAustralia.com
www.RawCanCure.com

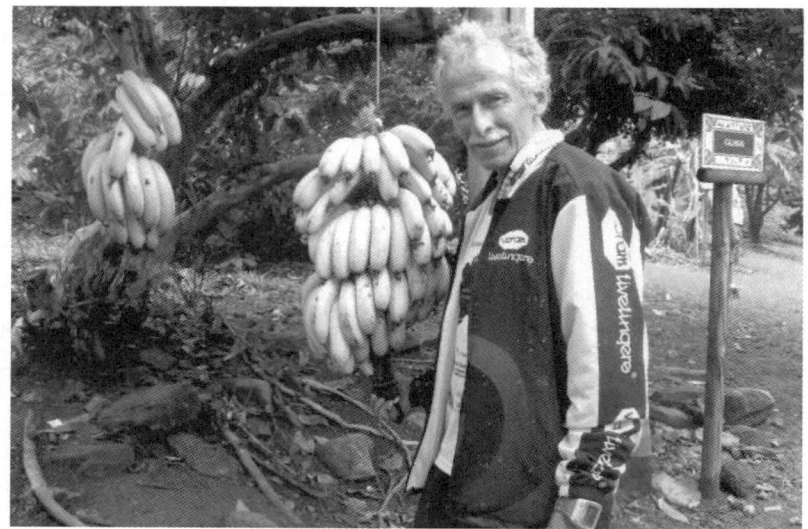
Banana bunch for lunch

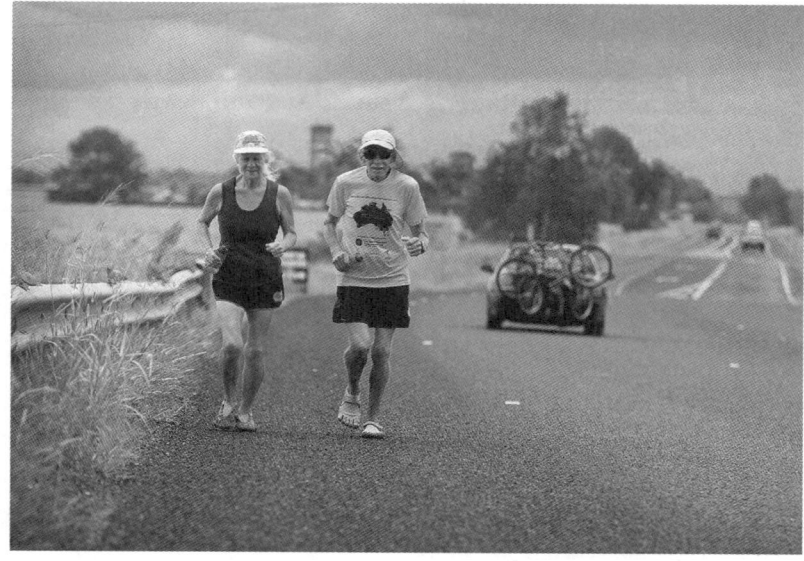
Storm brewing, QLD

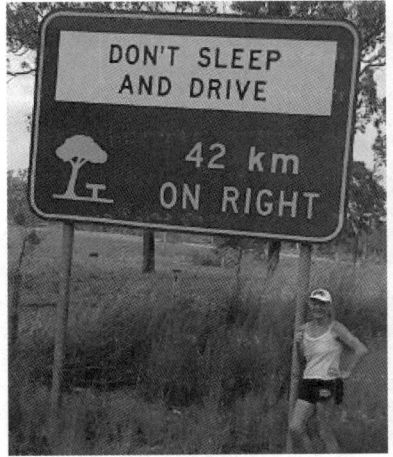 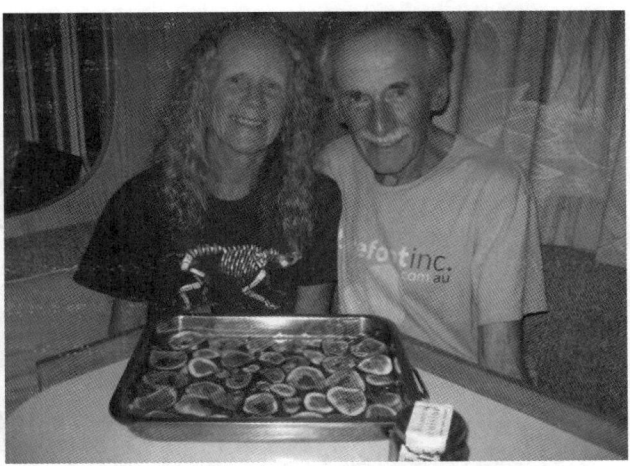

A 42km sign for us Fresh figgy pudding (Photo courtesy Marleen Kilkelly)

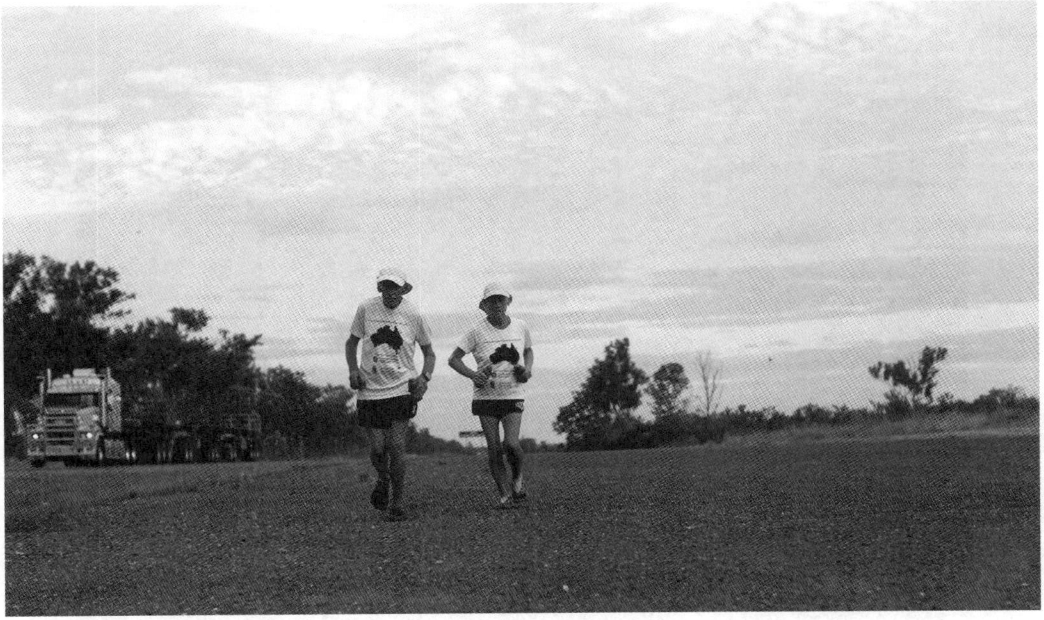

Avoiding the trucks, NT (Photo courtesy Myke Tran)

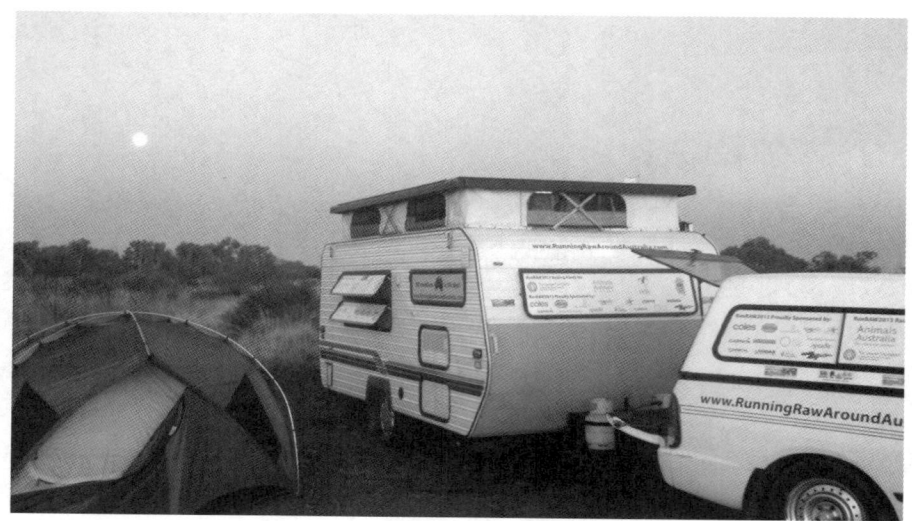

Moonset, QLD (Photo courtesy Narelle Chesworth)

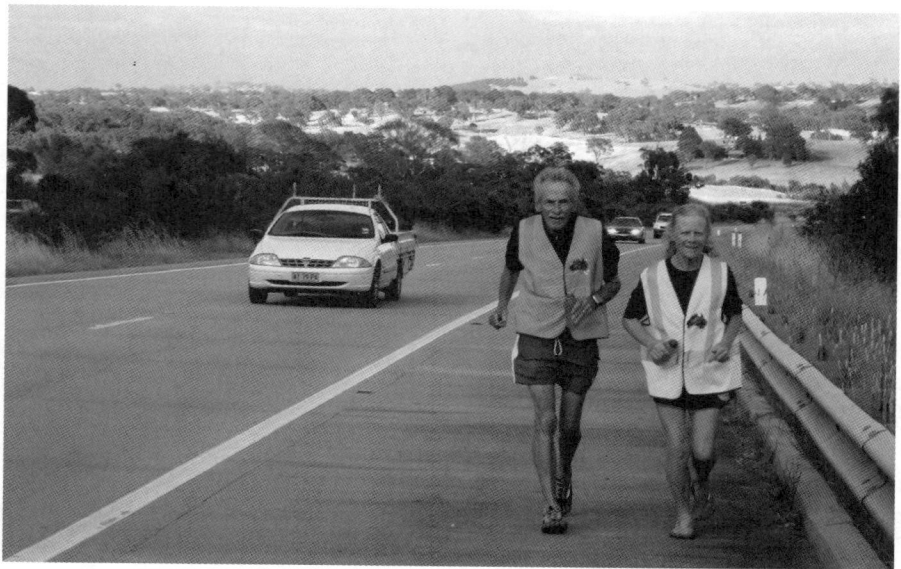

Uphill on The Great Divide, NSW (Photo courtesy Ping Chan)

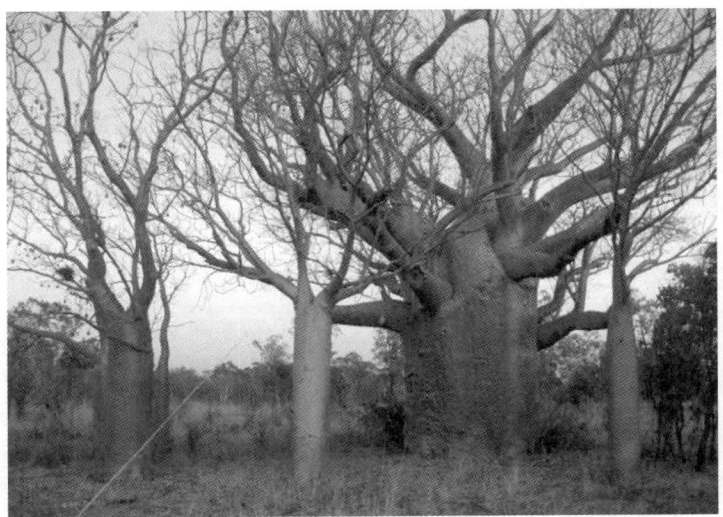

Boab forest, WA

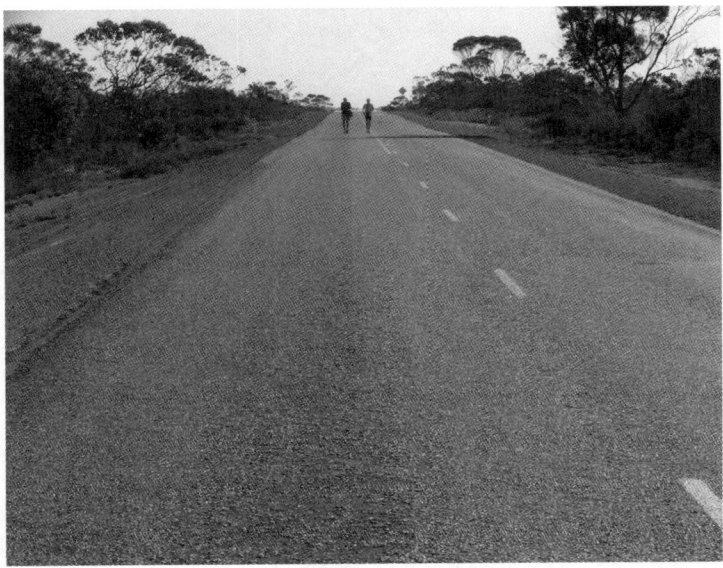

Running in the rain, WA (Photo courtesy Graeme Ward)

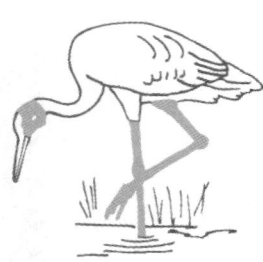

Be Published

Publish through a successful publisher.
Brolga Publishing is represented through:
- **National** book trade distribution, including sales, marketing & distribution through **Macmillan Australia**.
- **International** book trade distribution to
    - The United Kingdom
    - North America
    - Sales representation in South East Asia
- **Worldwide e-Book distribution**

For details and inquiries, contact:
Brolga Publishing Pty Ltd
PO Box 12544
A'Beckett St VIC 8006

Phone: 0414 608 494
markzocchi@brolgapublishing.com.au
ABN: 46 063 962 443
(Email for a catalogue request)